COMMUNITY HEALTH NURSING

COMMUNITY HEALTH NURSING

K. Madhav Naidu

genNEXT Publication

Community Health Nursing

Rs. 890

ISBN: 978-81-908675-1-1

Published in 2010 in India by
Gennext Publication
23 Main Ansari Road, Darya Ganj,
New Delhi-110002
E-Mail:GenNextpublication@hotmail.com
Phone: 23282060

Printed at: Singhal Print Media, Delhi

Contents

Preface

Present book is about community nursing theory, knowledge and skills. It is based on our research into education for primary health care, community nursing roles, practice and policy in India, together with many years of teaching community and public health. This book also draws on the knowledge, research and expertise of leading and emerging researchers, academics and experts of the field to develop a comprehensive exploration of the theory, knowledge and skills required for successful and effective community nursing practice in a range of practice settings. I have written this book because despite international literature being available, little current material has been available to inform teaching and practice in community nursing in India. I wanted to write a book that would be useful for undergraduate and post graduate nursing students, as well as practitioners already working in the field.

This book is based on the premise that community nursing is an area of specialty nursing practice and that nurses require a specific body of knowledge to work effectively in a community setting. Community nursing practice, as it is described here, has a breadth that is beyond a medical model approach. It is not just health teaching or sick care provision in a different place; rather, it encompasses a social model of health, and has been generated from community models of practice, whether services are being provided for individuals, families, groups or whole communities. Community nurses work with many different client groups, community settings and types of agencies, and they often possess additional areas of specialty knowledge. These added specialities can sometimes splinter community nursing and obscure the distinctive body of knowledge and expertise that the field represents. Because this knowledge is often not articulated, expertise in community nursing practice often goes unrecognized and remains unacknowledged, which is typical of much of the taken-for-granted knowledge in nursing. We wanted to describe the body of knowledge that comprises the expertise of community nursing. Thus this book aims to bring together theory, knowledge, skills and issues that are common to practice across all community nursing roles, regardless of the specialty area and population groups served.

1

Introduction

In the history of public health, 19th century makes a turning point. Several reformers notably Frank (1745-84) and Edvin Chadwik (1800 - 1890) in England published reports focusing the attention of government and people on the need for sanitary reforms.

A movement known as sanitary awakening started in England in the 20th century. The broad foundation of public health viz., safe drinking water, clean environment were held in all civilization.

Public health began to make rapid growth during 20th century. The role of nurse also began to expand along these lines. A remarkable development in public health was the successful control at many communicable diseases. Medicine and nursing began to link themselves to social sciences for a better understanding at these newer health problems.

On the international scenario the birth of WHO in 1946 gave impetus to the strengthening at medical and nursing services. All over the world a new era dawned signing positive health. There was shift of emphasis from the sick to the well person, from the individual to the community. Health has been recognised as a fundamental right of all human being. The term public health, preventive medicine and social medicine were found inadequate and were replaced by community health, which is much broader in the scope of public health or preventive medicine.

WHO set a goal at health for all by 2000 AD and prescribed primary health care at reasonable level and that health care to be attained by all by the year 2000 AD. The concept of community health has also permeated into nursing and gave birth to the concept of community nursing. Community health has been integrated into basic curriculum at nursing in 1958 by the Indian Nursing Council. The recent development in the concept of primary health and the goal at health care for all by 2000 AD has attached the nursing component at the health care system in the country. It has led to restructuring the pattern at rural health services. Every nurse has her responsibility in her area of work in whatever capacity she works in relation to community health services.

HEALTH

According to the World Health Organization's (WHO) definition of health, "Health is a state of complete physical, mental and social well-being, not merely the absence of disease." The WHO, a specialized agency of the United Nations, introduced the idea of considering health as a global issue, and brought nations and experts together to better develop the health of the world. In fact, health can be defined in positive and negative ways. The negative definition is absence of disease or illness while positive definition is the state of well-being. This is considered common sense, passed from generation to generation as part of the cultural heritage. The terms disease, illness and ill health are used interchangeably by laypeople and even by health care professionals. Disease and illness do not mean the same thing, although there is large degree of overlap in their definitions.

Disease: Disease is the objective state of ill health, normally verified by accepted proof. For example, a woman is diagnosed to have cervical cancer when a microscopic analysis shows evidence of changes in cell structure. Though she may not have experienced any symptom of the disease, she is considered to have the disease.

Illness: Illness is the subjective experience of loss of health. General malaise, tiredness, sleeplessness, aches and indigestion are examples of illness. Sometimes when patients visit doctors with the above problems, the doctors are unable to give a definite diagnosis because no abnormalities have been detected in the physical examination. Yet the patient feels unwell.

Ill health: Ill health is an umbrella term used to refer to the experience of disease plus illness. For example, a patient complains of acute abdominal pain with the doctor's diagnosis of appendicitis.

Some of the other definitions of health are as follows:

1. Health means wellness, the opposite of illness
2. The condition of being sound in body, mind or spirit, especially freedom from physical disease or pain
3. Health is a positive state of well being that is felt physically, mentally, socially and spiritually.

4. Health is a way life, requiring knowledge of body, functions and how to keep fit, and the will to cultivate healthy habits including diet and exercise.
5. Health is related to a person's self realization, relationships with others and feeling of giving a worth while contribution to the society.
6. Health is an individual responsibility, and if a person makes no effort to be healthy, no one can provide him with health.
7. Health is a positive quality of life which helps us to live life to its fullest and serve our fellowmen to the best of our ability.

Different Concepts of Health

C. Herzlich studied a group of middle-class Europeans and discovered that they described health in different ways.

- As a state of well-being and the absence of illness.
- As something to have, an inner strength or resistance to ill health.
- As a state of doing and being able to fulfil the maximum potential for life.

From the above, it was found that middle class people have a positive view of health. However, manual laborers can have rather different concepts of health, because they pay more attention to functional status or ability rather than the quality of being fit and active. For example, a mother is considered healthy if she is able to take care of the family, and a worker is healthy if s/he is able to earn a living.

You should note that because different people may hold different views, there is no right or wrong or model answer regarding the concept of health. If you look at the WHO definition of health from 1984, you will be able to differentiate differences between past and more recent definitions. "Health is the extent to which an individual or group is able, on the one hand to realize aspirations and satisfy needs; and, on the other hand, to change or cope with the environment. Health is therefore, seen as a resources for everyday life, not as an object of living; it is a positive concept emphasizing social and personal resources, as well as physical capacities (WHO, 1984).

Concept of Disease

There have been many attempts to define disease. Webster defines disease as " a condition in which body health is impaired, a departure from a state of health, an alteration of the human body interrupting the performance of vital functions". The Oxford English Dictionary defines disease as "a condition of the body or some part or organ of the body in which its functions are disrupted or deranged". From an ecological point of view, disease is defined as maladjustment of the human organism to the environment". From a sociological point of view., disease is considered a social phenomenon, occurring in all societies and defined and fought in terms of the particular cultural forces prevalent in the society. The simplest definition is, of course, that disease is just the opposite of health - i.e., any deviation from normal functioning or state of complete physical or mental well -being - -since health and disease are mutually exclusive. These definitions are considered inadequate because they do not give a criterion by which to decide when a disease state begins, nor do they lend themselves to measurement of disease.

WHO has defined health but not disease. This is because disease has many shades ("spectrum of disease") ranging from in apparent (sub clinical) cases to severe manifest illness. Some diseases commence acutely (e.g., food poisoning), and some insidiously (e.g., mental illness, rheumatoid arthritis). In some diseases, a "carrier" state occurs in which the individual remains outwardly healthy, and is able to infect others (e.g., typhoid fever). In some instances, the same organism may cause more than one clinical manifestation (e.g., streptococcus). In some cases, the same disease may be caused by more than one organism (e.g., diarrhea). Some diseases have a short course, and some a prolonged course. It is easy to determine illness when the signs and symptoms are manifest, but in many diseases the borderline between normal and abnormal is indistinct as in the case of diabetes, hypertension and mental illness. The end -point or final outcome of disease is variable - recovery, disability or death of the host.

Distinction is also made between the words disease, illness and sickness which are not wholly synonymous. The term "disease" literally means "without ease" (uneasiness)- disease, the opposite of ease - when something is wrong with bodily function. "Illness" refers not only to the presence of a specific disease, but also to the individual's perceptions and behaviour in response to the disease, as well as the impact of that disease on the psychosocial environment "Sickness" refers to a state of social dysfunction. Suffer has suggested the following Usage: Disease is a physiological/psychological dysfunction; Illness is a subjective state of the person who feels aware of not being well; Sickness is a state of social dysfunction, i.e., a role that the individual assumes when ill ("sickness role").The clinician sees people who are ill rather than the diseases, which he must diagnose and treat. However, it is possible to be victim of disease without feeling ill, and to be ill without signs of physical impairment. In short, an adequate definition of disease is yet to be found - a definition that is satisfactory or acceptable to the epidemiologist, clinician, sociologist and the statistician.

Factors Affecting Health

The individual and group health is determined by:

1. Human biology
2. Environment
3. Way of living
4. Economic status
5. Health Services

Human Biology: Hereditary characteristics that is height, weight, colour of the skin, blood groups etc. are determined by gene which are coming one from mother and one from father. The genetic constitution of man is land at the time of conception. So the state of health therefore depends partly on genetic constitution inherited by the individual. There are inherited diseases like diabetes, cleft palate, epilepsy and hypertension etc. or genetic defects.

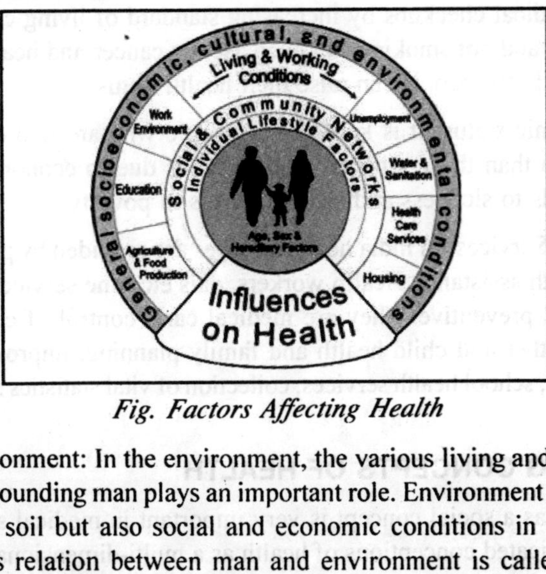

Fig. Factors Affecting Health

Environment: In the environment, the various living and non living things surrounding man plays an important role. Environment implies air, water and soil but also social and economic conditions in which man lives. This relation between man and environment is called "Human ecology". The man's environment is divided into three major components.

- Physical Environment: This is the part of man's external environment e.g.: water, air, housing, climate, soil, nutrition etc. Man has altered everything in his physical environment due to air pollution, water pollution, excessive novice, radiation hazards are main and man has become ill health
- Biological Environment: This is the living component of man's external environmental. It consists of plants, animals, insects, bacteria and virus with which man is in constant relationship. When the delicate balance is disturbed man's health is affected.

Social Environment: This pertains to man in relationship with his fellow human beings. The social environment is quite broad and ill defined. It is composed of customs, habits, income, occupation, religion, standard of living, human behavior, availability of health services, and social and political organizations. Maladjustment may result in problems like drug addiction, alcoholism, crime, violence, suicides, divorces, mental illness, hypertension, peptic ulcer etc. When man has controlled physical and biological environment and also social environment, the health and well being of the individually maintained.

Way of living: Health may not be given by one-person to another parson. It depends upon the way of living, the level of personal hygiene education and the life style of the people. People must maintained the rules of hygiene, eating, balanced diets, healthy habits, immunization and periodic medical checkups by increasing standard of living can control tuberculosis and not smoking can decrease the cancer and heart disease. By way of life the people can raise their health status.

Economic status: It is known that people who are rich enjoys the better health than those who are poor. This is due to economic status. Poverty leads to sickness and sickness leads to poverty.

Health Services: In India health services are provided by physicians, nurses, health assistants, Health workers, dais etc. The services are both curative and preventive. They are medical care, control of community diseases mother and child health and family planning, improvement of environment, school health services, collection of vital statistics and health education.

CHANGING CONCEPTS OF HEALTH

Health as a social concept is very important in medical sociology. More complicated conceptions of health as a multi-dimensional concept have emphasized not only physical health status, but aspects of overall well-being. Life expectancy slowly and steadily increased during the course of the 21st century resulting in a change in the concept of health for both individuals and society. This has been primarily the consequence of the reduction of infant and early childhood mortality and the control of major infectious diseases. Fear of dying has been replaced by the dedication to survival, health, and production, and science and technology have contributed much to creating this pattern of thinking.

Lawrence Henderson recognized adaptability as a basic biological phenomenon. The relation between nutritional requirements and homeostatic mechanisms is significant. Beyond a certain threshold, the latter cannot prevent impairments resulting from undernutrition, but the establishment of this threshold involves a complex process. In addition to being an end for each person, health is also regarded as a means for society.

These ideas seem embodied in the World Health Organization's (WHO's) definition of health: "a state of complete physical, mental and social well-being and not merely the absence of disease of infirmity." The main and perennial problem is how to translate the ideal into practical reality. Recognition of health as a right has strengthened the acceptance of its role as a determinant of development. An important cluster of determinants of health and disease stems from the health services, and these have changed in both concept and in practice, particularly following World War 2. Health care, being a basic need, was conceived as a service to be provided, even imposed by the central authorities, to those entrenched in their traditions.

Currently, there is movement from paternalism to community participation. It has become essential to catalyze the community for it is a vast potential source of cooperation in carrying out activities for disease prevention and cure throughout the world. A series of circumstances have supported the renaissance of the primary health care movement in the world.

The contributing factors – the bases for actual or forthcoming changes in health services – are identified. Regarding nutrition, in the last 30 years there has been a rebirth of nutrition as a social problem. Through system analysis, the determinants of chronic undernutrition have been identified, and from such an examination, malnutrition emerges as a problem of overall development. At this time the coverage of programs aimed at the social sectors – health, education, population, food subsidies, housing – is neither sufficient nor efficient. Many societies need to institute

Community

Community means a group of people living in a certain locality such as a village, who have common interests. They meet and react with one another. They may have different interests also and not get on well with one another. Some are rich, others poor, some eat too much. Other may go hungry, some have power and influence and may like to give orders. Others have no power and suffer injustices. The best kind of community is one in which every one cares about all the other members of the community. As a health worker you will be working with the community to help them in solving their problems especially to be healthier in every way.

Community Health

Community health includes the state of health of the members of the community, the problems affecting their health and the health care provided for the community. In community health work we help people to find out and think about their health problems and what can be done to improve the health of the whole community. Then we work together with the people and others in the health team to plan and carry out the problems of health care.

Qualities of Community Health Nurse

As a health worker living and working in a community, you may at first feel a stranger. You will realise that people are watching what you do, what you say and how you react to them. If your appearance, words and behaviour displease or shock people, if you seem to be proud and different or have a habit of gossiping, then you will not be accepted by the community and can do no effective work there. Student health worker need guidance and help in how to behave acceptably. There is a code of ethics for nurses published by the International Council of Nurses which May also guide the Health worker. In brief it is as follows:

- Have respect for life, dignity and rights of people, and serve them all without regard to race, religion, Colour, age, Sex, Politics or Social Status.
- Have respect for the values, customs and spiritual beliefs of people.
- Do not pass on personal information except to the right person.
- Keep up a high standard of work and personal conduct.
- Maintain a good relationship and Co-Operation with Coworkers in the health team, and community.

Important Points to Practice

- Always be neat and clean in appearance, and walk with purpose and good posture. This will make you feel good and make a good impression on others.
- Take special care of your own health of body and mind, and set a good example in your personal life and habits practice what you teach.
- Be Cheerful and enthusiastic in your work, and keep a sense of humour.
- Be disciplined in your use of time keep up punctuality, cleanliness and order. Have respect for property other than your own.
- Be obedient to your superior officers (with intelligence) and uphold their authority. Show them proper respect, and use correct channels of communication. Keep to service rules.
- Try to understand other people and the reasons for what they do and say. Be tactful, patient, sympathetic and kind in your attitude to them.
- Always be ready to help people with concern and care, but refuse to receive bribes.
- Develop good friendships and interests apart from your work. Try to have a hobby and healthy relaxation.
- Use every chance to go on learning, by reading books and journals and news papers. Also learn from people who cane helpful to you personally and to improve your work.
- Be disciplined in your spiritual life, in order to have resources to help others in distress of spirit.

PRIMARY HEALTH CARE

Many people, even health professionals, confuse Primary Health Care with a number of other concepts. First of all, Primary Health Care is not Primary Medical Care (or primary care), nor is it primary nursing. These terms should not be used interchangeably. The two documents that laid down the foundation for PHC were the Alma-Ata Declaration and the Ottawa Charter.

In recent decades, it was found that traditional Western medicine fails to address health issues in developing countries, as well as chronic conditions in developed countries. It was due to the fact that some of these diseases are related to socioeconomic factors such as poverty or affluent lifestyles. These provided a background to the conference hosted jointly by the World Health Organization (WHO) and the United Nations Children's Fund (UNICEF) at Alma Ata, the USSR, in 1978. The conference expressed the need for urgent action by all governments, all health and development workers, and the world community to protect and promote health of all the people of the world.

PHC was described by participants of the WHO Primary Health Care conference at Alma Ata 1978 as:

Essential health care based on practical, scientifically sound and socially acceptable methods of technology made universally accessible to individuals and families in the community through their full participation and at a cost that the community and country can afford to maintain at every stage of their development in the spirit of self-reliance and self-determination. It is the first level of contact with individuals, the family and the community with the national health systems bringing health care as close as possible to where people live and work, and constitutes the first element of a continuing health care process. (WHO-UNICEF 1978, Primary Health Care, Alma-Ata, USSR, WHO, Geneva)

PHC is, in fact, more than the above statement. It includes the prevention of disease and the promotion of health. It also states that care should be available, affordable, accessible and acceptable to the individual and the community. It emphasizes three levels of prevention: at the primary (prevention of disease), secondary (early detection) and tertiary level (rehabilitative and maintenance stage).

Moreover, it addresses three levels of care: the primary level of care (General practitioner), the secondary level of care (local non-specialist hospital) and the tertiary level of care (teaching and specialist hospitals). Macdonald (1992) stated that PHC is part of the search for a new model of health care which incorporates the advantages of modern medicine but which seeks to include a wider vision of health and health care into its system.

The WHO introduced the idea of considering health as a global issue. In order to promote the health of all people in the world, nations in the developing world are encourage to share the expertise of the developed nations, emphasizing non-exploitative healthcare among nations.

The philosophies that underpin PHC are equity, justice, self-determination, community participation and multi-disciplinary approaches.

PHC solves the real causes and fundamental problems causing ill health. It combines the best ideas in technical medicine. It is culturally appropriate and an inexpensive means of maintaining health and tackling diseases.

Primary Health Care includes the following:

- Health Education
- Promotion of a quality food supply and proper nutrition
- An adequate supply of safe water and basic sanitation
- Maternal and child health care
- Family planning
- Immunization against the major infectious diseases
- Prevention and control of locally endemic diseases
- Appropriate treatment of common diseases and injuries
- Provision of essential drugs

Essential Components of Primary Health Care

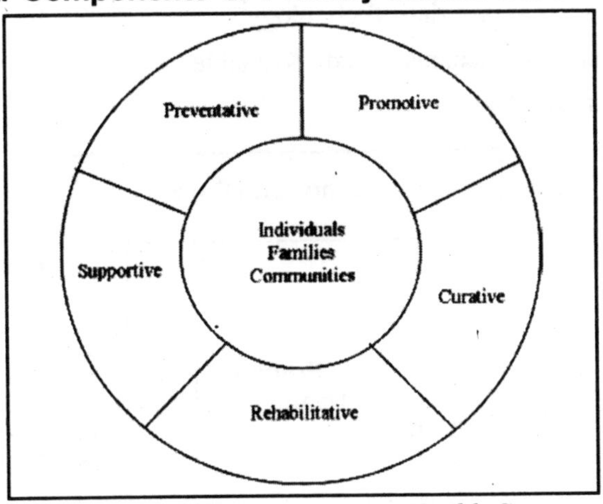

Fig. Components of Primary Health Care

The Declaration of Alma Ata outlined the 8 essential components of primary health care such as principles of,

Equitable Distribution

Health services must be shared equally by all people irrespective of their ability to pay and all (rich or poor, urban or rural) must have access to health services. Primary health care aims to address the current imbalance in health care by shifting the centre of gravity from cities where a majority of the health budget is spent to rural areas where a majority of people live in most countries.

Community Participation

There must be a continuing effort to secure meaningful involvement of the community in the planning, implementation and maintenance of health services, beside maximum reliance on local resources such as manpower, money and materials.

Intersectoral Coordination

Primary health care involves in addition to the health sector, all related sectors and aspects of national and community development, in particular agriculture, animal husbandry, food, industry, education, housing, public works, communication and other sectors.

Four Cornerstones in Primary Health Hare

1. Active community participation
2. Intra and Inter-sectoral linkages
3. Use of appropriate Technology
4. Support Mechanism made Available

Elements of PHC

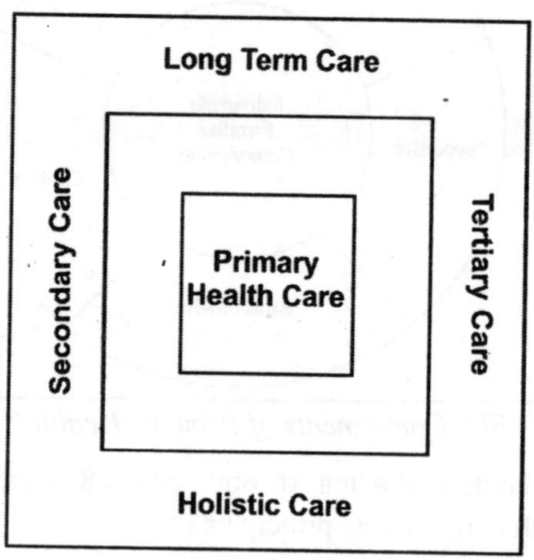

Fig. Elements of PHC

E-education for health L-locally endemic disease control E-expanded program of immunization M-maternal and child health E-essential drugs N-nutrition T-treatment of communicable disease s-safe water and sanitation

ROLE OF NURSE IN PROMOTING PRIMARY HEALTH CARE

About a decade ago, nursing literature that focused on the practical or applied aspects of health promotion in nursing practice was scarce. Nursing texts and nursing curricula typically followed the medical or disease model focusing on the treatment and diagnosis of disease. Most nurses enter nursing schools that do not specifically educate them about health promotion. The skills they acquire in nursing school are often related to acute care. Those who have not studied public health nursing may find themselves particularly disadvantaged in the area of health promotion.

Nurses are in the ideal and best position to assume the role of health promoter as our expertise and knowledge receives high credibility from the public. Nurses are often in close and frequent contact with patients, families, caregivers and the community. However, our expertise is not fully substantiated if we only confine ourselves to roles related to traditional patient care without positively influencing the health-promoting behaviours of our clientele.

Today, nurses should never limit their nursing responsibilities to what was learned in nursing school. Nurses need to work proactively to be sure that our roles are also seen as health promoters and prevention specialists. Nurses need to see their roles as holistic and expand their view of nursing. We must learn other new skills that are considered integral to contemporary nurse practice. Nurses must be multi-disciplinary. The skills they need to acquire include emergency care, illness assessment, psycho-social nursing, counselling, behavioural science, health promotion, statistical analysis, advocacy, presentation skills, political activity and knowledge, marketing, publicity, family intervention and community needs assessment. Today, nurses should see themselves as prime movers for change. We need to be alert to trends and changes in all sectors of society and understand how these could affect the health of the population.

Nurses working in acute care often have the misconception that health promotion is the responsibility of community health nurses. In fact, there are various avenues for health promotion in hospitals. Examples are patient and caregiver education and counselling services, clinical rehabilitation programmes, self-help groups and community wellness services. Moreover, health promotion initiatives such as improving and encouraging occupational and safety practices in hospitals and participating in staff wellness programmes are considered extremely valuable.

Nurses serve as role models for many of the people with whom they come in contact. Through their own behaviour, nurses influence the behaviour of others. The nurse's role as a model is not confined to influencing the health related behaviour of clients. Nurses also serve as role models for other health care professionals. It is understandable that the role modeling function is of primary importance. Therefore, the issue needs to be addressed in nursing curricula that prepare nursing students for that special role in their careers.

HEALTH FOR ALL

It was historic moment when the World Health Organisation, in May 1977, resolved that the main social target of governments and the W.H.O. in the coming decades should be the attainment by all citizens of the world of a level of health that will permit them to lead a socially and economically productive life.

This global initiative, first of its kind in the annals of mankind, culminated in the objective of Health for all by the year 2000 as the social goal of all nations. Though the objective of the W.H.O. itself set out in the preamble of its constitution, is "the attainment by all the peoples of the highest level of health to all people - a level that enables them to work productively and to participate actively in the social life of the community in which they live such that the individual and family needs are adequately met.

The joint WHO/UNICEF International conference in 1978 at Alma Ata endorsed the call for HFA and proclaimed Primary Health Care as the strategy to achieve HFA. The Alma Ata conference further declared that "existing gross inequality in the health status of people especially between developed and developing countries as well as within the countries is politically, socially and economically unacceptable". The primary health care approach is based on five cardinal principles viz., equitable distribution of health resources, community participation, focus on prevention, intersectoral cooperation and appropriate technology.

It is to be noted that though the goal of HFA is universal, the levels of health aimed at and the strategies are not uniform for all countries. Similarly though the Primary Health Care Approach is equally valid for all countries, the problems addressed at the level would differ between and among developed and developing countries depending on the political, social, economic, geographic and other factors.

India as a signatory to the Alma Ata declaration is committed to attaining the goal of HFA. Our National health Policy enunciated in 1983 reflects this commitment by the emphasis laid on providing uniform and comprehensive primary health care services through reorganization of the health service infra-structure, thorough overhaul of the current systems of education and training of health personnel and complete integration of all plans of health and human development sectors. It has laid down the goals for health and Family Welfare Programmes.

In India, the concept of Primary Health Care is beset with the following problems and constraints.

- Inadequate financial allocation to health care delivery.
- Lack of quitable distribution of resources both geographically and in terms of levels of care.
- Poor coordination and linkages of health with other sectors of development and among different sectors of health.
- Lack of appropriate manpower policy.
- Poor management practices and use of inappropriate technology.
- Lack of community privatization of health care posing a threat to public services.
- The increasing privatization of health care posing a threat to public services.

The National Health Policy does address the above issues by stating the problems in very general terms but did not give any specific directions nor set any time frame for solutions.

HFA is holistic concept calling for efforts in education, housing, communications and industry as well as in health. In other words social justice in health and other fields as land reforms and wages is essential opportunity, in the ultimate analysis. Hence a broad based movement of radical redistribution of economic and political power and deep transformation of ideas, attitudes and values are called for to achieve HFA. Thus measures for poverty alleviation and social justice hold the key to HFA in India. The other areas needing urgent action are:

- Programmes promoting community participation.
- Transformation of ideas, attitudes and values among professionals and administrators.
- Increased budgetary allocation for health sector.
- Steps to consolidate the primary health care system, to provide back-up support of higher levels and to strengthen epidemiological services.

After the above overview of the goals, achievements, problems and prospects, we wish to point out that the philosophy and concept of HFA have to be understood in the correct perspective.

Development programmes should focus more on quality of human resources, on human well being and on productivity. Access to health services, education food security and clean environment are the basic prerequisites for HFA. To ensure these for all people may be a distant dream, but a dream which we should strive to realize.

HEALTH PROMOTION

In the past decade, health promotion has been a highly fashionable term. Until 1980, health promotion simply referred to health education. According to Green & Kreuter (1999), health promotion is the combination of educational and environmental supports (organizational, political and economic) for actions conducive to health. Tones (1994) defined health promotion as any combination of educational, legal, fiscal, economic, environmental and organizational interventions designed to facilitate the achievement of health and the prevention of diseases. To conclude, health promotion refers to 'health enhancing activities'. The activities can focus on individuals, groups or the whole population. Health promotion is not just confined to health professionals and health care services but everyone in different sectors of society.

Health promotion is broadly categorized into 3 major categories, namely health education, prevention and health protection.

Health education: Health education is considered the core component of health promotion. Health education activity provides adequate, accurate and reflective information and knowledge to recipients. Recipients are influenced and able to make their own rational decisions through the empowerment process. A top down approach to health education is inappropriate. Instead, information is provided according to the recipients' needs, with providers and recipients learning from each other.

Prevention: Prevention reduces the risk of occurrence of a disease process, illness, injuries, disability, handicap or some other unwanted events. There are three levels of prevention, namely primary, secondary and tertiary. Examples include healthy lifestyle, immunization, health screening, maternal and child health, rehabilitation programmes and sexuality education. Prevention programmes can be done on face-to-face basis or through mass media.

Health protection: Health protection consists of regulations, policies, or voluntary practices that are aimed at improving the living and working environment and prevention of ill health. For example, the proposed new ordinance for a total ban on smoking in restaurants and most indoor public areas aims to reduce heart disease and lung cancer in the population. Automobile seat belt legislation ensures that passengers are protected from injuries in case of motor vehicle accidents. Policy on mandatory food labeling enables consumer to make healthy and rational choices on food. Health promotion is concerned with the whole of life. Various terms such as holistic, ecological, systems, interdisciplinary and intersectoral grasp this dimension.

Health Promotion Approaches

According to Naidoo & Wills, there are five different approaches to health promotion:

The medical approach: It aims at freeing clients from disease. In this approach, clients remain passive recipients led by experts or professionals. The crucial value is patient compliance. Examples are patient's compliance with medical treatments; these include drug compliance or compliance with medical interventions.

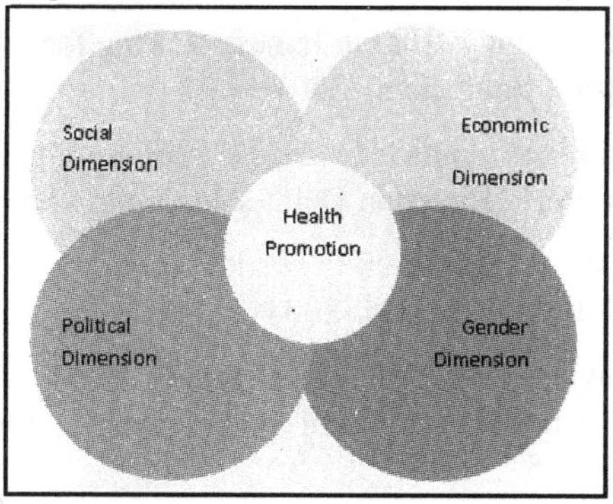

Fig. Health Promotion Approaches 19

The behavioural change approach: It implies that clients are responsible for their own health. This approach aims at attitude and behaviour change leading ultimately to changes in lifestyle. The value of the approach is a healthy lifestyle, which is determined by the health promoter. For example, programmes on healthy eating to prevent heart disease.

The empowerment approach: It aims to work with clients or the community to meet their perceived needs. Health workers advocate for clients, allow for discussion, facilitate for them and give them the freedom to choose, and support clients' decisions. The health promoter facilitates client empowerment. An example is when dealing with controversial sex issues such as pregnancy termination or premarital sex; the sex educator provides adequate information and facilitates in-depth discussions with the client. This approach provides clients with the freedom to make their desired choice based on rational thinking. Health professionals then respect their choices.

The social change model: It aims to address inequalities in health that are based on class, race, disabilities, disease or gender. This is a top down approach using political action to change the physical and social environment. For example, everyone should have equal access to information, education, employment, services and facilities, and has the right to be treated fairly. In Hong Kong, anti-discrimination laws make it unlawful to discriminate against people on certain grounds. The mission of the Equal Opportunities Commission is to help individuals understand their rights and responsibilities under the legislation and provide redress for discrimination.

REFERENCES

Karon Saucier Lundy; Sharyn James; "Caring for the Public Health" Jones & Barlett Publishers –2001

Philis E Schubert ; Janice E (EDT)" Community Health Nursing: Caring in action"; Thomson Delmor learning; -2003

Patrician Carroll; "Community Health Nursing: A Practical Guide"; Thomson Delonar learning; -2004

Lloyd F Novick ; Gleen P Mays: Public Health Administration ; Principles for population based management" ; Jones and Bartlett Publishers;-2005

Dianne Watkins; Judy Edwards; Pam Gastrell; "Community Health Nursing" Frameworks for Practice"; Elsevier Health Sciences- 2003

Jenny little wood; "Current issues in Community Nursing" Primary Health Care in practice"; Elsevier Health Sciences ; 1999.

Kamalam S; "Essentials in Community Health Nursing Practice"; Jaypee Brothers, Medical Publishers (P) Ltd, New Delhi.

Marcia Stanhope & Lancaster Jeanette; " Community Health Nursing – Process and practice for promoting health"; The C V Mosby Co, St Louis Toronto, 184.

2

Family Health Care & Services

In the last twenty years of nursing the focus in caring for patients has changed dramatically. This change is due to the changing family. The family has changed due to changes in society. The single patient has changed from medical needs plus what the patient views as important including their family. In my own experience in nursing, years ago the patient was the primary focus only. Now it takes a family to heal a patient. For patients to improve their health or to maintain wellness we as nurses have to look at the whole picture. What is the whole picture? The whole picture is what it takes to achieve a basic balance in the lives of our patients. Our goal as nurses is to meet the needs of our clients. This goal has two key points that years ago were different. We now consider the needs of the patient and those involved with the patient. As healthcare has evolved, nursing now understands that the basic needs of the patient and family must be met in order to promote a positive outcome.

FAMILY HEALTH SERVICES

The term "Family Health" Covers a very broad field. It is one of the major activities of the world health organization. It is divided into the following sub-areas:

a. Maternal and child health services.

b. Family planning services.

c. Nutrition.

d. Health education.

The purpose of the Family Health Program is to improve the health of women, children (including children with special health care needs) and families based on their health needs from birth to early childhood, during the school age and teen years, through young adulthood and the childbearing years including pregnancy. The Family Health Program has the responsibility to develop capacity and infrastructure to assure that health care systems "work" for mothers, children and families. The Family Health Program has maternal and child health professionals who provide their expertise, guidance, and technical assistance to local public health departments and other providers as well as to consumers with the intent to advance the health of women, children and families in Wisconsin.

MATERNAL AND CHILD HEALTH SERVICES

The MCH Program works with local public health departments, community based organizations, state-wide organizations and other providers to provide and or assure quality health services are delivered to mothers, children, and families. Primary areas of focus include: Increasing healthy birth outcomes; Promoting and assuring comprehensive primary care for children ages birth to 21, including children with special health care needs; Promoting healthy lifestyles among school-age youth, ages 6-21, including children with special health care needs; Assure access to safe, healthy child care up to age six, including children with special health care needs; Preconception, pregnancy-testing, and family planning/ reproductive health services. Maternal health includes the physical, mental and social well-being of women during pregnancy and delivery. Of the 150 million women who become pregnant each year, it has been estimated that more than 600,000 die annually from pregnancy-related causes.

With regard to maternal and reproductive health, the important elements of the programme include:

- Provision of antenatal care, including at least three antenatal care visits, iron prophylaxis for pregnant and lactating mothers, two doses of tetanus toxoid vaccine, detection and treatment of anaemia in mothers, and management and referral of high-risk pregnancies.
- Encouragement of institutional deliveries or home deliveries assisted by trained health personnel.
- Provision of postnatal care, including at least three postnatal visits
- Identification and management of reproductive tract infections, including sexually transmitted infections.

The Need for MCH Services

There are four main reasons why mother and child health care must be given top priority in terms of providing health services:

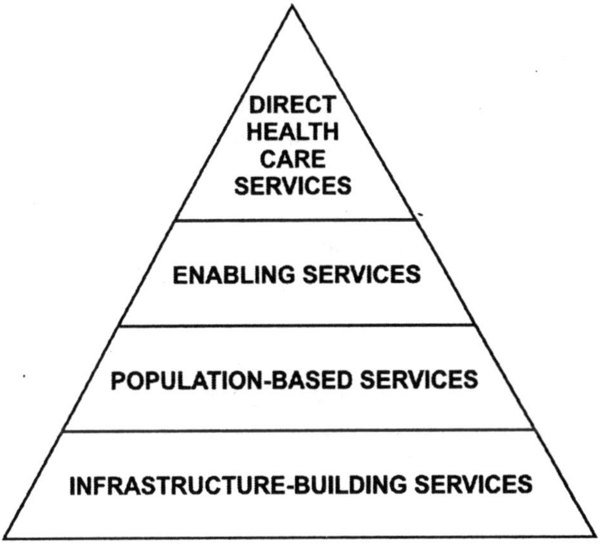

Fig. MCH Services

1. Mothers & Children below the age of 15 yrs., make up the majority of the population.
2. Mother and children constitute a "Special risk" or vulnerable group.
3. By improving the health of mothers and children we improve the health of the family & community.
4. Ensuring child survival is a future investment for the family & Community.

Objectives of MCH Care

The Objectives of MCH care have been defined as below:

1. Reduction of Material, perinatal, infant and child mortality & Morbidity.
2. Promotion of reproductive health.
3. Promotion of physical and Psychological development of the child and adolescent within the family. The ultimate objective of MCH care is life long health.

Role of Nurses in MCH Care

The functions are explained under four headings as follows:

1. Direct Care Provides:
   a. Antenatal Care i.e., Care of the women during Pregnancy.
   b. Intranatal Care i.e., care of women at the time of delivery.
   c. Post Natal care i.e., cares of the women after delivery.
   d. Child care: i.e., child survival activities i.e.,
      — Immunization.
      — Promotion of breast feeding.
      — Growth monitoring.
      — Weaning.
      — Oral rehydration.
      — Birth spacing.
2. Health Communication and Education:

   The groups that require priority attention are:
   — Dais.
   — Mothers.
   — Family.
3. Supervision and management:

   The Community health Nurse will have to supervise the work of dais, ANMS& Female workers. That means supervision of records, individual conference and counselling.
4. Research & Evaluation:

Research & Evaluation influence the Welfare of mothers and children.

FAMILY PLANNING SERVICES

The issue of family planning all over the World has attracted attentions due to its importance in decision making about population growth and development issues. In this wise, Geographers have become increasingly alarmed by the precipitous rise in its effects on population growth through out the World. The World Health Organisation defined Family Planning as the practice that helps individuals or couples to attain certain objectives such as avoiding unwanted pregnancies, bringing about unwanted babies at the right time, regulating the interval between pregnancies, controlling the time at which birth occurs in relation to the ages of the parents and determining the number of children in the family.

Onokerhoraye also defined family planning as the provision of birth prevention information services and appliances. It also involves teaching men and women about their bodies and teaching them how to prevent births usually with contraceptives but sometimes also with abortion or sterilization.

Various works and researches have also been done on perceptions and attitudes of people on family planning, but major emphases had always been placed on the role of women and the female gender approaches in many cases. In spite of the introduction of family planning services as means of curbing fertility rate, the population still rises because of the attitudes of the people involved. Hatcher opined that family planning is now seen as human right basic to human dignity. People and governments around the world understand this. Their work further showed that family planning helps women protect themselves from unwanted pregnancies. Since the 1960s family planning programmes have helped women around the world avoid about 400 million unwanted pregnancies. As a result, many women's lives have been saved from high-risk pregnancies and unsafe abortions.

However, most available works still point to emphasis being placed on the women fold at the detriment of the men counter part. In line with the postulates of the Central Place Theory, health and family planning facilities can be conceived as constituting a hierarchical system with secondary health and family planning facilities occupying an intermediate position.

More than 45 years ago, India became the first country in the developing world to initiate a state-sponsored family planning program with the goal of lowering fertility and slowing the population growth rate. Since the program's inception, fertility levels have declined throughout the country, at varying paces in different regions; overall, the total fertility rate decreased from 6.4-;6.6 lifetime births per woman in the early 1970s to 3.4 births per woman in the mid-1990s.

Since the 1960s, however, the Indian population has continued to grow by approximately 2% annually and has more than doubled in size, from 439 million in 1961 to an estimated 930 million in 1996. The population is expected to grow beyond 1.5 billion before it stabilizes.

Despite the decline in fertility, the reproductive health situation in India remains poor: Although the rate of infant mortality declined from more than 200 infant deaths per 1,000 live births in the 1960s to approximately 74 per 1,000 live births in the 1990s, maternal mortality ratios (550 deaths per 100,000 live births) remain among the highest in the world. Moreover, two-thirds of Indian women go through pregnancy and childbirth without seeing a trained birth attendant, and obstetric and gynaecologic disorders are widely prevalent and remain largely untreated and silently borne. The AIDS pandemic has added another dimension to the poor reproductive health scenario. Finally, contraceptive choice and quality of care within the Indian program remain problematic.

Role of Nurses in Family planning

Family planning is a national programme. The main role of a health worker or nurses in family planning services are:

1. Education and Counselling.
2. To assist the Physician.
3. To promote the concept of small family and child spacing.
4. To spread information to all eligible couples about family planning methods.
5. To arrange for clinical and surgical services.
6. To ensure an adequate supply of Contraceptives.

NUTRITION

Man kind eats to satisfy the feeling of hunger. Nutrition plays an important role in the promotion and maintenance of health and in the prevention of disease in order to keep well our bodies, need nourishment. Just as a plant will not grow without water sun shine and proper manure, human beings also need food stuffs of different kinds of nourish to the body. Malnutrition and under nutrition are the greatest international health problems of the present day. A sound knowledge of nutrition is therefore essential for all community health workers. Nutrition deals with the way in which the human body receives and uses all the substances or materials necessary for its growth and development and for keeping it is good condition.

Man kind eats to satisfy the feeling of hunger. Nutrition plays an important role in the promotion and maintenance of health and in the prevention of disease in order to keep well our bodies, need nourishment. Just as a plant will not grow without water sun shine and proper manure, human beings also need food stuffs of different kinds of nourish to the body. Malnutrition and under nutrition are the greatest international health problems of the present day. A sound knowledge of nutrition is therefore essential for all community health workers. Nutrition deals with the way in which the human body receives and uses all the substances or materials necessary for its growth and development and for keeping it is good condition.

Definition

Nutrition may be defined as the Science of food and its relation ship to health. It is concerned primarily with the part played by nutrients in body growth and development and maintenance. The word nutrient or "food factor" is used for specific dietary constituents such as proteins, Vitamins and minerals. Dietics is the practical application of the principles of nutrition, it includes the planning of meals for the well and sick. Good nutrition means "maintaining a nutritional status that enables us to grow well and enjoy good health.

Relation of Nutrition to Health

A person who does not eats the right foods or does not eat enough is malnourished and we call this s malnutrition also means that a child is less clever than he should be. The trouble may start even before birth if his mother does not have the right foods when she is pregnant. The malnourished child does not play but sits doing nothing. He is slow in learning to walk and talk. At school he is hungry, sleepy, dull and very slow to learn The children are slow in passing mile stones.

SCHOOL HEALTH PROGRAMMES

The school health services are important dimension of community. The reasons are, large number of young people in the total population, due to rapid growth and development, for early detection of nutritional and communicable diseases, due to group living.

The main objectives of School Health Programmes are as follows:

- The promotion of positive health.
- The prevention of disease.
- Early diagnosis, treatment and follow up of defects.
- Awakening health consciousness in children.
- The provision of healthful living.

Aspects of School Health Services

Some aspects of school health services are as follows:

- Health Appraisal of school children & School personnel.
- Remedial measures and follow up.
- Prevention of communicable diseases.
- Healthful school environment.
- Nutritional Services.

- First aid and emergency care.
- Mental Health.
- Dental Health.
- Eye health.
- Health Education.
- Education of Handicapped children.
- Proper maintenance and use of school health records.

Health Appraisals

Health Appraisal consists of periodic medical examination of school children and also teachers & other school personal. The School Health committee (1961) in India recommended medical examination for the children who are newly entered in the school and there after every 4 years. The physical examination include - test for Vision, hearing, speech, blood, urine, and faeces.

Children frequently suffer from dental diseases i.e., dental Carries. So at least once a year, a dental examination should be conducted.

Teachers & School personals are some of source of infection like pulmonary tuberculosis, So they should also be examined.

Daily Morning Inspection helps the teachers in detecting those children who need medical attention, these children have symptoms such as unusually flushed face, any rash or spots on the body, sore throat, rigid neck, nausea, vomiting, red or watery eyes, Headache, symptoms of acute cold, chills or fever, diarrhoea, body pain, Head lice, skin infections like scabies, etc.

Remedial Measures and Follow Up

After medical examination they should be given appropriate treatment and follow up. Special clinics should be conducted.

Prevention of Communicable Diseases

This can be done by National Immunization programme. A record of all immunization should be maintained as part of school health records when the child leaves the school, the health record should be accompanied with him.

Healthful School Environment

A healthful school environment is necessary for the child to grow best as emotionally, socially & personally. The school authority should follow same standards towards location, site structure, class room, furniture doors and windows, lighting, water supply, eating facilities and lavatory for the school.

Nutritional Services

If the child is physically weak, he may be mentally weak also. So the child can't take full advantage of schooling. In India the nutritional disorders are malnutrition, Vitamin, Iron and Calcium deficiencies. To prevent these disorders the midday school meal, applied nutrition programme, Vitamin A prophylaxis (Against blindness) programmes should be implemented.

First Aid and Emergency Care

The School teachers should be well trained during teacher training programme or in service training programmes in order to give first aid and emergency care for the pupils in school premises.

Mental Health

The School is the right place for shaping the child's behaviour and promoting mental health. The mental health of the child affects the physical health and learning process. Some of the school children problems are drug addiction, Juvenile delinquency and maladjustment. The school teacher plays an important role helping the child to attain positive mental health.

Dental Health Service

A school health programmes for dental examination at least once in a year should be provided for the children to prevent dental diseases & maintain dental hygiene.

Eye Health Services

The eye health services are to be provided in school to detect the refractive errors, treatment of squint, eye infections such as trachoma.

Health Education

In school Health services the most important element is health education towards environmental health, personal hygiene and family life.

Education of Handicapped Children

The ultimate goal is to assist the handicapped child and his family members, and the child will be able to reach his maximum energy to lead a normal life as possible.

School Health Records

In school, there should be a cumulative record for every student. Such record contains identifying data, i.e., date of birth, parent's name & Address, past health history & findings of physical examination & Screening tests and record of services provided. These records are useful to analyse and evaluate the school health programmes & provide a useful link between the school, home & the community.

Role of the Community Health Nurse

The nurse provides care to students and staff who have been injured or who present with acute illnesses. Care may involve treatment of health problems within the scope of nursing practice, communication with parents for treatment, and referral to other providers. The nurse uses the nursing process to assess, plan, implement, and evaluate care for students with chronic health conditions. This care should begin with the development of a nursing care plan (also known as an individualized health care plan) that should include an emergency action plan.

The nurse is responsible for medication administration and the performance of health care procedures that are within the scope of nursing practice and are ordered by an appropriately licensed health care provider. The nurse also assists faculty and staff in monitoring chronic health conditions. As the scope of nursing practice expands to utilize the increasingly complex technology needed to provide up-to-date care for clients, the nurse's body of knowledge grows through personal professional development.

In addition to providing health services directly, the nurse must take into account the nature of the school environment, including available resources. As the health care expert within the school, the nurse assesses the overall system of care and develops a plan for assuring that health needs are met. This leadership role includes developing a plan for responding to emergencies and disasters and training staff to respond appropriately. It also involves the appropriate delegation of care within applicable laws. Delegation to others involves initial assessment, training, competency validation, supervision, and evaluation by the nurse.

In order to address potential health problems that are barriers to learning or symptoms of underlying medical conditions, the nurse often engages in screening activities. Screening activities may include vision, hearing, postural, body mass index, or other screening. Determination of which screenings should be performed is based on several factors, including legal obligations, the validity of the screening test, the cost-effectiveness of the screening program, and the availability of resources to assure referral and follow-up.

FAMILY AS A UNIT OF COMMUNITY HEALTH SERVICE

Family can be said to be the basic unit in community health service. For families and communities to stay healthy, they need access to primary health care providers, like nurse practitioners. In many communities, there are not enough physicians, which can make it difficult for families to reach services that are important for the prevention and treatment of common health conditions. Family and community health programs try to improve families' well-being by improving access to nurses and other health-care providers.

Family is a system of relationships existing between parents and children's. It is a group of persons whose relations to one another's are based upon consanguinity. From the perspective of children, the family is a family of orientation: the family serves to locate children socially, and plays a major role in their enculturation and socialization. From the point of view of the parents, the family is a family of procreation the goal of which is to produce and enculturate and socializes children. However, producing children is not the only function of the family; in societies with a sexual division of labour, marriage, and the resulting relationship between two people, is necessary for the formation of an economically productive household.

Functions of the Family

Every member of a family contributes to the family unit as a whole, and every family unit contributes and adds to society. A well-known functionalist named Talcott Parson was able to break down the functions of the family into an easy to understand theory. He stated that the main functions of the family were, to ensure that new babies actually survive to become adult members of that society, to regulate sexual activity, to ensure that children are satisfactorily socialized into the norms and values of society, to provide economic support for other family members, to satisfy our emotional needs for love and security, and finally, to provide us with a sense of place and position in our society. In summary, the main function of the family is to provide for the basic needs of each other.

Some of the major functions of family can be enumerated as:

- The regulation of sexual behaviour and reproduction.
- Care and training of children.

- Co-operation and division of labour.
- Primary group satisfactions.
- It also helpful for socialization, race perpetration. Regulation and satisfaction of sex needs with economic functions.

The functions of family are affectional, economic, recreational, protective, religious and educational.

FACTORS INFLUENCING FAMILY HEALTH

The health status of a family is dependant upon many factors. In the main, you can think of different communities as being of different social classes. A person's social status is almost directly related to that person's health and the social group that you belong to will have a potential affect on your health and life chances.

NURSING PROCESS IN FAMILY

In the ever-changing world of technology in the healthcare setting, it is important not to overlook the family as a very important part of caring for the patient. The family is an extension of the patient and one is dependent on the other members for providing emotional and physical support. The family is the most important element in achieving and maintaining a society. There needs to be learning from within the family for individuals to be members of a society. A family is important to bring about a state of happiness and meaning in life to an individual and for future development and growth.

Family health nursing is an important focus of healthcare in 2008, as healthcare has shifted form patient centered care to family centered care. The days of extended lengths of stay, and short patient visits with only the most immediate family members are gone. Even the dynamic of the family itself has changed resulting in a shift in healthcare culture.

In the 21st century, families consist of a diverse group of individuals, with various heads of household, and living in a broad range of homes. Of course, a patient may not consider those living in the household to be "family," as today's family consists of whom the patient recognizes to be in his or her inner circle.

Families today may consist of married, divorced, or co-habitating individuals of various sexual orientations. Families may or may not have children. For families with children, various methods are available in which to have a child-natural conception, sperm banks, surrogate mothers, or adoption. Families dramatically vary in culture, race, and ethnicity with less concern for maintaining their individual heritage. More commonly now, grandparents, siblings, aunts, uncles, and others are raising or helping to raise children in the family. As people are living longer and requiring increasing care after hospitalization, the family can play an integral part in this care. Families are considered a valuable resource for information regarding the patient. They can provide information to assist in the care of the patient and planning his or her care after discharge.

The nurse needs to evaluate the health of the family to determine how it will influence the patient's progress. Many studies reveal that family health and the health of the family members are strongly correlated. Berkley and Hanson suggest the health of the family is dependent upon the balance between the stressors the family experiences and the strengths the family displays. How a family deals with stress is important to the cohesiveness of the structure.

Nursing is seen as a process, which includes:

Recognition: This process is initiated by the recognition of a need. This is based on nursing observation, perception and judgement.

Assessment: Having recognized that a need exists, an assessment of the possible courses of action is made. The nurse must decide what action should be taken and whether she is capable of taking such action.

Intervention: The nurse carries out activities decided upon as being most effective, in order to fulfil the recognised need. This phase contains all the tasks, procedures and practices which are performed by nurses. This is also the phase which has received the greatest attention both in the teaching and practice of nursing.

Evaluation: The Nurse should know the effectiveness of the nursing intervention. It demands a similar range of perceptual and judgment skills as the recognition phase.

Organization: It is the ability on the part of the nurse to organise nursing activity and to recognise the place of that activity in relation to others also involved in caring for the patient or client.

PRINCIPLES AND TECHNIQUE OF HOME VISITS

The basic principles in family visits are:

Meet the family: It is first necessary to meet the family, in order to establish contact with family members. Obtain consent for a base line survey of the health situation.

Identification of health problems: Various approaches may be used to identify family health problems and health needs, they include:

- Base - line survey.
- Scrutinizing the records.
- Specific questions regarding diseases common in the area.
- Questións regarding births, deaths, disability, failure to work etc.

Setting Priorities for health problems: Four standards are used for setting priorities among health problems.

- Frequency with which the problems occurs (prevalence)
- Seriousness of the problem for individuals and society.
- Urgency of the problem.
- Feasibility or susceptibility to control the problem within the financial resource limitations.

Planning and problem solving: Having recognized that a problem or need exists, the community health nurse must decide what action should be taken by the health team. Planning involves questions of setting objectives, and defining solutions to the problem.

Intervention of Implementation: The community health nurse carries out activities decided upon as being most effective in order to fulfil the recognized need.

Evaluation: Evaluation will measure the extent to which the problem has been solved or the need met. Evaluation provides "Feed back" that can lead to programme modification, which will make the programme more effective.

EQUIPMENTS

No home visit should be made without bag or kit. There are two separate kits. One is for deliveries (Delivery kit) and the other for general nursing and for prenatal and postnatal visits.

Delivery Kit

The UNICEF kit is widely used for deliveries and is most suitable. The equipment is contained in an aluminium box or leather bag. The contents of UNICEF delivery kit are:

- Plastic bag containing plastic apron and sheet, with soap, nail brush and towel in a water proof bag- 1

- Kidney trays -2
- Lotion bowls -2
- Pairs of artery forceps -2
- Pairs of dissecting forceps -1
- Pair of Scissors -1
- Bowl lifting forceps -1 pair
- Gloves -1 pair
- Instrument box (Containing syringe and needless) -1
- Complete set of enema can with tubing, catheter & clip -1
- Urethral Catheter -1
- Mucus extractor -1
- Spring balance -1
- Clinical Thermometer -1
- Rectal Thermometer -1
- Stock of cotton for making boiled swabs - sufficient
- Sterile gauze pieces for card dressing, mouth wipes, cord binders -sufficient.
- Antiseptic lotion (Dettol bottle) -1
- Prescribed drugs
- Fetoscope -1
- Measuring tape -1
- Notebook, pen/pencil, Paper bags

Community Health Nursing Bag

Various contents of Nursing bag of a community health nurse are:

- Soap, nail brush and towel in water proof bag -1
- Complete set of enema can -1
- Urinary Catheter (Rubbers) -2
- Clinical Thermometer -1
- Rectal Thermometer -1
- Scissors -1
- Artery forceps -2
- Dressing forceps -1

- Gallipot -1
- Kidney tray -1
- Bag of sterilised dressings -1
- Measuring Tape -1
- Fetoscope -1
- Bag of Sterilised swab sticks -1
- Spring balance -1
- Rubber gloves -1
- Large cotton bag -1
- Any prescribed drugs (spirit, gentian violet etc.)
- Cord and perineal dressings
- Mucus sucker -1
- Cord ligatures -1
- Eye antiseptics -1
- Small cut sized papers for giving medicines
- Pen, Pencil note book or dairy

EQUIPMENT CARE

Regular care of equipment is most important to prevent any possibility of errors and infection by carrying contaminated articles from house to house, to preserve the equipment for use as long as possible, and to put it to the best possible use. It should be remembered that the contents of the kit should be clean and in good condition but not necessarily Sterile. The following practices are recommended for different types of equipment:

Bag: If the bag is of metal, it should be well washed with soap and water or boiled water. If it is of leather, it can be dried in the sun. The cotton lining must be clean and boiled & replaced. As outer pocket can be made for keeping soap, towel and news paper.

Rubber goods: All should be well washed in soap and water and rinsed. Tubes and catheters must be hung to drain. Plastic apron and sheeting should be hung in the shade to dry. Gloves should be dried with clean cloth, both inside and outside and aired for a few hours. Rubber goods should be sterilized put them in boiling water and boiling them for ten minutes.

Thermometer: It should be soaked in an antiseptic solution, after washing with soap and water.

Bottles: All bottles should emptied once a month, after the corks are removed. The bottles & the corks should be boiled. Clean, well marked labels should be affixed on the bottles giving the contents and dosage before filling them up.

Enamelware and Stainless Steel: Boil such ware for 20 minutes, dry with a clean towel while the ware is still hot. In an emergency, it may be flamed (for this, rinse the bowl with a little spirit, then set fire to it with a match, being careful to do this only where there is no danger of setting fire to anything else).

Cord Ligatures: Remove the screw from the bottles and boil the bottles, the top and the threads for twenty minutes. Then place threads into (Spirit) bottle & use sterile forceps. Replace the cork and screw it tightly.

Eye Antiseptic: If a silver nitrate preparation is used, it must be renewed every week. It is very important that this bottle be well labelled. Now a day, freshly prepared lotion of penicillin 1/100 is generally used.

Instruments: All instruments should be washed well with cold water after use, boiled for 20 minutes and dried with a clean towel before being replaced. Do not boil the scissors. These can be thoroughly washed with soap & water, flamed or put in an antiseptic solution before use. A little oil can be added at the joints and blades after several uses to keep scissors sharpened and being rusted.

Dry Dressing and swabs: There are several methods of sterilizing dressing and swabs:

- Arrangements can be made with the local hospitals or primary health centres to sterilize dressing.
- The swabs and dressings can be packed in small cotton bags and then be placed in lined tins and autoclaved in the usual way.
- Swabs can be baked in the tins. The bottom and top of this must be perforated & the lid let open during baking.

Blood Pressure Machine: The Cotton arm band should be separated from the rubber bag and then washed and ironed in the usual way.

Stethoscope: The chest piece may be immersed in soapy water or an antiseptic solution. The kit must be placed in a safe and clean place and not locked away, as it must be available at all times. The delivery bag should be completely disinfected after each use. If the same bag is also used for nursing care, empty the bag completely and boil all boilable articles. Soak other equipment in antiseptic or soapy water. Wash the bag after completion, wash your hands well.

WORKING WITH FAMILIES IN PREVENTION OF DISEASE AND PROMOTION OF HEALTH

From the early beginnings of humanity, the family has developed to form, the most important unit of our society today, and that which has the most marked effect on its members. The influence of the family stands in a peculiarly central, crucial position. It faces inward to the individual, outward toward society, preparing each member to take his place in the wider social group by helping him to internalize its values and traditions as part of himself.

From the first cry at birth to the last words at death, the family surrounds us and finds a place for all ages, roles and relationships for both sexes. It has enormous creative potential, including that of life itself, and it is not surprising that, when it becomes disordered, it possesses an equal potential for terrible destruction. So strong is the influence of this basic unit on the individual that it could be argued that 'the family' is instrumental in determining the success or failure of that person's life. While the importance of the family is widely acknowledged, recent changes in societal norms have created a need to re-visit the conventional concepts of what comprises a family unit. Half a century ago the majority of families consisted of two parents who were married to each other and had between them produced a varied number of children. Relationships were also maintained with extended family members who were related by blood or law.

In the current era, however, there are a large proportion of people involved in non-traditional family forms which include single parent or step-parent households, cohabitation of unmarried couples and an increasing incidence of long-term homosexual partnerships. People with a blood or legal tie may not therefore necessarily live together, or see each other on a regular basis. Recognition as a family member can more realistically be seen in terms of feelings of affinity, obligation, intimacy and emotional attachment.

Research indicates that those involved in intimate relationships lead 'fuller' lives and judge such relationships to be rewarding, but there is also a destructive potential within family dynamics, particularly in disruptive situations which create disorder. One of the most difficult and stressful situations to which any family may be exposed is the experience of loss. Loss in this instance is used to mean 'the separation from something which is, in some way, part of the individual's being or which belongs to the individual'. That 'something' may be a person, removed by death, or the breakdown of a relationship. It may also be the loss of a faculty, or body image, loss of independence or status, of money or material possessions or the loss of role such as mothering or fathering. When the family is faced with a diagnosis of rapidly progressive terminal illness 'loss' is a predominant feature. Bowen outlined the disruptive impact of death or impending loss on a family's functional equilibrium and described the emotional shock waves that can reverberate throughout an entire family system long after the loss of an important family member.

Ninety per cent of the care of dying people in the last year of their lives takes place in the home, and the care is usually provided by the unpaid relatives and friends of the patient with support from community health and social services. Despite the fundamental role that the family plays in the care of the patient at home, and the obvious need for support from professionals, the concept of 'family nursing' is not seen as central to community nursing. Assessment of family dynamics is carried out informally, without proper recording or analysis of data, and family interventions are often haphazard and disorganized. The widespread application of the Roper model for nursing within Scotland may in some part be responsible for this trend, because while the model emphasizes the importance of seeing the person within a social context, the actual framework lends itself to a more individualized approach to nursing, and has no obvious facility to address the needs of the family as a unit.

FAMILY HEALTH RECORDS

Record and Reports are necessary to collect information and they are useful for:

- Assessing the health of the family.
- Collecting statistics, which are very important to health authorities.
- Attention of the doctor or other members of the health team to specific needs of individuals or families, and for follow up services.
- Information of Supervisors in assessing work done.
- Assessing need for various drugs, transport etc., based on numbers and types of patients.

- A tool for health education of individuals, families and communities.
- Evaluating progress of the health programmes for replacing.

Records to be maintained in the sub-centre include:

- Area Records, with general information about each area.
- Family folders and individual's health cards.
- Eligible couple register and record of contraceptives distributed.
- Maternal and child health records (Including antenatal care, child care, Nutrition and immunizations).
- Records of distribution of iron and folic acid, also Vitamin A solution.
- Vital events Register (Births and deaths).
- Stock register for receipt, issue and balance of drugs, contraceptives, stationery etc.
- Records of medical care and referrals.
- Inventory of furniture, linen and equipment.
- Records of meetings with Village Health Guides and dais, co-workers and supervisors.
- Monthly reports and other periodic reports as and when required.
- Daily dairy.
- Maps, Charts, Graphs.

RECORD MAINTENANCE

1. Record must be kept carefully and in clean conditions, safe from rats and insects.
2. It is important that records are not lost or mislaid. They are confidential and should be shown only to authorized persons.
3. Have a good system of filing, family folders, including records of individuals. Should be divided into localities and filed in order of house numbers. It is also useful to have a register or index cards filed in alphabetical order according the heads of the families.
4. Records must be readily available and should be kept up to date.

WRITING OF RECORDS AND REPORTS

Remember that the delivery of health services is not complete until details are written up in the correct register or record. The last half an hour of each day's work should be reserved for completing the records. In writing records and reports, following points should be kept in mind:

- Write them promptly, and keep them up to date.
- Write legibly, to be understood by others.
- Keep sentences short and clear.
- Be accurate and complete in important details.
- Replace records in their proper place.
- Consult your supervisor in ease of difficulty in completing records and wring reports.

Daily Dairy

It is not practicable for the health worker to take registers and large record books while carrying out village visits, yet memory is unreliable. Therefore a notebook called dairy should be carried and used constantly and the information written up in the proper record on return to the health centre. The purpose of dairy is:

- For immediate record of day's activities by the health worker. E.g.: Home Visits, Immunizations, Vitamin A administration, health teaching, etc.
- To record the name and address of persons to whom preliminary help has been given, and follow up to be done or referral if needed.
- To record observations during visits and matters needing to be reported to the supervisors or PHC authorities.

The information should be neatly, correctly, and honestly written.

Monthly Report

At the beginning of each month the health worker has to complete the report forms and submit one copy to her supervisor keeping one copy in her file at the health centre. The report includes detailed information of work carried out by herself, Villages Health Guides and Dais during the previous month, under the following Headings:

- Immunization.
- Communicable diseases.

- Vital Events.
- Family planning.
- Maternal and child health (Including deliveries, care of the under five and nutrition supplements supplied)
- Environmental Sanitation.
- Treatment of minor elements (patient numbers, and referrals)
- Health education activities
- Home visits.
- Other activities.

REFERENCES

Alexander H, MacDonald E. Evaluating policy-driven multi-agency partnership working: A cancer prevention strategy group and a multi-agency domestic abuse group. Presentation to the United Kingdom Evaluation Society Annual Conference, December 2001.

Anderson L, Shinn C, Fullilove M et al. The effectiveness of early childhood development programs: A systemic review. Am J Prev Med. 2003;24(S3): 32-46.

Angus et al, (1995), Sustainable Health Care for Canada, Queen's-University of Ottawa Economic Projects, Ottawa (available at www.cprn.org), and Auer et al. (1995).

Baranowski T, Perry CL, Parcel GS. In: Glanz K, Lewis FM, Rimer RK, (Eds.). How individuals, environments and health behaviour interact. Health Behaviour and Health Education: Theory, Research and Practice, 2nd ed. San Francisco: Jossey-Bass Inc.; 1997. p. 153-178.

Best A, Stokols D, Green LW, Leischow S, Holmes B, Buchholz K. An integrative framework for community partnering to translate theory into effective health promotion strategy. Am J Health Promot. 2003;18(2): 168-176.

Best A, Moor G, Holmes B, Clark PI, Bruce T, Leischow S, Buchholz K, Krajnak J. Health promotion dissemination and systems thinking: Towards an integrative model. Am J Health Behav. 2003;27(S3): S206-S216.

3

Health Administration in India

Every country has its own health problems depending upon the standard of living of its people, size of the population, geographical location of the country, etc. India is a vast country with an area of 3.2 million square kilometres and a population of 1027 million (2001). The health problems of such a vast country must also be large in magnitude. The health problems of India may be classified as below:

- Communicable Disease Problems
- Nutritional Problems
- Environmental Sanitation Problems
- Medical Care Problems
- Population Problems

NATIONAL HEALTH POLICY

The Ministry of Health and Family welfare evolved a National Health Policy in 1983 in view of the national commitment to attain the goal of Health for all by the year 2000. The health strategies suggested include restructuring the health infrastructure, development of health manpower, research and health development. The broad recommendations of health policy are:

- To establish one health sub centre for every 5,000 rural population (3,000 in tribal and hilly areas) with one male and female health worker.
- To establish one primary health centre for every 30,000 rural population (20,000 in hilly and tribal areas).
- To establish Community Health Centres, each serving a population of one lakh.

- To train village Health Guides selected by the community for every village or 1,000 rural population.
- To train traditional birth attendants or Dais in each village.
- Training of various categories of other staff, e.g. multipurpose workers.

These schemes are expected to ensure the availability to adequate infrastructure and medical and paramedical manpower to take us nearer the goal of universal provision of primary health care as envisaged in the National Health Policy. The National Health Policy laid down specific goals to be achieved by 1985, 1990, 1995 and 2000 AD. The National Health Policy has given a new direction to health planning in India, making primary health care the central function and the main focus of the national health system. The goal of national health planning in India was to attain health for all by the year 2000.

Since then there has been significant changes in the determinant factors relating to the health sector, necessitating revision of the policy, and a new National Health Policy -2002 was evolved.

HEALTH SERVICES ORGANIZATION

The health services organization in the country extends from the national level to the sub-centre level in the remote rural areas. Broadly, four levels of health organization may be distinguished:

- National
- State
- District
- Local

These roles played by them are described below:

NATIONAL LEVEL

The administration at the Centre consists of the Ministry of Health and Family Welfare, headed by a Minister, the Minister for Health and Family Welfare. The Union Health Ministry has 2 main departments

- The Department of Health,
- The Department of Family Welfare.

The Secretary to the Govt. of India, in the Ministry of Health and Family Welfare is in overall charge. He is assisted by a special Secretary who heads the Family Welfare Department.

The Director General of Health Services (DGHS) is the chief technical adviser to the Government on all matters relating to medical care and public health.

The responsibility of the Union Health Ministry consists mainly of policy making, planning, guiding, co-ordinating and evaluating. The functions of the Union Health Ministry have been set out in the 7th Schedule of Article 246 of the Constitution of India under 2 heads

- The Union List
- The Concurrent List.

The functions specified in the Union List are

- Administration of International Health
- Administration of Central Institutes
- Promotion of research; drugs control
- Census operations
- Regulation of labour and co-ordination with the States.

The functions specified in the Concurrent List are the responsibility of both the Union and State Governments. These are:

- Prevention of spread of communicable diseases
- Prevention of food adulteration
- Control of drugs and poisons
- Vital statistics
- Labour welfare and economics and social planning.

Central Council of Health

The Central Council of Health was set up by a Presidential Order in 1952 to promote coordinated and concerted action between centre and the states in the implementation of health programmes and measures pertaining to health.

A similar council also exists for family welfare. In recent years, these two councils have been meeting jointly to take coordinated decisions. The Central Council of Health and Family Welfare also make recommendations to the Central Government regarding distribution of grants-in-aid and review the work done through the utilization of these grants.

STATE HEALTH ADMINISTRATION

There are at present 28 States and 6 Union Territories and the national capital territory of Delhi in India. The States are independent in matters pertaining to the provision of health services to people living within their jurisdiction. Consequently, each State has evolved its own pattern of health administration.

But in each State there is a Minister of Health and Family Welfare elected by the people and Directorate of Health Services (known in some States as the Directorate of Health and Family Welfare).

The State Health Ministry is headed by a Minister of Health and a Deputy Minister of Health. In some States, the Health Minister is also in-charge of other portfolios. The Health Secretary is usually a senior Officer of the Indian

ADMINISTRATIVE SERVICE

The Health Directorate is headed by the Director of Health Services (or Director of Medical and Health Services as it is known in some States) who is assisted by a team of Joint Directors, Deputy Directors and Assistant Directors. The Deputy and Assistant Directors may, be of two types - regional and functional. The Regional Directors Inspect all the branches of public health within their jurisdiction irrespective of their specialty.

The Functional Directors are usually specialists in a particular branch of public health such as nursing, family planning, tuberculosis, leprosy, malaria, MCH, etc. A recent development in many States is the appointment of a Director of Medical Education.

The State Health Directorate is responsible for formulating and evaluating plans; directing the execution of approved plans and programmes.

THE DISTRICT PATTERN

The District in India is the pivot of the administrative structure. In some States (e.g. West Bengal), the district health organization is headed by a single Chief, the Chief Medical Officer of Health who is responsible for all community services in the district.

In some States (e.g. Andhra Pradesh, Madhya Pradesh), there are 2 Chiefs - District Medical Officer (DM0) or Civil Surgeon who is in-charge of medical services and the District Health Officer or District

Health and Family Welfare Officer who is in-charge of health and family welfare.

MUNICIPALITIES

The following types of local self- government Institutions are generally found in the urban areas

- Town Area Committees (in areas with population ranging between 5,000 and 10,000)
- Municipal Boards (in areas with population ranging between 10,000 and 2 lakhs).
- Corporations, (with population above 2 lakhs). The health organization in a Corporation is headed by a Health Officer, assisted by Deputy and Assistant Health Officers, Sanitary Inspectors and an army of sanitation staff.

  The services provided comprise sanitation and public health, MCH, control of foods and food sanitation and collection of vital statistics.
- The Municipal Boards are headed by elected Presidents. The services provided are usually confined to sanitation and public health because of limited financial position.

DECENTRALISED STATE ADMINISTRATION

The present structure of local self- government in the State is based on a three-tier structure, known as the Panchayat Raj.

The three levels are:

1. Village level: Gram Sabha, Gram or village Panchayatraj and Nyaya Panchayat
2. Block level: Panchayat Samiti
3. District level: Zilla Parishad..

Village Level

Gram sabha is the basic unit of the system of Panchayati Raj, It is an assembly of all the adults of the village. The meetings of the Sabha are held twice a year.

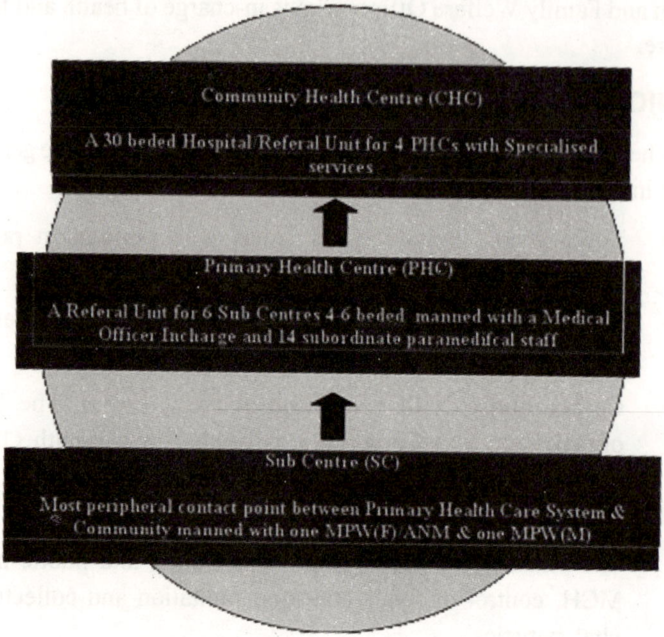

Fig. Village Level

Gram panchayat is the executive organ of the Gram Sabha. It is headed by a President known as Sarpanct or Mukhiya and the members comprise 10 to 30. Members of the Panchayat an elected by the adults of the Gram Sabha and they hold office for a period of 3 to/years.

The functions of the Panchaya cover the entire field of civil administration. e.g., sanitation, street lighting, control o disease, adult literacy, youth clubs Mahila Samitis, etc. The Panchaya Secretary helps the Panchayat in it; various activities,

Nyaya panchayat is the judicial organ of the Gram Sabha There is one Nyaya Panchayat for a group of 5 village Panchayats. The Nyay; Panchayats try civil cases and minor criminal offences. They are empowered to impose fines up to Rs. 100/-.

There are two health functionaries at the village level, namely (a) the Health Guides, and (b) trained Dais.

Health Guides: In India, about 72.2 per cent of the population live in rural areas. They are hardly covered by health services. It is now realised that a wide range of illnesses can be treated or prevented at the village level by a person with a relatively simple training or preparation. He has been called a village Health Guide (formerly known as community health worker or community health volunteer).

The scheme to train village health guides was initiated in the country on 2nd October 1977. These are voluntary health workers selected by the local community and trained locally for, 3 months at the primary health centre and sub centre.

After training, they are given a Manual which gives them detailed instructions of what they should do and a medical kit containing medicines worth Rs.600 a year. The Health Guides (now mostly women) provide the first contact between the community and the official health system. It is proposed to train one health guide for every 1000 rural population.

During the year 1981 the scheme was made 100 per cent centrally sponsored under family welfare programme. Now, since April 2002 the scheme is state sponsored. At present 3.23 Lakh village health guides are working in the country. Each VHG is paid an honorarium ofRs.50 per month.

The village health guides perform vaccinations. They give advice on simple health education measures. They give advice on the construction of latrines, garbage disposal and disinfection of water supplies. They refer cases to the nearest primary health centre where and when necessary.

They provide primary health care services with greater emphasis on child survival and MCH programme. Their work is supervised by the Community Health Nurses and Health Assistants.

Evaluation reports indicate that the health guides' scheme has been accepted and welcomed by the community. and co- operation, two social education organizers, an overseer with a public health bias, 10 village level workers and some auxiliary staff.

Block Level

The Block consists of about 100 villages and a population of about 80,000 and is provided with; Panchayat Samiti. This Samiti consists of all Sarpanches (heads) of the village panchayats in the Block; MLAs, MPs residing in the Block area, representative; of scheduled castes and tribes. The Block Development Officer is the ex-officer (secretary of the Panchayat Samiti. The Panchayat Samiti supervises and give; technical assistance and guidance to the village Panchayats engaged in development work. The Samiti also acts as an agent of the State Government, which provides money for developmental projects.

District Level

The instrument of local self-government at the District level is the Zilla Parishad. The members of the Zilla Parishad include all heads of the Panchayat Samitis in the district, MPs, MLAs, representatives of scheduled castes and tribes and co- operative societies. The Collector is a non-voting member. The Zilla Parishad is a supervisory and co-ordinating body. Its functions and powers vary from State to State. In Gujarat, control of primary health centres is exercised by the Zilla Parishads through the District Health Officer.

The Govt. of India in 1977 launched a scheme known as "Rural Health Service" - on the principle of "placing people's health in people's hands". It is based on the recommendations of the Shrivastav Committee in 1975. One of the main recommendations of the committee is to create a band of voluntary workers (e.g., community health workers) who will function as an interface between the local community and the national health system at the peripheral level.

The rural health scheme was subsequently modified in the light of the National Health Policy, which was approved by Parliament in 1983 to achieve the goal of "Health for All by the year 2000". The rural health infrastructure to deliver the rural health care, as it exists today.

The Tenth Five Year Plan, covering the period 2002 to 2007, represents another step in the evolution of development planning in India. There is a visible shift in the focus of development planning from the mere expansion of services to planning of enhancement of human well being.

PRIMARY HEALTH CENTRE

The Primary health Centre plays an important role in the health care delivery system (PHC). It is an institution for providing comprehensive health care which includes preventive, promotive and curative services under one roof. Medical officer or the health officer governs the functions of the primary health centre.

The programme of establishing primary health centres and sub centres with 4 to 6 beds at each PHC in a community development block having a population of 60,000 to 80,000 was launched as an integral part of the community development programme in the year 1952. Since then 5499 PHC and 49300 sub centres have been established until 1980.

The population coverage of PHC has been increased up to 1 lakh and more. The population coverage of sub-centre is about 10,000. PHC are upgraded with 32 to 40 bed hospitals during the sixth five-year plan. The primary health centre and sub-centre provide an infrastructure for the delivery health services in the rural areas of the country.

Functions of the Primary Health Centre

- Medical care
- MCH and family planning
- RCH
- Environment sanitation.
- School health services.
- Control of communicable diseases.
- Collection of vital statistics
- Health education.

Nursing services in the Primary health centre

Health services for the mother

- Antenatal care
- Delivery care
- Postnatal care

Child health services

- Under five clinics
- Adequate nutrition
- Immunization
- Health teaching

Family planning

NATIONAL PLANNING

Planning is a concept of recent origin. The object of national planning is to give a social and economic content to political freedom. Health planning which is a new term in health vocabulary is an important part of national planning. Heath planning is based on the health needs and health demands of the population.

The goal of health planning is the achievement of the optimal level of health. Nurses have their own contribution to make to health planning, because they are responsible for implementing many aspects of the health programme.

PLANNING COMMISSION

In March 1950, the Government of India had set up a Planning Commission to promote a rapid rise in the standard of living of the people by efficient exploitation of the resources of the country, increasing production and offering opportunities to all for employment in the service of community.

Health, being an important contributory factor to national development, the Planning Commission gave due importance to health and established a separate Division in the Planning Commission for the formulation of the health programmes to be included in the nations Five Year Plans. A Bureau of Planning was also constituted in 1965 in the Union Health Ministry to secure better coordination between the Centre and State Governments. For purposes of planning. the health sector has been divided into the following sub-sectors:

- Control of communicable diseases
- Medical education, training and research.
- Medical care including hospitals,
- Dispensaries and primary health centres.
- Public health services.
- Family Planning Indigenous system of medicine.

All the above sub-sectors have been given due consideration in the nation's Five Year Plans. However, the emphasis has changed from Plan to Plan depending upon the felt-needs of the people and technical considerations. The Health Plan is implemented at various levels - national, state, district, block and village.

ACHIEVEMENTS

As a result of the five year plans, considerable improvement has taken place in the field of health. A brief account of the achievements, has laid down specific goals to be achieved by year 2005, 2007, 2010 and 2015.

FIVE YEAR PLANS

The Tenth Five Year Plan, covering the period 2002 to 2007, represents another step in the evolution of development planning in India.

There is a visible shift in the focus of development planning from the mere expansion of services to planning of enhancement of human well-being.

The targets of Tenth Five-year plan for the plan period and beyond are:

- Reduction in the decadal rate of population growth between 2001 to 2011 to 16.2 percent
- Reduction in infant mortality rate to 45 per thousand live births by 2007 and 28 by 2012.
- Reduction in maternal mortality ratio to 2 per thousand live births by 2007 and 1 by 2012.

SOCIAL WELFARE SERVICES

Social welfare services are intended to cater to the weaker sections of the population. These include women, children, handicapped, aged, scheduled castes and tribes.

MINISTRY OF WELFARE

The Ministry of Welfare. Govt. of India, has been formed by pooling subjects related to welfare of the disabled, programmes of social defence, welfare of the scheduled castes and tribes and minorities.

The welfare of women and child development is looked after by a separate Department of Women and Child Development set up in the Ministry of Human Resources Development.

WELFARE PROGRAMME

1. Welfare of the disabled: The number of disabled persons in the country has been estimated to be around 120 lakhs. The Ministry of Welfare is implementing programmes for the early detection, treatment, education and rehabilitation of disabled persons, namely the blind, the deaf, the orthopaedically handicapped, the mentally retarded, spastics and the leprosy cured patients.
2. Social defence: Problems of family and social disorganization are manifest in the form of delinquency, juvenile vagrancy, drug addiction, alcoholism and crimes of various types. In order to control these problems, programmes of social defence have been launched by the Government, mainly within the framework of specific legislation and allied measures.
3. Women and child development: The Department of Women and Child Development in the Ministry of Human Resource Development has two bureaux: (i) Nutrition and child

development, and (ii) Women's welfare and development. The Central Social Welfare Board and the National Institute of Public Cooperation and Child Development assist the Department in its functions.

4. Central Social Welfare Board: The Central Social Welfare Board was set up in 1953. It surveys the needs and requirements of social welfare organizations in the country. All welfare schemes sponsored by the Board are implemented through voluntary agencies such as Mahila Mandals. The Mahila Mandals receive grants up to the extent of 75 per cent for approved activities. Some of these activities are:

   - Nutrition Programmes. These are feeding programmes to children in the age group 0-6 years, nursing and expectant mothers.
   - ICDS Project: In the Fifth Five Year Plan highest priority had been accorded to child welfare programmes. The most important scheme in this field was the Integrated Child Development Services (ICDS) for children in the age group 0-6 years, nursing and expectant mothers, etc. Under the scheme, a package of services consisting of supplementary nutrition, immunization, health check- up, referral services, nutrition and health education and non-formal pre- school education was delivered. There are now 4131 ICDS projects operating in selected blocks in the country. A Child Development Project Officer is directly in-charge of each ICDS project. The focal point for delivery of services is an anganwadi.
   - Other Activities: Numerous other- services are rendered such as organizing Working Women's Hostels, Foster Care Homes, services to physically handicapped persons, welfare services for the Aged and socio-economic projects.

VOLUNTARY ORGANIZATIONS

Besides the Central and State Governments, more than 10,000 voluntary organizations are also, engaged in social welfare activities. Important organizations are:

- The Indian Red Cross Society.
- Bharat Sevak Samaj.
- The Kasturba Memorial Fund.

- Lions Club.
- Ramakrishna mission.
- The Hindu Kusht Nivaran Sangh.
- Tuberculosis Association of India.
- Indian Council for Child Welfare.
- Family Planning Association of India.
- All India Women's Conference.
- The All India Blind Relief Society.

SPECIAL COMMUNITY HEALTH SERVICES

Industrial Nursing

The care of healthy people is the principal function of an occupational health service. This is quite unlike the care of sick people in a hospital setting. Doctors and nurses who are accustomed to the background of illness-oriented or curative medicine may not be quite successful in an occupational setting unless they are oriented to work in the care of healthy groups.

The aim of occupational health service is to keep the people at work healthy and to prevent them from falling ill. The whole emphasis is on prevention of ill-health and promotion of health. It is useful to consider at this juncture the basic functions of an occupational health service:

- To identify occupational hazards.
- To advise on the control of occupational hazards.
- It is not the role of an occupational health service to become deeply involved in routine medical treatment (except to give initial treatment for injuries and illnesses of sudden onset).
- To recognize at an early stage occupational or other disease and to screen vulnerable groups if advisable.
- To give advice about the placement of people in suitable work.
- To provide general advice and supervision of conditions at work which may influence health such as general and food sanitation.
- To undertake health education.
- It will be seen from the above list that most of the functions are preventive.

ROLE OF NURSES IN OCCUPATIONAL HEALTH SERVICES

Nurses will have to function within the framework of the above listed functions, which are mostly preventive in nature. Accordingly the role of nurses will include the following:

- She will assist the medical officer at examination of employees.
- She will take an intelligent interest to protect and improve the physical and mental health of all workers.
- She will attend to daily treatment of minor injuries, and assist the doctor when necessary.
- She must have good knowledge of first aid
- She must be able to identify, assess and advise management on the control of any health hazards affecting employees
- She may have to run an immunization clinic, antenatal clinic or school health clinic
- She has to conduct health education in all situations
- She may undertake home visiting and propagate the ideas of health and family welfare.

The occupational health nurse must have a strong bias towards preventive medicine. One nurse can deal with between 500 to 2000 work people. She should attend refresher in-service training courses from time to time.

COMMUNICABLE DISEASE PROBLEMS

Communicable diseases continue to be a major problem in India, whereas they have been largely controlled in the developed countries such as USA and UK. It has been estimated that nearly 54 per cent of deaths in India are due to communicable diseases.

MALARIA

Till 1950, malaria was considered to be a major health problem of India. An estimate of the disease in 1953 showed an annual incidence of 75 million cases, and 8 lakhs deaths. The National Malaria Control and Eradication Programmes launched in 1953 and 3958 respectively gave a deathblow to malaria; by 1971, the incidence of malaria declined to just over one million cases and no deaths. The disease, which was on its way to eradication reappeared. In 1976, the incidence of malaria arose to a peak of 6.47 million cases (of which 7, 42, 247 were falciparum cases) with 59 deaths.

The Govt. of India introduced a modified plan of operation from 1977 to tackle the situation effectively. Efforts are now being made to contain the disease. By 1984 the incidence of malaria was brought down to 2.1 million cases, since then the epidemiologlcal situation has not shown any great improvement. It seems to have reached a plateau, which is causing concern. By the end of 2001, about 2.05 million cases of malaria (with about 1 million cases of falciparum malaria) and 1015 deaths were reported from different states.

TUBERCULOSIS

Tuberculosis may be said to be leading communicable disease of India today. Four people per 1.000 populations have bacteriological confirmed disease. It has been estimated that there are at least 14 million cases of pulmonary tuberculosis in the country, of which at least 3.5 million are sputum positive. The number of deaths from tuberculosis is often quoted as 500,000 each year. About 2 to 2.5 million cases of pulmonary tuberculosis are added every year.

DIARRHOEAL DISEASES

Diarrhoeal diseases constitute one of the major causes of morbidity and mortality, especially in children below 5 years of age. They are responsible for about 6.27 lakh deaths each year. Outbreaks of diarrhoeal diseases (including cholera) continue to occur in India due to poor environmental conditions. The type of cholera that is now widely prevalent in India is "El Tor Cholera". It is milder infection as compared to older "classical cholera".

ACUTE RESPIRATORY INFECTIONS

Acute respiratory diseases are one of the major causes of mortality and morbidity in children below 5 years of age. It is estimated that about JL3.6,. per. cent hospital admissions and 13 percent in patient deaths in paediatric wards are due to ARI

LEPROSY

Leprosy is widely prevalent in India. With 5.59 million estimated cases India accounts for about 64 per cent of the global burden (0.9 million) of the disease and 87 per cent of the Region's registered cases. At present the reported prevalence rate is about 3.73 per 10,000 population.

Out of these cases about 18.5 per cent are children below the age of 15 years. The proportion of multibacillary cases among total cases is about 33.9 percent.

The deformity rate among total active cases is approximately 2.7 per cent. Presently all the districts in the country provide free Multi drug treatment (MDT) services.

FILARIA

Filariasis is another communicable disease problem of India. Although widespread in the country, the disease is heavily concentrated all along the east coast parts of Madhya Pradesh and Uttar- Pradesh. Surveys indicate that 454 million people are living in filarial areas.

There are 2 types of filarial Infection in the country - W. bancrofti, and B. malayi. Filariasis due to W. bancroftiis the more widely prevalent infection that due to B. malayi is restricted to certain areas in Kerala. Assam, Orissa, Madhya Pradesh, Chhattisgarh and West Bengal.

SEXUALLY TRANSMITTED DISEASE

Syphilis and gonorrhoea constitute the major problem. The exact population at a risk is not known.

AIDS

The problem of AIDS is increasing in magnitude every year. Since AIDS was first detected in the year 1986, the cumulative number has risen to 8220 by the end of July 1999. About 87.3 thousand cases are seropositive for HIV in the count

OTHERS

Enteric fever, helminthic infestations, viral hepatitis, kala-azar, meningitis and Japanese encephalitis are among the other important communicable disease problems in India. The tragedy is that most of these diseases can be either easily prevented or treated with minimum input of resources.

MALARIA

The 1994 resurgence of malaria compelled the Government of India to appoint an Expert Committee on Malaria to identify the problem areas and to suggest specific measures against the different paradigms of malaria. Thus the Malaria Action Programme (MAP) was evolved and is being implemented. The objectives of this new Malaria Action Programme are:

- Management of serious and complicated malaria cases.
- Prevention of mortality with particular reference to high risk groups
- Reduction of morbidity
- Control of outbreaks and epidemics
- Reduction of falctparum
- Incidence and containment resistance malaria
- Maintenance of low incidence status.
- The recent resurgence of malaria in many parts of the country necessitated the need to strengthen the health promotion component of the programme.
- It has been decided to observe Anti Malaria Month before the onset of monsoon i.e. month of June every year.

NATIONAL FILARIA CONTROL PROGRAMME

A National Filaria Control Programme was launched in 1955. To begin with, 22 filaria survey units and 13 control units were set up 'in different parts of the country to get a correct picture of the extent of filariasis in the country. As a result of these surveys, it is now estimated that about 412 million people are living in filarial areas. The main activities under the N.F.C.P are:

- Anti-mosquito and anti-larval measures in endemic area
- Establishment of filaria clinics for the detection and treatment of positive microfilaria cases.
- Provision of underground drainage in hyper endemic cities and towns.

Achievements

- Since June 1978, the operational component of the NFCP has been merged with the urban malaria scheme, but research and activities continue to be with the Director, National Institute of Communicable Diseases, Delhi.
- At present 206 filaria control units are functioning in the country. 199 filaria clinics are functioning in the rural areas.
- Besides, 12 Headquarters Bureaux and 3 Regional filaria training and research centres are also functioning in the country.
- During the Eighth Five Year Plan, it was envisaged to distribute anti-filarial drugs through primary health care delivery system in the rural areas of endemic states.

- As a consequence of continued research, it is now known that the Annual Single dose mass drug Therapy with antifilarial drug helps in reducing transmission to a very significant level.
- Accordingly the Directorate of NMEP developed a Pilot Project for introduction of this strategy in 13 endemic districts in 7 states namely Andhra Pradesh, Bihar, Kerala, Orissa, Tamil Nadu, Uttar Pradesh and West Bengal for 5 years to cover 40 million population.
- Initially it was introduced in south Arcot Vallali district in Tamilnadu in 1996. In Kerala, Orissa UP and West Bengal, the strategy has been introduced in 1997
- The strategy is being well received by community. The operational modalities include door-to-door drug delivery in Tamilnadu and Kerala through booth system in other states. The day mass drug therapy is given is called Filaria Day.

The national Tuberculosis Control Programme is a centrally sponsored programme. The activities of N.T.C.P. comprise:

- Early detection and domiciliary treatment of T.B. cases.
- BCG vaccination of infants and children.
- Isolation facilities, especially for those who require surgery or emergency treatment.
- Training and Demonstration.
- Rehabilitation
- Research.

A District Tuberculosis Control Programme was evolved in 1962 as a new approach to the community control of Tuberculosis. Early detection of T.B. cases by all primary health centres in the district and other hospitals and agencies, domiciliary treatment of all sputum positive cases and B.C.G. vaccination of all those below 20 years of age are the main concern of the District T.B. Control Programme. National T.B. Control Programme has been accorded high priority by the government with the inclusion of NTCP in the 20-point programme, there is expansion of essential activities under the programme. Short-term chemotherapy has been introduced in 292 districts and is being introduced in more districts in a phased manner.

Revised National Tuberculosis Control Programme has been introduced in the country as a Pilot Project since 1993 covering 2.35 million population. The second phase was expanded to 17 more places covering about 13.85 million population. At present it is in third phase covering about 450 million population. The objective of this strategy is to achieve at least 85 percent cure rate of infectious cases through DOTS to detect at least 75 per cent estimated cases through quality sputum microscopy; and involvement of NGOs in information, education and communication activities. DOTS is given by peripheral health staff such as MPWs or through voluntary workers such as teachers, anganwadi workers, dais, ex-patients, social workers etc. They are known as DOT agent.

ORAL REHYDRATION THERAPY

Diarrhoea is one of the leading cause of child mortality. Oral Rehydration Therapy started in 1986-87 is being implemented through RCH programme. Supplies of ORS packets to the states are being organized by central Government. Twice a year 150 packet of drugs are provided as part of drug kit supplied to all sub-centres in the country. The programme emphasises the rational use of drugs for the management of diarrhoea. Adequate nutritional care of the child with diarrhoea and proper advice to mothers on feeding are two important areas of this programme.

ACUTE RESPIRATORY DISEASE CONTROL

The standard case management of ARI and prevention of death due to pneumonia is now an integral part of RCH programme. Peripheral health workers are being trained to recognize and treat pneumonia. Cotrimoxazole is being supplied to the health workers through the CSSM drug kit. Prevention and control of vitamin A deficiency in children is estimated that a large number of children suffer from sub- clinical deficiency of vitamin A. Under the programme, 5 doses of Vitamin A are given to all children under three years of age. The first dose (1 lakh units) is given at nine months of age along with measles vaccination. The second dose (2 lakh units) is given along with DPT/OPV booster dose. subsequent three doses (2 lakh units per dose) are given at six months intervals.

NATIONAL LEPROSY ERADICATION PROGRAMME

The main objective of the programme is early detection of leprosy cases and their treatment (domiciliary) with multi- drug therapy to control- the spread of leprosy. There are two kinds of units functioning in the country -

- National Leprosy Control Units and
- Survey, Education and Treatment (SET) Centres.

Leprosy control units are established in highly endemic areas in other areas, SET Centres are established. The SET Centres are attached to the primary health centres. A Leprosy Control Unit covers a population of 4 lakhs and is headed by a medical officer under whom 20 Para-medical workers (PMWs) work, at the rate of one PMW for 20.000 population, two non-medical supervisors for 10 PMWs. The SET centre covers a population of 25,000 and is looked after by a PMW who works under the guidance of the medical officer of the primary health centre. Mobile Leprosy Treatment Units provide services to leprosy patients in the non- endemic districts.

Each MLTU consists of one medical officer, one non-medical officer, one non-medical supervisor, two para medical workers and a driver. At present the existing infrastructure is as follows.

Leprosy Control Unit or Modified Leprosy Control Units (LCU/ MLCU) 778. Urban Leprosy Centre (ULC) 907. SET Centres 5744, Temporary Hospitalization Ward (THW) 290, Reconstructive Surgery Unit (RSU) 75, Sample Survey cum Assessment Unit (SSAU) 40. Mobile Leprosy Treatment Unit (MLTU) 350. During 1997 the government of India decided to implement Modified Leprosy Elimination Campaign (MLEC) in all the states/UTs. Till the end of May 1998. 22 States/UTs have implemented MLEC. The strategy comprise short orientation training in leprosy to health staff including medical officers, health workers and volunteers; creating public awareness about leprosy; and house to house search for a period of six days for suspected cases of leprosy.

NATIONAL AIDS CONTROL PROGRAMME

National AIDS Control Programme was Launched in India in the year l987. The Ministry of Health and Family Welfare has set up National AIDS Control Organization (NACO) as a separate wing to implement and closely monitor the various components of the programme, The aim of the programme is to prevent further transmission of HIV, to decrease morbidity and mortality associated with HIV infection and to minimize the socio- economic Impact resulting from HIV infection. The national strategy has the following components:

- establishment of surveillance centres to cover the whole country;
- identification of high risk group and their screening;
- issuing specific guidelines for management of detected cases and their follow-up

- formulating guidelines for blood bank, blood product manufacturers, blood donors and dialysis units
- information education and communication activities by involving mass media and research for reduction of personal and social impact of the disease
- control of sexually transmitted disease; and condom programme.

BLOOD SAFETY PROGRAMME

National and State/UTs level Blood Transfusion Councils have been set-up in the country. Professional blood donation has been prohibited in the country since 1st January 1998. Only licensed blood banks are permitted to operate, and voluntary blood donation is encouraged. The strategy is to ensure safe collection, processing, storage and distribution of blood and blood products. Zonal blood testing centres have been established to provide linkage with other blood banks affiliated to public, private and voluntary sector.

As per national blood safety policy, testing of every unit of blood is mandatory for detecting infections like HIV, hepatitis B. malaria and syphilis. In the country 1233 blood banks have been licensed to supply blood. 815 blood banks have been modernized with provision of adequate facilities of equipment and development of appropriate manpower, 40 blood component separation units have been established. Besides district level and small blood banks with independent HIV testing facilities, 154 zonal blood-testing centres and 9 HIV Reference Centres are functioning in the country. HIV Test Kits are supplied up to district level blood banks.

STD CONTROL PROGRAMME

STD control is linked to HIV/AIDS control, as behaviours resulting in transmission of STD and HIV are same. HIV is transmitted more easily in the presence of another STD. Hence, early diagnosis and treatment of STD is now recognized as one of the major strategies to control spread of HIV infection. STD control programme has been in operation in India since 1946.

The programme is based on specialized facilities offering clinical services for diagnosis and treatment of STD and relies on the health seeking behaviour of individuals with STD. Patients with STD form a special group for health education and individual counselling. The facilities currently providing STD control are - 5 Regional STD Reference centres, skin leprosy STD clinics in medical colleges and 504 STD clinics usually located at district hospitals.

NATIONAL FAMILY WELFARE PROGRAMME

IODINE DEFICIENCY DISORDERS CONTROL PROGRAMME

A national goitre control programme was launched in 1962, based on iodized salt. After 20 years of operation, it was found that the prevalence of goitre had remained the same. Reassessment of the problem by the ICMR showed that goitre is widely prevalent in the country, besides the traditional Himalayan belt of endemic goitre. As a result, a major national programme - Iodine Deficiency Disorder (IDD) Control Programme was initiated in which nation- wide, rather than area-specific use of iodized salt is being promoted. It was decided as a national policy to fortify all edible salt in a phased manner by the end of 8th plan. The essential components of a national IDD programme are use of iodized salt in place of common salt, monitoring and surveillance, manpower training and mass communication.

NATIONAL WATER SUPPLY AND SANITATION PROGRAMME

National water supply and sanitation programme was initiated in 1954 with the object of providing safe water supply and adequate drainage arrangements for the entire rural and urban population of the country. The Central Government is providing long-range loans to States for implementing urban water supply schemes; and outright grants equal to half of the cost for implementing the rural water supply schemes.

MINIMUM NEED PROGRAMME

The Minimum Need Programme (MNP) was introduced in the first year of Fifth Five Year Plan. The objective of the programme is to provide certain basic minimum needs and thereby improve the living standards of the people. It is the expression of the commitment of the government for the "social and economic development of the community particularly the underprivileged and underserved population". The programme includes the following components:

- Rural Health
- Rural Water Supply
- Rural Electrification

- Elementary Education
- Adult Education
- Nutrition
- Environment Improvement of Urban Slums
- Houses for landless labourers

20-POINT PROGRAMME

In addition to the Five Year Plans and Programmes, in 1975. the government of India Initiated a special activity. This was the 20-point Programme-described as an agenda for national action to promote social justice and economic growth. At least 8 out of 20 points are related directly or Indirectly, to health.

QUALITIES AND FUNCTIONS OF A PUBLIC HEALTH NURSE

Nursing differs from other professions its humanitarian aspects. The nurse first has interest in people, and in understanding human behaviour, has concern over human and ability to empathize are basic qualities required of a nurse. A good nurse has a friendly disposition, earnest, charitable, resourceful, operative and takes responsibility with native. Minimum essential skills of a nurse are observation, communication, leaving besides supportive and essential skills. She must have abilities to like interpretations, make judgments and take decisions.

Nursing calls for a pleasure of self-discipline not only of lotions but of other aspects of behaviour and action. The community nurse must be prepared to play a much wider role than is offered by her work in hospitals. There is much greater element of decision-making. Management skills, administration of programmes, teaching and acting as a team leader, as well as a member of the health team are all important. Perhaps the most crucial requirement is that the nurse must be prepared to learn from the people, and share leadership with them when it is necessary and to plan with them.

FUNCTION OF A COMMUNITY HEALTH NURSE

The functions of a community health nurse have been classified broadly under the following heads:

- Administration
- Communication

- Nursing
- Teaching
- Research

Administration

The nurse is responsible for the day-to-day assignment of the nursing staff and supervision of these personnel. She provides direction and leadership to those whom she supervises. She is responsible for planning, implementation and evaluation of a practical plan of nursing administration within the primary health centre and its associated sub centres.

Communication

This involves ability to maintain good working relationship with members of the health team, related agencies and the community. She is a link between the patient, the family and the doctor. She participates in the staff and community meetings.

Nursing

She provides comprehensive nursing care to individuals and families. This includes family care of the pregnant women, before, at the time of and after delivery, care of the newborn, the premature, the infant, toddler, the school child, nutrition and family planning.

Teaching

Teaching comprises:

- Knowledge and skills of methods of individual
- Group teaching
- Preparation and use of simple teaching aids
- Training of dais and health workers;
- Participation in student training programmes.

Research

There is probably far more research relevant to nursing than nurses realise. A good deal of knowledge derived from sociology and psychology is relevant to public health nursing, viz. infant feeding and weaning, mother and child relationship, nursing needs and practices in the community, utilization of the existing nursing services, job analysis of nursing personnel in the team, etc.

FAMILY HEALTH SERVICES

The term "family health" covers a broad field. It is one of the major activities of the World Health Organization. It is divided into the following sub-areas:

- Maternal and child health
- Family planning
- Nutrition
- Health education

The broad objectives of the family health services are:

- to reduce maternal and child mortality and morbidity rates
- spacing of children
- to solve the problems of malnutrition at the family level
- to educate all members of the family In the basic requirements of healthy living)

This section studies the care of mothers and children. The other aspects of family health are considered in the following topics

MATERNAL AND CHILD HEALTH

THE NEED FOR MCH SERVICES

There are four main reasons why mother and child health must be given top priority in terms of providing health services. Mothers and children below the age of 15 years make up the majority of the population in almost all countries. In developing countries, they comprise nearly 65 per cent of the total population (in India 64 per cent).

By virtue of their large numbers, their needs in terms of health care are greater Mothers and children constitute a "special risk" or vulnerable group - in terms of illnesses and deaths, connected with pregnancy and childbirth in the case of mothers; and growth and development in the case of children. By improving the health of mothers and children, we improve the health of the family and community, and Ensuring child survival is a future Investment for the family and community.

A WHO Expert Group (1976) defined mother and child health services as the promotive, preventive, curative and rehabilitative care for mothers and children.

OBJECTIVES OF MCH CARE

The objectives of MCH care have been given below:

Reduction of maternal, perinatal, health is an important function of the primary health centres in India. There should be special clinic days and time set apart for this work. The services of specialists should be enlisted as and when necessary. That is, the school health clinic should be linked up with the PHC and higher levels of health care.

Immunizations: The school offers excellent opportunities for Immunisation for children. Immunization by 1990 was part of a global effort coordinated by the World Health Organization. The national immunization schedule is given below.

School sanitation: The school should be a model of good sanitation. There should be adequate, safe drinking water facilities preferably supplied by a tube well. Urinals and privies should be provided - one urinal for 60 students and one sanitary latrine for 100 students. Arrangements should be separate for boys and girls. Vendors other than those approved by the school health authority should not be allowed inside school premises. A healthful school environment is necessary for the best emotional, social and personal health of the pupils.

Nutritional services: A child, who is physically weak because of poor nutrition cannot be expected to take full advantage of schooling. The community health nurse may be required to administer the following nutrition programmes: (a) Midday school meal(b) vitamin A prophylaxis programme - administration of a large dose (200,000 IU) of vitamin A orally to children every 6 months up to the age of 6 years or so.

First Aid: In every school, a fully equipped First Aid Box should be at hand. The emergencies commonly met with in schools are: (a) accidents (b) Injuries (c) medical emergencies like abdominal pain, epileptic fits, fainting, etc.

Health Education: Health education has an important role to play in the promotion of both individual and community health. Health education in schools should not be reduced merely to teach the children a set of rules of hygiene. Participation of children in community health programmes (e.g., construction of wells, latrines, vaccination campaigns, etc) should be encouraged, whenever possible. The hygiene of skin, hair, teeth and clothing; the importance of exercise, sleep, nutrition and good habits; the need for Immunization, safe water, control of flies and other/insects are some of the topics on which health- education may be profitably-Imparted.

School Health Records: The health record of each student should be properly maintained. The record should contain:

- Identifying data - name, date of birth and address
- Past health history
- Record of findings of physical examination and screening
- Record of services provided.

These records, besides providing Information on the health aspects of school children, also serve as a useful link between the home, school and community.

CAUSES OF POOR HEALTH

Poor health persists as a major problem in many developing countries, including India. The causes responsible for this situation need to be understood in effective measures are to be undertaken to improve health. The causes of poor health in India may be enumerated as below:

1. Environmental causes:
    - Lack of safe drinking water
    - Lack of basic sanitation
    - Crowded,
    - Unsanitary living conditions
    - Pollution of water, food, soil and air
2. Socio-economic causes:
    - Poverty
    - Illiteracy
    - Ignorance
    - Prejudicial customs, traditions,
    - Beliefs and cultural patterns
    - Inadequate nutrition
    - Lack of personal hygiene
    - Rapid population growth
3. Others:
    - Uneven development of health
    - Care services and nursing care
    - Inadequate primary health care

HOME VISITING

Home visiting is the backbone of public health nursing. The purpose of home visiting is:

- To carry out simple nursing care in the home
- For the prevention of disease
- Promotion of health of the members of the family.

PRINCIPLES OF HOME VISITING

- Home visiting should be made according to the needs of the people
- It should be part of a planned visiting programme
- Collect background Information: regarding the family In particular an community in general - that is Information regarding the family size occupation, Income, religion resources, customs and cultures.
- Identify the health problems of the family
- Use safe technical skills, and nursing procedures
- In health teaching; be sure of what you discuss, i.e. scientific soundness
- The approach to the family should be kind and courteous with a view to gain their confidence

PLANNING AND EVALUATION

Planning is an art and science. The purpose of planning is to achieve definite objectives within a specified time and within the available resources.

- First make survey and prepare a map of the area with details of topography location of villages, population, road etc. Collect all the background information of the community. Prepare family folders and Individual cards.
- Identify the families or individuals in need of home visiting. These are usually the antenatal and postnatal cases, infants, toddlers, chronically sick and those who are unable to attend a treatment centre.
- On the first visit, the public health nurse should introduce herself to the family and explain the purpose of the visit. The talk should be informal giving plenty of opportunity to ask questions and raise discussion.

- Take the nursing bag. Treat minor illnesses. Advise hospitalization where necessary. Undertake immunization where necessary. Give health instruction on personal and environmental hygiene.
- Follow up: This is' the most important part of home visiting, to find out how far the instructions given were followed; and to give credit for what they have done.
- Evaluation Try to evaluate what has been achieved against the goals. The questions to be raised are:
- How far the visit has been useful?
- What have been the difficulties?
- What more needs to be done?

BAG TECHNIQUE

The Bag

- The bag should be made of canvas, leather or light metal.
- It should be such that it can be carried by the hand or on the shoulder.
- The bag should have outside pockets for keeping a note-book, tape measure, newspaper or plastic sheet, towel, soap in a soap dish, and a nail brush.

Bag Technique

As the same bag may have to be used in several homes, every effort should be made to keep the bag as clean as possible.

- First spread the newspaper or plastic sheet on a flat surface in a clean area and place the bag on it. It should be kept away from children and animals.
- Wash hands with soap and water each time before opening the bag.
- Remove only what is needed.
- Carry out the nursing procedure.
- Wash and boil all the Instruments after finishing the work; wash hands, open the bag and replace them in the bag. When this is not possible, place them in a separate bag.
- Bum the soiled dressings.

- Fold the used newspaper with used side inside, and keep it in the outer pocket.

Equipment

No home visit should be made without bag or kit. There are two separate kits - one for deliveries (Delivery Kit) and the other for general nursing and for prenatal and postnatal visits.

- Delivery Kit: The, UNICEF kit is widely used for deliveries and is most suitable. The equipment is contained in an aluminium box.
- Nursing Bag: If no separate bag is supplied, the nurse should Improvise, using a tin with an air-tight lid, or a plastic bag. As the equipment may have to be carried by hand for long distances and for long periods, the tin or bag should be as light as possible and should contain only essential articles. Unless the whole container can be completely disinfected, a separate cotton lining should be used. The nurse must also carry separately (not in her kit) a pen or pencil, a notebook or diary in which to note down observations and enter records before leaving the patient's home.

NUTRITIONAL PROBLEMS

Malnutrition is widely prevalent in India. The specific nutritional problems are:

PROTEIN-CALORIE MALNUTRITION

This is due to deficiency of calories and proteins in the diet. A large number of children are victims of kwashiorkor and marasmus in India

ENDEMIC GOITRE

About 71 million people are estimated to be affected by endemic goitre (i.e., swelling of the thyroid gland in the neck) and other iodine deficiency disorders. This condition is due to iodine deficiency.

VITAMIN DEFICIENCIES

Deficiency of vitamin A is an important public health problem in India especially in the age group, 3 to 5 years. About 12.000 to 14,000 children are estimated to go blind every year.

The knowledge of the roles of community health nursing, scope and concept and health problems in India and health strategies in India is essential. A greater emphasis is made on disease control programme, preventive medical care and five year plans and twenty point programme, emphasising health care system in the central state level and primary health care centre and sub-centre level.

REFERENCES

Billings J. Community development: A critical review of approaches to evaluation. J Adv Nurs. 2000;31(2): 472-480.

Birch S, Stoddart G, Beland F. Modeling the community as a determinant of health. Can J Public Health. 1998;89(6): 402-405.

Bryant T. Role of knowledge in public health and health promotion policy change. Health Promot Int. 2002;17(1): 89-98.

CART Project Team. Community action for health promotion: A review of methods and outcomes 1990-1995. Am J Prev Med. 1997;13(4): 229-239.

Coday M, Klesges LM, Garrison RJ, Johnson KC, O'Toole M, Morris GS. Health opportunities with physical exercise (HOPE): Social contextual interventions to reduce sedentary behaviour in urban settings. Health Educ Res. 2002;17(5): 637-647.

Cook A, Jardine A, Weinstein P. Using human disease outbreaks as a guide to multilevel ecosystem interventions. Environ Health Perspect. 2004; 112(11): 1143-1146.

Cummins SK, Jackson RJ. The Built Environment and Children's Health. Pediatr Clin North Am. 2001;48(5): 1241-1252.

Deschesnes M, Martin C, Jomphe-Hill A. Comprehensive approaches to school health promotion: how to achieve broader implementation? Health Promot Int. 2003;18(4): 387-396.

Donaldson C C, Halma L, Gall N, (2002) "Setting Priorities and Allocating Resources in Regional Health Authorities: A Report from Two Pilot Exercises Using Program Budgeting and Marginal Analysis".

Ebrahim S, Smith GD. Exporting failure? Coronary heart disease and stroke in developing countries. Int J Epidemiol. 2001;30(2): 201-205.

Edwards N. Population health: Determinants and interventions. Can J Public Health. 1999; 90(1): 10-11.

4

Determinants of Health

The health of both the individual and the general population is determined by the social, biological, physical and behavioural factors. Biological determinants are inherent or acquired. The genetic heritage can be a factor for the disease or any other ailments. Behavioural determinants of the health are much-studied factors, it has been seen that a particular class of diseases is found to occur in a group or association having similar personality traits. Social factors are again one of the most important determinants of health. It is often seen that people who mingle well and have social groups are better known people about the different aspects of health. Whereas the people who remain isolated and are not social do not have sufficient knowledge about health and other factors.

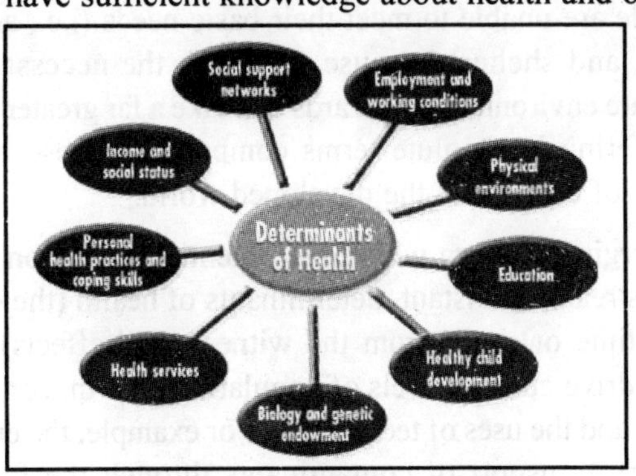

Fig. Determinants of Health

Many factors combine together to affect the health of individuals and communities. Whether people are healthy or not, is determined by their circumstances and environment. To a large extent, factors such as where we live, the state of our environment, genetics, our income and education level, and our relationships with friends and family all have considerable impacts on health, whereas the more commonly considered factors such as access and use of health care services often have less of an impact.

The determinants of health include:

- The social and economic environment,
- The physical environment, and
- The person's individual characteristics and behaviours.

ENVIRONMENT

An environmental determinant of health is usually any kind of external agent that can be physical, chemical, biological, social or cultural that can cause a change in the health status of an individual or a group of individuals. The determinants of health help in detecting the causes for the diseases and as such help in the process of getting cure for that.

Factors in our natural environment (e.g. air, water quality) and human-built environment (e.g. housing, workplace safety and road design) play a role in individual and public health.

Hundreds of millions of people suffer from respiratory diseases caused by biological and chemical agents in the air, both indoors and outdoors. According to the World Health Organization (WHO), over one billion people are unable to meet their basic needs (i.e., adequate food, clean water, and shelter) because they lack the necessary income or land. These are environmental hazards that take a far greater toll on human life and suffering in absolute terms compared to those environmental determinants of concern in the developed world.

An emerging concern with great potential impact on public health relates to upstream, or distant, determinants of health (the exposures are far apart in time or space from the witnessed ill-effects) including as policies that drive current levels of population growth, consumption and waste issues, and the uses of technology. For example, the environmental, transboundary transport of contaminants through the food chain has resulted in global chemical contamination.

Other transboundary issues include acid precipitation, ozone, greenhouse gasses, and hazardous wastes. Global ecological integrity (i.e., the ability of life-support systems to sustain themselves in the presence of polluting forces) and global change (including concerns about climate change from global warming, ozone depletion, and the loss of biodiversity) have given people reason to adopt the WHO maxim: "Think globally, act locally." Reducing wastes and consumption at the local level can have positive effects on the entire earth's ecosystems.

AIR QUALITY

Emissions from motor vehicles, industry, heating and commercial sources, as well as tobacco smoke or household fuels, pollute the air we breathe. Evidence shows that air pollution at current levels in cities is responsible for a significant burden of disease, mortality, hospital admissions and exacerbation of symptoms, especially in relation to cardiovascular disease. Very young children and pregnant woman are especially vulnerable to air pollutants. WHO estimated that in children aged 0-4 years, throughout the European Region, around 700 deaths occur annually from acute respiratory infections that can be attributed to PM10 exposure.

FOOD SAFETY

Food can be contaminated with chemical or microbiological agents. The strict regulations and measures applied in European countries mean that food is generally safe, but ingestion of contaminated food may still present an important route of exposure. Children are at particular risk of illness, as their bodies are developing and they generally consume more food on a body weight basis than adults. In most countries adult intake levels of chemicals in food have been 10-30% of the provisional tolerable weekly intake (PTWI) levels, sometimes higher. The data on intake among children are very patchy. The total intake seems to be lower than in adults, but per kg body weight the intake is higher.

CHEMICAL SAFETY

The number of existing chemicals is very large, and for many of them the health risks are not known. Chemicals can reach our body through different routes (e.g. food, air, water) and cause a variety of health effects. Due to the many ways in which chemicals are used and released, the many exposure routes involved, and the different mixtures of chemicals present, the public health relevance of chemicals can be extremely difficult to assess. Children are especially sensitive to lead exposure. Elevated blood lead levels (>10ug/l) have been associated with toxicity in the developing brain and nervous system of young children, leading to lower intelligence quotient (IQ). Levels have significantly reduced since the mid-80s, but many children still have levels that may harm their health.

WATER AND SANITATION

Safe drinking water and sanitation are essential for health. Microbial contamination can lead to outbreaks of waterborne diseases. Chemical contamination of drinking water occurs less frequently but may also have health impacts, generally chronic and long-term. In the eastern part of the Region, the percentage of homes with an adequate supply of piped and safe water remains rather low (ranging from 58% to 80%), albeit rising. There are important disparities between urban and rural areas: only 30-40% of rural households in Asian countries have access to safe drinking water.

OCCUPATIONAL HAZARDS

Every day at the workplace, employees face health and safety hazards such as accidents, dust, chemicals, noise, violence or stress. The effects range from premature deaths and injuries to occupational diseases such as for example cancer and respiratory disease. In recent years, a slightly decreasing trend was visible in the standardized incidence rates of work injuries among young workers. A clear decrease could only be noted in a few countries, indicating that overall progress is not adequate.

UV AND IONIZING RADIATION

Various types of radiation can cause negative health effects. Solar radiation is beneficial for our body as a source of vitamin D, however, excessive exposure may pose a threat to health. Ultraviolet (UV) radiation causes premature ageing of the skin and may lead to the development of malignant melanoma. Radon is a gas emitted by certain types of soil and building materials, and can cause lung cancer. Children are those most at risk from excess exposure to UV radiation, e.g. due to still developing skin protection mechanisms. Worldwide, the incidence of melanoma has been increasing, also in younger age groups. Moreover, many people increase their exposure through artificial sources in solariums. Raising awareness and encouraging skin protection are the most effective preventive strategies.

HOUSING

Several environmental factors present indoors can cause negative health effects. Examples of such factors are indoor air quality (polluted for example by use of solid fuels), noise, humidity and mould growth, temperature, presence of hazardous substances (for example asbestos, lead and radon), hygiene and sanitation, and overcrowding. An unsafe household can cause unintentional injuries such as falls, drowning, poisoning, fires and choking.

The amount of people living in homes with self-reported problems of dampness varies greatly among countries, ranging between 10% and 30%. Solid fuel use in homes in the WHO Region in 2004 varied from below 5% to over 70%. The geographical pattern shows a gradual increase from west to east of the Region.

MOBILITY AND TRANSPORT

Transport can directly lead to health problems (injuries and death), but also indirectly (through air pollution, noise and climate change related to emissions from traffic, but also through reduced physical activity). Increased motorized transport can lead to more road traffic injuries, which are the main cause of death among people, especially males, and a major cause of physical disability, especially among the youngest. Motorized transport is also an important factor in the reduction of physical activity, such as for example walking and cycling. Low levels of physical activity contribute to the ongoing epidemic of overweight and obesity.

ACTS REGULATING THE ENVIRONMENT

Over the years, together with a spreading of environmental consciousness, there has been a change in the traditionally-held perception that there is a trade-off between environmental quality and economic growth as people have come to believe that the two are necessarily complementary. The current focus on environment is not new-environmental considerations have been an integral part of the Indian culture. The need for conservation and sustainable use of natural resources has been expressed in Indian scriptures, more than three thousand years old and is reflected in the constitutional, legislative and policy framework as also in the international commitments of the country.

Even before India's independence in 1947, several environmental legislation existed but the real impetus for bringing about a well-developed framework came only after the UN Conference on the Human Environment (Stockholm, 1972). Under the influence of this declaration, the National Council for Environmental Policy and Planning within the Department of Science and Technology was set up in 1972. This Council later evolved into a full-fledged Ministry of Environment and Forests (MoEF) in 1985 which today is the apex administrative body in the country for regulating and ensuring environmental protection. After the Stockholm Conference, in 1976, constitutional sanction was given to environmental concerns through the 42nd Amendment, which incorporated them into the Directive Principles of State Policy and Fundamental Rights and Duties.

Since the 1970s an extensive network of environmental legislation has grown in the country. The MoEF and the pollution control boards (CPCB i.e. Central Pollution Control Board and SPCBs i.e. State Pollution Control Boards) together form the regulatory and administrative core of the sector.

A policy framework has also been developed to complement the legislative provisions. The Policy Statement for Abatement of Pollution and the National Conservation Strategy and Policy Statement on Environment and Development were brought out by the MoEF in 1992, to develop and promote initiatives for the protection and improvement of the environment. The EAP (Environmental Action Programme) was formulated in 1993 with the objective of improving environmental services and integrating environmental considerations in to development programmes. Other measures have also been taken by the government to protect and preserve the environment.

LEGISLATION FOR ENVIRONMENTAL PROTECTION IN INDIA

Water

Water quality standards especially those for drinking water are set by the Indian Council of Medical Research. These bear close resemblance to WHO standards.

Water (Prevention and Control of Pollution) Act, 1974

The Act prohibits the discharge of pollutants into water bodies beyond a given standard, and lays down penalties for non-compliance. The Act was amended in 1988 to conform closely to the provisions of the EPA, 1986. It set up the CPCB (Central Pollution Control Board) which lays down standards for the prevention and control of water pollution.

Water (Prevention and Control of Pollution) Cess Act, 1977

This Act provides for a levy and collection of a cess on water consumed by industries and local authorities. It aims at augmenting the resources of the central and state boards for prevention and control of water pollution. Following this Act, The Water (Prevention and Control of Pollution) Cess Rules were formulated in 1978 for defining standards and indications for the kind of and location of meters that every consumer of water is required to install.

Air

Air quality standards especially those for drinking water are set by the Indian Council of Medical Research. These bear close resemblance to WHO standards.

Air (Prevention and Control of Pollution) Act, 1981

To counter the problems associated with air pollution, ambient air quality standards were established, under the 1981 Act. The Act provides means for the control and abatement of air pollution. The Act seeks to combat air pollution by prohibiting the use of polluting fuels and substances, as well as by regulating appliances that give rise to air pollution.

National Ambient Air Quality Standards (NAAQS) for major pollutants were notified by the CPCB in April 1994. These are deemed to be levels of air quality necessary with an adequate margin of safety, to protect public health, vegetation and property (CPCB 1995 cited in Gupta, 1999). The NAAQS prescribe specific standards for industrial, residential, rural and other sensitive areas.

The Air (Prevention and Control of Pollution) Rules formulated in 1982, defined the procedures for conducting meetings of the boards, the powers of the presiding officers, decision-making, the quorum; manner in which the records of the meeting were to be set etc. They also prescribed the manner and the purpose of seeking assistance from specialists and the fee to be paid to them.

Complementing the above Acts is the Atomic Energy Act of 1982, which was introduced to deal with radioactive waste. In 1988, the Motor Vehicles Act, was enacted to regulate vehicular traffic, besides ensuring proper packaging, labelling and transportation of the hazardous wastes. Various aspects of vehicular pollution have also been notified under the EPA of 1986. Mass emission standards were notified in 1990, which were made more stringent in 1996. In 2000 these standards were revised yet again and for the first time separate obligations for vehicle owners, manufacturers and enforcing agencies were stipulated. In addition, fairly stringent Euro I and II emission norms were notified by the Supreme Court on April 29, 1999 for the city of Delhi.

Forests and Wildlife

The Wildlife (Protection) Act, 1972

The WPA (Wildlife Protection Act), 1972, provides for protection to listed species of flora and fauna and establishes a network of ecologically-important protected areas. The WPA empowers the central and state governments to declare any area a wildlife sanctuary, national park or closed area.

There is a blanket ban on carrying out any industrial activity inside these protected areas. It provides for authorities to administer and implement the Act; regulate the hunting of wild animals; protect specified plants, sanctuaries, national parks and closed areas; restrict trade or commerce in wild animals or animal articles; and miscellaneous matters. The Act prohibits hunting of animals except with permission of authorized officer when an animal has become dangerous to human life or property or so disabled or diseased as to be beyond recovery (WWF-India, 1999). The near-total prohibition on hunting was made more effective by the Amendment Act of 1991.

The Forest (Conservation) Act, 1980

This Act was adopted to protect and conserve forests. The Act restricts the powers of the state in respect of de-reservation of forests and use of forestland for non-forest purposes (the term 'non-forest purpose' includes clearing any forestland for cultivation of cash crops, plantation crops, horticulture or any purpose other than re-afforestation).

General

Environment (Protection) Act, 1986

This Act is an umbrella legislation designed to provide a framework for the co-ordination of central and state authorities established under the Water (Prevention and Control) Act, 1974 and Air (Prevention and Control) Act, 1981. Under this Act, the central government is empowered to take measures necessary to protect and improve the quality of the environment by setting standards for emissions and discharges; regulating the location of industries; management of hazardous wastes, and protection of public health and welfare.

The Environment (Protection) Rules, 1986

These rules lay down the procedures for setting standards of emission or discharge of environmental pollutants. The Rules prescribe the parameters for the Central Government, under which it can issue orders of prohibition and restrictions on the location and operation of industries in different areas. The Rules lay down the procedure for taking samples, serving notice, submitting samples for analysis and laboratory reports. The functions of the laboratories are also described under the Rules along with the qualifications of the concerned analysts.

The National Environment Appellate Authority Act, 1997

This Act provided for the establishment of a National Environment Appellate Authority to hear appeals with respect to restriction of areas in which any industry operation or process or class of industries, operations or processes could not carry out or would be allowed to carry out subject to certain safeguards under the Environment (Protection) Act, 1986.

Factories Act, 1948 and its Amendment in 1987

The Factories Act, 1948 was a post-independence statute that explicitly showed concern for the environment. The primary aim of the 1948 Act has been to ensure the welfare of workers not only in their working conditions in the factories but also their employment benefits. While ensuring the safety and health of the workers, the Act contributes to environmental protection. The Act contains a comprehensive list of 29 categories of industries involving hazardous processes, which are defined as a process or activity where unless special care is taken, raw materials used therein or the intermediate or the finished products, by-products, wastes or effluents would cause material impairment to health of the persons engaged and result in the pollution of the general environment

Public Liability Insurance Act (PLIA), 1991

The Act covers accidents involving hazardous substances and insurance coverage for these. Where death or injury results from an accident, this Act makes the owner liable to provide relief as is specified in the Schedule of the Act. The PLIA was amended in 1992, and the Central Government was authorized to establish the Environmental Relief Fund, for making relief payments.

National Environment Tribunal Act, 1995

The Act provided strict liability for damages arising out of any accident occurring while handling any hazardous substance and for the establishment of a National Environment Tribunal for effective and expeditious disposal of cases arising from such accident, with a view to give relief and compensation for damages to persons, property and the environment and for the matters connected therewith or incidental thereto.

INTERNATIONAL AGREEMENTS ON ENVIRONMENTAL ISSUES

India is signatory to a number of multilateral environment agreements (MEA) and conventions. These are:

- Convention on International Trade in Endangered Species of wild fauna and flora (CITES), 1973
- Montreal Protocol on Substances that deplete the Ozone Layer (to the Vienna Convention for the Protection of the Ozone Layer), 1987
- Basel Convention on Transboundary Movement of Hazardous Wastes, 1989
- UN Framework Convention on Climate Change (UNFCCC), 1992
- Convention on Biological Diversity, 1992
- UN Convention on Desertification, 1994
- International Tropical Timber Agreement and The International Tropical Timber Organisation (ITTO), 1983, 1994

PATHOGENIC FACTORS

Infectious diseases are caused by pathogens which are the organisms too tiny to see without a microscope. Most pathogens belong to one of four major groups: bacteria, viruses, fungi, or protozoa.

BACTERIA

Microbes belonging to the bacteria group are made up of only one cell. Bacteria inhabit a variety of environments. Psychrophiles, or cold-loving bacteria, can live in the subfreezing temperature of the Arctic. Thermophiles are heat-loving bacteria that can live in extreme heat, such as in the hot springs in Yellowstone National Park. Extreme thermophiles, or hyperthermophiles, thrive at 235 degrees Fahrenheit near volcanic vents on the ocean floor. Many bacteria prefer the milder temperature of the healthy human body.

Like humans, some bacteria (aerobic bacteria) need oxygen to survive, but others (anaerobic bacteria) do not. Amazingly, some can adapt to new environments by learning to survive with or without oxygen.

Like all living cells, each bacterium requires food for energy and building materials. There are countless numbers of bacteria on Earth - most are harmless and many are even beneficial to humans. In fact, less than 1 percent of them cause diseases in humans. For example, harmless anaerobic bacteria, such as Lactobacilli acidophilus, live in human intestines, where they help to digest food, destroy disease-causing microbes, fight cancer cells, and give the body needed vitamins. Healthy food products, such as yogurt, sauerkraut, and cheese, are made using bacteria.

Certain bacteria give off toxins that can seriously affect our health. Botulism, a severe form of food poisoning, affects the nerves and is caused by toxins from Clostridium botulinum bacteria. Under certain circumstances, however, bacterial toxins can be helpful. Several vaccines that protect us from getting sick are made from bacterial toxins. One type of pertussis vaccine, which protects infants and children from whooping cough, contains toxins from Bordetella pertussis bacteria. This vaccine is safe and effective and causes fewer reactions than other types of pertussis vaccine.

VIRUSES

Viruses are among the smallest microbes, much smaller even than bacteria. Viruses are not cells. They consist of one or more molecules of DNA or RNA, which contain the virus's genes surrounded by a protein coat. Viruses can be rod-shaped, sphere-shaped, or multisided. Some look like tadpoles.

Unlike most bacteria, most viruses do cause disease because they invade living, normal cells, such as those in the human body. They then multiply and produce other viruses like themselves. Each virus is very particular about which cell it attacks. Various human viruses specifically attack particular cells in the body's organs, systems, or tissues, such as the liver, respiratory system, or blood cells.

Although types of viruses behave differently, most survive by taking over the machinery that makes a cell work. Briefly, when a single virus particle, a "virion", comes in contact with a cell it likes, it may attach to special landing sites on the surface of that cell. From there, the virus may inject molecules into the cell, or the cell may swallow up the virion. Once inside the cell, viral molecules such as DNA or RNA direct the cell to make new virus offspring. That's how a virus "infects" a cell.

Viruses can even "infect" bacteria. These viruses, called bacteriophages, may help researchers develop alternatives to antibiotic medicines for wiping out bacterial infections.

Many viral infections do not result in disease. For example, by the time most people in the United States become adults, they have been infected by cytomegalovirus (CMV). Most of these people, however, do not develop CMV disease symptoms. Other viral infections can result in deadly diseases, such as HIV infection, which causes acquired immunodeficiency syndrome (AIDS).

FUNGI

A fungus is actually a primitive vegetable. Fungi can be found in air, in soil, on plants, and in water. Thousands, perhaps millions, of different types of fungi exist on Earth. The most familiar ones to us are mushrooms, yeast, mold, and mildew. Some live in the human body, usually without causing illness. In fact, only about half of all types of fungi cause disease in humans. Those conditions are called mycoses.

Mycoses can affect skin, nails, body hair, internal organs such as the lungs, and body systems such as the nervous system. Aspergillus fumigatus, for example, can cause aspergillosis, a fungal infection in the respiratory system.

Some fungi have made our lives easier. Penicillin and other antibiotics, which kill harmful bacteria in our bodies, are made from fungi. Other fungi, like certain yeasts, also can be beneficial. For example, when a warm liquid like water and a food source are added to certain yeasts, the fungus ferments. The process of fermentation is essential for making healthy foods like some breads and cheeses.

PROTOZOA

Protozoa are a group of microscopic one-celled animals. Protozoa can be parasites or predators. In humans, protozoa usually cause disease. Some protozoa, like plankton, live in water environments and serve as food for marine animals, such as some species of whales. Protozoa also can be found on land in decaying matter and in soil, but they must have a moist environment to survive. Termites wouldn't be able to do such a good job of digesting wood without these micro organisms in their guts.

Malaria is caused by a protozoan parasite. Another protozoan parasite, Toxoplasma gondii, causes toxoplasmosis in humans. This is an especially troublesome infection in pregnant women because of its effects on the foetus and in people with HIV infection or other immune deficiency.

FOOD

Man kind eats to satisfy the feeling of hunger. Nutrition plays an important role in the promotion and maintenance of health and in the prevention of disease in order to keep well our bodies, need nourishment. Just as a plant will not grow without water sun shine and proper manure, human beings also need food stuffs of different kinds of nourish to the body. Malnutrition and under nutrition are the greatest international health problems of the present day. A sound knowledge of nutrition is therefore essential for all community health workers. Nutrition deals with the way in which the human body receives and uses all the substances or materials necessary for its growth and development and for keeping it is good condition.

Nutrition may be defined as the Science of food and its relationship to health. It is concerned primarily with the part played by nutrients in body growth and development and maintenance. The word nutrient or "food factor" is used for specific dietary constituents such as proteins, vitamins and minerals. Dietics is the practical application of the principles of nutrition, it includes the planning of meals for the well and sick. Good nutrition means "maintaining a nutritional status that enables us to grow well and enjoy good health.

A person who does not eat the right foods or does not eat enough is malnourished and we call this malnutrition, it also means that a child is less clever than he should be. The trouble may start even before birth if his mother does not have the right foods when she is pregnant. The malnourished child does not play but sits doing nothing. He is slow in learning to walk and talk. At school he is hungry, sleepy, dull and very slow to learn Children are slow in passing mile stones. Good nutrition is a basic component of health. The relation of nutrition to health may be seen from the following view points:

Growth and development: Good nutrition is essential for the attainment of normal growth and development. Not only physical growth and development, but also the intellectual development, learning and behaviour are affected by malnutrition. Mal nutrition during pregnancy may affect the foetus resulting in still birth, premature birth and small for the date's babies. He is under weight because of not having enough of the kind of foods needed for growth. Good nutrition is also essential in adult life for the maintenance of optimum health & efficiency. So nutrition affects the individual's health from birth to death.

Specific deficiency: Malnutrition is directly responsible for certain specific nutritional deficiency diseases. The commonly reported ones in India are kwashiorkor, marasmus, blindness due to Vitamin A deficiency, anaemia, beriberi, goitre etc., Good nutrition therefore is essential for the prevention of specific nutritional deficiency diseases and promotion of health.

Resistance to infection: Malnutrition predisposes to infections like tuberculosis. It also influences the course and out come of many clinical disorders. Infection, in turn, may aggravate malnutrition by affecting the food intake.

Mortality and Morbidity: The Indirect effects of Malnutrition on the community are even more striking a high general death rate, high infant mortality rate, high sickness rate and a lower expectation of life. Over nutrition, which is another form of malnutrition is responsible for obesity, diabetes, hypertension, cardiovascular and renal diseases, disorders of liver and gall bladder. More recent reports suggest that diet perhaps plays an important role in certain types of gas to intestinal cancers. It is now quite well acceptable that diet and certain diseases are interrelated.

SELECTION, STORAGE AND PREPARATION OF FOODS

Selection

The health worker should help family to plan the diet selecting foods for a mixed, well balanced diet:

- Select more than one kind of cereal grain. Raw milled rice and white flour should be avoided. Select parboiled milled rice and whole wheat flour which are much more nutritious.
- Select different kinds of pulses and nuts.
- Buy grains and pulses in fairly large quantities if possible, if necessary going to some place where they are cheaper.
- Select foods that are in season, plentiful and cheap.
- Select a different kind of vegetables for each day as far as possible. Buy fresh and make sure they are of good quality. Include some vegetables or fruit that can be eaten raw.
- Try to produce foods at home: Vegetables, fruits, milk, eggs etc.

Storage

- All foods should be kept in clean conditions safe from rats and other pests.
- Vegetables and fruits lose their nutrient value if kept too long. Try to buy frequently. Keep them cool, away from sunlight and where there is plenty of fresh air. Use while fresh.

Cooking

Cooking is an art. It is linked with dietary habits and cultural pattern of people. Different methods are used in different types of diets. The main purposes of cooking are:

1. To soften and break down the cellulose of plant foods and the connective tissue and fibres of animal foods, to make them more digestible.

2. To develop new flavours in food, either by the method of cooking or by adding spices other flavouring substances.
3. To destroy the harmful bacteria, worm eggs and parasites, so that the food is safe for human use.
4. It stimulates the digestive juices.
5. It introduces variety, i.e., many different types of dishes can be prepared with the same ingredients.
6. Good cooking increases the acceptability of food; where as bad cooking may lead to rejection of foods.

Cooking Methods

During the process of cooking, heat is applied to food in some way or other. The amount of heat and the form of heat depends upon the food to be cooked. Methods which may be used are boiling, simmering, stewing, steaming, frying, grilling, baking and roasting.

Boiling: Cooking in water at 100°C (212°F) is called boiling. For this the water must be bubbling freely, but steadily, all over the surface. Rice, dal, pulses, roots, tubers and other vegetables are cooked in this way. Boiling in excess of water may result in loss of Vitamins and minerals. So, minimum water should be used.

Simmering: It is a modification of boiling. It is cooking food in water just under boiling point. The temperature should be about 84°C. Meat and fish are best cooked by simmering because at high temperature, the fibres of meat are hardened.

Steaming: It is cooking food in the vapour which rises from boiling water. This may be done by placing the food container in a steamer above a pan of boiling water or pressure cookers. Because of increased pressure of steam, the temperature attained is higher than 100°C. This process is best to save nutrients, food and time.

Stewing: This is method differs from boiling, in that:

- Comparatively smaller amounts of liquid are used.
- Prolonged low degrees of heat is applied, usually about 200°F i.e., simmer food slowly with only a little liquid in a covered pan on top of the stove. The addition of onions, tomatoes or small cut vegetables and some condiments and herbs can make a meat stew appetising. In this method the nutrients are not lost. Stewing is used for cooking meat.

Frying: It is cooking food in very hot fat or oil. This is one of the quickest methods of cooking and should be done in an open pan. These are of two types:

- Shallow Frying: Shallow frying is suitable for cooking foods like eggs, sausages, dosai and pre-cooked foods.
- Deep frying: Food is completely immersed in large quantity of hot oil. E.g. Puri, pakoda, Vadai, cutlets etc. In deep frying oil should be sufficiently hot, otherwise food will absorb lot of oil and oil is free from moisture.

Roasting: Food is smeared with a little fat and exposed directly to heat or flame. Chicken or tender mutton may be cooked by this method and also large joints of meat and for root vegetables- dry roasting. E.g. Ground nuts. This causes only slight loss of nutrients.

Baking: It is cooking food by dry heat. It is done in a hot air oven. Food is enclosed by hot air, so that it gets heat from all sides. The cooking temperature may vary from 250°F to 500°F. Baking is an expensive and slow method of cooking. By this method Biscuits, Cakes, Bread are usually cooked.

Puffing: This is applying heat for a few seconds. It causes slight loss of thiamine only. Puffed rice, Bengal gram and peas are commonly used for snacks.

Grilling: It is cooking food by exposing it directly to very great heat either in front of a bright, hot fire or a special grilling plate. It is very quick method of cooking. Only tender foods can be cycled e.g.: Meat and fish, kebab, cheese, tomatoes, brinjal etc. Stoves heated by gas and electricity are usually fitted with plates which can be heated for grilling.

General Principles of Cooking

- Vitamin C is mostly lost in any kind of cooking especially by cooking for a long time. So you should not cook for a long time.
- Adding cooking soda to dal to hasten or to greens cause heavy loss of vitamin C. Therefore soda should not be used.
- Green leafy vegetables should be cooked in covered, quickly in a little boiled and salted water. Other vegetables should be covered.
- Vegetables should be eaten after thorough wash with salt water and clean water. Cut in to large pieces to prevent loss of vitamins.

- Add tamarind or other acids only at the end of cooking or vegetables become hard.
- Should not open the coverings while cooking food. Too much of opening may cause loss of vitamins.
- Should not wash the rice so many times before cooking, this may cause loss of vitamin B which is in the outer layer of rice.
- Should not pour too much water and remove it, may cause loss of nutrients.
- Use fresh vegetables for cooking to save nutrients.
- Using too much of oil also dangerous to health. Oil should be heated well before using.

Preservation of Foods

While fresh foods usually have a better taste, appearance and colour, it is useful to be able preserve foods and keep them longer. By preservation methods, growth of bacteria is slowed down. (Freezing is the best way to pressure foods at home but a refrigerator is costly). It is the best way but it is costly to preserve foods at a low temperature if possible.

- Cold storage: The home refrigerator has now made to store and preserve a variety of foods. Fruits and vegetables should be kept just above the freezing point i.e, 0°C or 31 - 33°F, meat and butter are kept at much lower temperature. There is no growth of food poisoning organisms at this low temperature.
- Drying or Dehydratation: Drying removes water and with out moisture micro-organisms can not grow. Vitamin C is destroyed but other nutrients are preserved. Milk, fruits, vegetables fish and meat may preserved by drying. Preserved fruits and vegetables can be used when out of season to supply nutrients such as iron and carotene. A simple dryer has been invented which could provide the basis for a cottage industry for preserved food.
- Smoking: Meat may be preserve with smoke. Smoke contains phenols which help in preservation.
- Salting and pickling: Salt is a preservative. By adding certain condiments mangoes, vegetables, meat and fish may be preserved.

- Making Jam: By boiling fruits and adding quantities of sugar, jam is made which the housewife can keep for some time.

ACTS REGULATING FOOD HYGIENE

There are a number of food laws being implemented by various Ministries/Departments. These are primarily meant for two purposes namely (1) Regulation of Specifications of food and (2) Regulation of Hygienic condition of Processing/Manufacturing. Some of these food laws are mandatory and some are voluntary. Various food laws operational in India are given below.

PREVENTION OF FOOD ADULTERATION ACT

Food is essential for nourishment and sustenance of human being. Hence, adulteration of food is required to be checked. Government of India has made law known as "The Prevention of Food Adulteration Act, 1954" which contains provisions for the prevention of adulteration of food. This Act prohibits manufacture for sale or sale, etc. of adulterated and misbranded food articles, adulterant, any article which is manufactured in contravention of Act or Rules there under, and any article of food without licence.

Main functionaries under the said Act are the Food (Health) Authority, Local (Health) Authority and Food Inspector. Act gives power to the Food Inspector to perform various acts including drawing of sample of food article from any food establishment so as to check the movement of adulterated or misbranded food articles. The Local (Health) Authority and the Food (Health) Authority are the supervisory authorities.

The Prevention of Food Adulteration Rules, 1955 which are framed by Government of India under the above Act provide by and large, standards for various types of food articles, colouring matter, preservatives, stabilizers, etc. which can be used in food articles, labelling and packing of various food articles and other provisions relating to sale of food articles.

The Ministry of Health and Family Welfare is responsible for ensuring safe food to the consumers. Keeping this in view, a legislation called "Prevention of Food Adulteration Act, 1954" has been enacted. The objective envisaged in this legislation is to ensure pure and wholesome food to the consumers and also to prevent fraud or deception. The Act has been amended thrice in 1964, 1976 and in 1986 with the objective of plugging the loopholes and making the punishments more stringent and empowering Consumers and Voluntary Organisations to play a more effective role in its implementation.

The subject of the Prevention of Food Adulteration is in the concurrent list of the constitution. However, in general, the enforcement of the Act is done by the State/U.T Governments. The Central Government primarily plays an advisory role in its implementation besides carrying out various statutory functions/duties assigned to it under the various provisions of the Act.

The laws regulating the quality of food have been in force in the country since 1899. Until 1954, several States formulated their own food laws. But there was a considerable variance in the rules and specifications of the food, which interfered with inter-provincial trade. The Central Advisory Board appointed by the Government of India in 1937 and the Food Adulteration Committee appointed in 1943, reviewed the subject of Food Adulteration and recommended for Central legislation. The Constitution of India provided the powers to Central Government for making such legislation as the subjects of Food and Drugs Adulteration are included in the concurrent list. The Government of India, therefore, enacted a Central Legislation called the prevention of Food adulteration Act (PFA) in the year 1954 which came into effect from 15 June, 1955. The Act repealed all laws, existing at that time in States concerning food adulteration.

THE FOOD SAFETY AND STANDARDS ACT, 2006

With the coming into effect of the Food Safety and Standards Act, 2006 (FSSA) enacted by Parliament in August 2006, the Prevention of Food Adulteration Act, 1954 will stand repealed, from the date on which Food Safety and Standards Act comes into force on such date as the Central Government may, by notification in the Gazette appoint.

Notwithstanding the repeal of the enactment and Orders specified in the Second Schedule, the standards, safety requirements and other provisions of the Act and the rules and regulations made there under and Orders listed in that Schedule shall continue to be in force and operate till new standards are specified under this Act or rules and regulations made there under.

Provided that anything done or any action taken under the enactment and Orders under repeal shall be deemed to have been done or taken under the corresponding provisions of this Act and shall continue in force accordingly unless and until superseded by anything done or by any action taken under this Act.

World Bank Assisted-Capacity Building Project on Food Safety As trade in food commodities expands globally, food safety can no longer be considered a mere domestic issue. The agreements under the WTO require the development of modern food control and safety programs by national Governments. The issue does not relate only to end product parameters but also to process control. In order to strengthen the food safety infrastructure in the country, a 5 year World Bank Aided Capacity Building Project for Food Safety and Quality Control of Drugs has been launched by the Central Government.

DRUGS AND COSMETIC ACT

In 1937 a Bill was introduced in the Central Legislative Assembly to give effect to the recommendations of the Drugs Enquiry Committee to regulate the import of drugs into British India. This Bill was referred to the Select Committee and the Committee expressed the opinion that a more comprehensive measure for the uniform control of manufacture and distribution of drugs as well as of imports was desirable. The Central Government suggested to the Provincial Governments to ask the Provincial Legislatures to pass resolutions empowering the Central Legislature to pass on Act for regulating such matters relating to control of drugs as fall within the Provincial sp here. Provincial Governments got the resolution passed from the Provincial Legislatures and sent them to the Central Government for getting through the Bill to regulate the import, manufacture, distribution and sale of Drugs and Cosmetics. Thereupon the Drugs and Cosmetics Bill was introduced in the Central Legislative Assembly.

SOCIO-CULTURAL DETERMINANTS

Most of the burden of disease affecting people and resulting in health problems in is the result of complex interactions between individuals and socio-economic and environmental determinants of their health. Current epidemiological trends in the health (such as mental health problems, asthma, injuries, inappropriate nutrition, obesity, and physical inactivity) reflect the impact of extensive socio-cultural shifts experienced over recent decades. Issues around economic disadvantage, cultural diversity and tolerance, the changing nature of work and family structures, family violence and homelessness challenge the health system to meet increasingly complex health needs in collaboration with other sectors.

The greatest burden of ill health is borne by those most disadvantaged in India. One of the dominant features affecting the health situation of all countries is the social gradient in health and disease. This gradient in health and disease is prevalent in all socioeconomic strata of society. On every rung up the socioeconomic disadvantage ladder from least to most disadvantaged, people experience more sickness, shorter life expectancy and poorer health. People of greater socioeconomic disadvantage experience worse health than those of higher socioeconomic status for almost every major cause of mortality or morbidity. Moreover, socioeconomic differences in health are evident for both females and males at every stage of the life course.

Social and economic disparities are one of the major public health challenges confronting India. A safe environment, adequate income, meaningful social roles, secure housing, higher levels of education and social support are all associated with better health and wellbeing. In addition to health behaviours, these social, cultural, economic and environmental factors comprise what we call population health determinants. The interaction of all these factors ultimately determines the health of individuals, families and communities. A wealth of evidence supports the strong association between poverty and ill health.

Socioeconomically disadvantaged adults who are less formally educated or poorly educated experience the highest rates of illness such as cardiovascular disease and diabetes. They also have the highest prevalence of risky behaviours such as smoking and hazardous use of alcohol. In addition, income inequality has a significant impact on population health. Specifically, income and wealth inequalities have been correlated with increased all-cause mortality. While our socioeconomic position connects us to the physical and social resources which can make our life better, the feelings of empowerment and status that go with the connection to these resources are also important. This second dimension is important because people who feel in control of their lives are also more likely to take control of their health. A lack of control over work and home life has powerful effects on our health. Like continuing anxiety, feelings of insecurity and social isolation, the psychosocial impact of a lack of control at home or at work accumulate during life and increase the chances of poor mental health, physiological wear and tear and premature death.

Psychosocial factors affect physical health through the stress response. Although the stresses of modern life rarely demand strenuous or even moderate physical responses, turning on the stress response diverts energy and resources away from many physiological processes important to long-term health maintenance. For brief periods, this stress response has minimal impact, however, if people feel tense too often or the tension goes on for too long, they become more vulnerable to a wide range of conditions including infections, diabetes, high blood pressure, heart attack, stroke, depression and aggression. The lower people are in the social hierarchy of countries such as India, the more common these problems become.

While many population health interventions target lifestyle factors where health gains can be made, the social influences on health behaviours must be considered in both the design and implementation of these interventions. The World Health Organisation identifies the need to understand the interaction between material disadvantage and social meanings. "It is not simply that poor material circumstances are harmful to health; the social meaning of being poor, unemployed, socially excluded, or otherwise stigmatised also matters." As well as income and education, other social factors are also known to affect the health of populations. For example, unmarried and divorced people, and men have consistently higher age-adjusted death rates than married people and women.

Additionally, social trends such as the increase in one-parent families, the ageing population and an increase in the age of people starting families are already influencing the economic environment and the health status of the population. Minority status also can influence health outcomes. This may be due to limited service knowledge, poor language skills, employment discrimination, an associated low socioeconomic living environment, and absence of social networks within minority migrant communities and refugees, as well as due to genetic determinants. For example, minorities experience interpersonal violence, institutional discrimination, or socioeconomic disadvantage, all of which have independent detrimental effects on health, regardless of the health indicator used. Social determinants of health are often beyond the control of the individual.

Addressing them through multidisciplinary efforts at the population level can assist in preventing illness and improving the overall health of the community. While universal access to healthcare is one of the social determinants of health, more important to the health of the population as a whole are the social and economic conditions that make people ill and in need of healthcare in the first place.

TRADITIONS, CUSTOMS & HABITS

Traditions

These are the ideas, habits and ways of behaviour passed on from one generation to another. In rural areas traditions are important for social life. Being a guide to conduct, they give a feeling of unity and security to the members of a community. Some of the Traditions may cause difficult to poorer families. E.g. the traditional marriage feast, which results in a heavy defect which the family can never repay.

Customs

This is a social phenomenon. It is a rule or norm of action. Customs are the long established habits and usages of the people. These are part of the traditions; customs are common ways of acting. They are strong traditions, which have been followed for several generations and have great influence on the behaviour of the people in the community. Customs plays a major part in regulating our social behaviour. They determine our culture, preserve it and transmit in from generation to generation. Some of the customs were learnt by imitation from other people.

All custom are not irrational. Customs, which appear to be irrational, are sometimes reformed or even abolished due to deliberate thought of the concerned people. Today the educated class of Indians does not follow many customs of the ancestors. Customs are important means of controlling social behaviour. That are powerful no one can escape their range. They regulate social life especially among illiterate peoples to a great extent. It develops social relationships among people. Enemies are turned into friends by customs. It is not easy to change customs- they are social norms, which every one in the community is forced to follow.

Habits

There are an individual phenomenon and in time may become customs. It means an acquired facility to act in a certain manner with out resort to deliberation or thought. In acquisition of habits makes an action. Easy and familiar. For e.g. Two meals a day, brushing the teeth, morning walking etc. All these are fail in the field of automatic behaviour. It becomes both psychologically and physiologically easy for as to act in habitual way.

Habit is learning. We learn to do an act in a particular way, i.e. socially acceptable. From earliest childhood one is taught entire rules of behaviour which involves the acquisition of habits. Habits are developed by individuals and in time may become customs. Repeating certain actions, until they are done with out any conscious effort forms habits. Habits are important in skill development and help us to do many things quickly, easily and well, without having to think about each step every time. Good habits of Hygiene, eating, sleeping etc should be taught to children.

Bad habits such as smoking, talking alcohol and drugs hard to break. One should remain master of one's habits never become a slave to them. Society may approve to some habits and disapprove of others, but society does not control the habits of the people Traditions and Habits affecting Health.

Traditions and Habits Affecting Health

The Health Worker needs to find out about the traditional beliefs and home cures in the community. It will be found that some of these are useful, some are harmless, but others are harmful. Useful cures can be encouraged, e.g. the use of tulsi leaves and eucalyptus leaves for coughs and colds, neem leaves in cases of chickenpox, and papaya seeds for intestinal worms. Harmless beliefs can be allowed e.g. for hiccup, a bit of broomstick is stuck to the forehead with saliva. Harmful habits and beliefs are to be discouraged by patient health education, e.g. passing faeces on open ground, branding a newborn baby with red hot iron, and use of cow dung on burns, wounds or ulcers.

SOCIAL PROBLEMS

Drug addiction: It is defined as a state of Periodic or chronic intoxication detrimental to the individual and society produced by the repeated intake of habit forming drug.

To call a person a drug addict the following criteria must be satisfied:

- Psychological dependence.
- Physical dependence
- Development of tolerance

Reasons for drug dependence are:

- Curiosity and natural tendency to experiment with drugs.
- Disturbed home environment i.e. broken families, destructed families and disturbed families.
- An escape phenomena from tensioned and frustrations in life for e.g. unemployment.
- Impact of culture.
- Ignorance regarding of habit forming nature of the drugs.
- Lack of communication i.e. generation gap.

Management includes:

- Identification of drug addicts and their motivation for
- Detoxification.

- Hospitalization.
- Rehabilitation.

Simultaneously with medical treatment, changes in environment are important. The patient must affect a complete break with his group. Prevention measures include education of target groups and the general public through TV, radio, leaflets and posters.

Dowry system: Dowry started as an innocent custom a symbol of love from parents to their daughters on the eve of her marriage. But it has in recent years grown into a social evil with many instances of beside - burning and suicides. Under the dowry prohibition act, 1986 the minimum punishment for taking or abetting the taking of dowry has been raised to 5 years imprisonment and a fine of Rs. 15000.

Unmarried mothers: We do not have accurate statistics regarding unmarried mothers in India. Social customs and traditions in India, the problem of unmarried mothers in India must be insignificant. Such mothers have a multiplicity of needs not only for medical termination of pregnancy but also for understanding and warmth and guidance all of which nursing can provide.

Handicapped: The handicapped are blind, deaf, and dumb, orthopaedically handicapped, leprosy affected, mentally retarded, and emotionally and socially handicapped. The rehabilitation services are available for handicapped in India are as follows:

- Medical care facilities
- Education for blind, deaf and orthopaedically handicapped
- Vocational tanning 4. Job placement and sheltered work shops
- Pensions, scholarships and allowances for the education and training of the handicapped.

During the fifth five year plan there is provision for establishment of four national institutes for the blind the deaf and orthopaedically handicapped and mentally retarded. Social problems may start with individual problems such as alcoholism, prostitution, venereal disease or delinquency. When these problems affect a large number of people they become social problems and a danger to the welfare and safety of the whole community.

Many social problems are due to the population growth, which leads to overcrowding especially in city slums. We then have problems of housing, sanitation, communicable diseases, poverty and crime. It will be seen that many of the social problems are connected with community health. In order to solve social problems, there is a need to coordinate activities in the areas of social welfare and assistance, community health services, and laws to control social evils.

Delinquency: Juvenile delinquency refers to the criminal offences by children and youth. In an adult the delinquent act is called a crime. There is a high rate of delinquency and crime in the city: in market places, bus stands, railway stations and near cinemas and hotels. Thefts are common, also burglary (breaking into steal) and sexual offences. Juvenile delinquency often starts with a breakdown of family life, and lack of affection, also of controls in the home. The child fails to socialize. He does not learn to accept the norms and values of society. It may be due to poverty that the child runs away to the city. He may steal money for food, smoking and drinking. Some are confused by seeing films or reading magazines which show a different way of life than that of the village.

With the widening gap between the 'haves and 'have-notes the individual with a hunger for more money or possessions often steals to satisfy that hunger. Later he gets drawn into a criminal group. There are even big crime organizations, which are able to carry on successfully, using bribes and threats to get what they want and escape the law. Anti-social practices of this type are a serious danger to the welfare of society.

Prostitution: This is an ancient social evil. It is more common in urban areas. The causes for a girl becoming a prostitute may be similar to those causing boys to become delinquents. Sometimes it is because of shame when she gets pregnant without being married. It may be because she wants money to dress well, or to give financial help to the family. Another reason girls become prostitutes are kidnapping, or someone in the trade promising a job in the city. Soon the unfortunate girl is imprisoned to the men who pay for this. The Government of India has passed 'The Suppression of immoral Traffic Act' to control prostitution. Raids are made on brothels and girls taken to jail, but it is not difficult for the brothel-keeper to pay and get her back. Rehabilitation programmers are needed to help these girls and limit this problem.

Beggary: As in the case of prostitution, in the case of begging also there are organizations in the cities, which kidnap or lure children to make them beg in the streets. Sometimes children are maimed (made into cripples) in order to get more money from the sympathetic public. This kind of beggary brings a lot of money to the organizers. In other cases beggary is a family profession. In general the public think of alms giving as a virtue. The social problem of begging can be ended only when there is a social change n the attitude to begging.

Alcoholism: Moderate drinking is not a problem, but excessive drinking and addiction to alcohol is a social problem. The person who is addicted may do harm to his family, and leave them without money. His work suffers or his job is lost. He may harm others also when drunk. Because of the harmful results of drinking alcohol to the individual to his family and to the society. Gandhi promoted prohibition, but for various reason this is now dropped by most of the states of India.

SOCIAL STRATIFICATION

It is the horizontal division of society into higher and lower social units. These divisions called social strata include the caster and class groups. It is the division of society into permanent groups or categories linked with each other by the relationship of superiority and subordination. Some individuals and groups are rated higher than other on the basis of opportunities and privileges that they enjoy. For e.g. In India doctor and engineers are rated higher than teachers. Status and role, economic and political groups are also factors in social stratification.

Caste

It is a collection of families or group of families bearing a common name, membership of which is hereditary, imposing on its members certain restriction in matter of social interaction. It is a hereditary type of social group. The Hindu's social order is based on the caste system. Membership is by birth. The group or caste has a common name and traditional occupation. The members have to marry with in their own group, or else be treated as outcast. The rules about food and drink are very strict. The society is divided into various castes with a well developed life of their own.

The status of a person does not depend on his wealth but on the traditional importance of the caste in which he had born. Status is determined not by vocation but by birth. There are regular caste councils to regulate and control the conduct of all caste members. Their rules over all caste members work powerfully which keeps the people in their proper places. In our society, the classes are divided into high and low. Brahmins in India stand at the apex of the social ladder.

In contrast to high position enjoyed by Brahmins, the sudras was subject to lowest treatment. Member of upper classes must not travel the in the company of sudras. If sudras violate the rules, they must undergo severe punishments. Ever the well is polluted if a low caste man draws water from it. Sudras could not study the sacred literature. A person born in a caste remains in it for life and dies in it. Members of a particular caste are expected to follow the caste occupation. They can't change to other occupation. Generally the impure castes are made to live on the outskirts of the city. To help them up the social ladder, they are given opportunities and reservations in education and jobs. There is an "unsociability offences Act" to control the ill- treatment of untouchables.

Social Class

It is one or two or more broad groups of individuals who are ranked by the members of the community, in socially, superior and inferior position. The members of the upper class are superior. Whereas the members of lower class are servants and mode of living is manual labour. In modern communities wealth is the primary determinant of social stratification. There is an intimate relation between the social class and the occupation, which indicates the mode of life and general social standing. The members of class possess common interests; they're brought into consciousness by the need of defence against the common enemy. Social class is a section of a community different from other sections because of social status. Social status may be because of birth or race.

In the modern society social status may be related to any of the following: income, occupation, education, political power, economic power, or religious power. Those who share a common status are grouped in a social class, and they feel belonged in that class. The 'upper class' includes those with greater wealth and property. Besides status, they often have power over the 'lower' class, and power may be misused. The poor are exploited and become still poorer. There is a gap between the rich and the poor, which is becoming wider. The 'middle class' in Indian society is growing in size and strength. This is a strata between the upper and lower classes. It is based on economic factors and includes doctors, college professors, business managers, office workers and factory workers. A middle-class consciousness and culture is developing in modern India.

Mobility

People in society continue to move up and down the status scale. It is called social mobility. It is to be distinguished from migration which is a movement in geographical space. Mobility has been classified as Horizontal mobility and Vertical mobility. Horizontal mobility refers to change of residence or job without status change. E.g. transfer of teacher from one school to another. Vertical mobility refers to movement in any or all of the three areas of living; class, occupation and power. Mobility may be downward or upward. This term can mean a change in social status, or a change of place, e.g. from rural to urban area.

In India today, large numbers of rural people migrate to the cities. They go in search of work, or to beg in order to live. If he finds a way to earn money, he may move up from lower class to middle class. Suppose a Brahmin moves from his village to the city. He will probably lose the superior social status he had before. In the urban community there is much more social mobility than in the rural community.

Independent India has adopted the principles of equality, freedom and justice. The Government planning and legislation are slowly bringing about social change. Education, influence of foreign cultures, politics and inter-group conflicts are other reasons for social change and social mobility. For example, when a certain social group accepts Family Planning the smaller number of children gets a better education, and later some may get top positions in society. In this way a whole group may move up in social status.

MARRIAGE SYSTEM

Marriage is an institution which admits adult's men and women to family life. It is a stable relationship and in which men and women is socially permitted to have children. The right to have children implying the right to several relations.

Types of Marriages

- Polyandry: In this system, one wife has many husbands.
- Fraternal polyandry: One wife is regarded as the wife of all brothers who have relation with her.
- Polygyny: One husband is having two or many wives at a time.
- Monogamy: One man marries are woman at a time.
- Experimental marriage: Two people, before they settle down to a life of permanent union, may be allowed to lead matrimonial life temporarily in order to find out if they can settle down permanently or not.
- Companionate marriage: This is the marriage of two persons on the understanding that if there are no children, the marriage may be dissolved by mutual consent.

The family is not an organized group. Members are joined into a group because of marriage and kinship. They are related to one another, share the family home, and a common kitchen. The family begins with marriage. In most families there is one man to one woman; this is monogamy type of society. Polygamy (two or more wives) is practiced in some societies, e.g. Muslim. They way in which man and woman come together (mate) also vary. In India it is usual for the elders or parents to arrange the marriage of their children. Usually the couple must be of the same religion and caste. It is also the tradition in India for elder sisters to be married first, then brothers.

In Modern society, often there are 'love marriages', in which the man and woman marry their own choice of partner. This type may be interacts, even inter-racial marriage. In some societies, marriage is a social contract, in others a religious sacrament. Registration of the marriage makes it legal. If the marriage breaks up, one or other partner may get a divorce. Broken marriages have a very bad effect on the children, and are not good for the society. We should do all we can to help in keeping good relationship between husbands and wives. This is most important for the total family and community welfare.

FAMILY STRUCTURE

Contemporary society generally views family as a haven from the world, supplying absolute fulfilment. The family is considered to encourage "intimacy, love and trust where individuals may escape the competition of dehumanizing forces in modern society from the rough and tumble industrialized world, and as a place where warmth, tenderness and understanding can be expected from a loving mother, and protection from the world can be expected from the father. However, the idea of protection is declining as civil society faces less internal conflict combined with increased civil rights and protection from the state. To many, the ideal of personal or family fulfilment has replaced protection as the major role of the family. The family now supplies what is "vitally needed but missing from other social arrangements".

The family is the simplest group capable of maintaining itself. It is, therefore, we may say, the primary social structure. Because it contains both sexes and all ages it is capable of reproducing itself, and so of reproducing society. For the same reason it contains practically all social relations in miniature. It has therefore often been called, and rightly, "the social microcosm". The relations of superiority, subordination, and equality, which enter so largely into the structure of all social institutions, are especially clearly illustrated in the family in the relations of parents to children, of children to parents, of parents to each other, and of children to one another. Comte, for this reason, claimed that the family was the unit of social organization, not the individual. However this may be, it is evident that families do enter, as units, very largely into our social and industrial life. While the tendency may be to make the individual the unit of modern society, it is nevertheless true that the family remains the simplest social structure in society, and from it, in some sense; all other social relations whatsoever are evolved.

The Modern family has 'decreased control of the marriage contract. Women in modern family have attained an increasing degree of economic independence. In modern family the woman is not the devotee of man, but an equal partner in life with equal rights. It is a smaller family. It is no longer a joint family. It is secular in attitudes.

Types of Families

Nuclear Family: The nuclear family consists of father, mother and children. By tradition, father is the earning member and mother stays at home to care for the family. In a modern family these roles may change. When mother has a better job and earns more than father, there is often conflict, and children become insecure and may become delinquents.

Joint Family: The joint family consists of a number of married couples and their children who live together in the same household. If it is a matriarchal family (For example in Kerala) the bridegroom comes to the bride's home and the senior female of the household is the head of the family. In a patriarchal family, the wife has to stay in her husband's home and her social status is very low. There are often problems related to dowry and property.

Three Generation Family: In three generation family young couples continue to live with their parents and have their own children.

Functions of the Family

Different functions of a family are:

Protection: At birth, the young child is totally dependent upon adults for all its needs. Survival would be difficult without adequate care given by the family members. In fact, the family looks after not only the children but all the other members too. Caring for and giving protection to the children, the sick and the old is an important function of the family.

Emotional bonding: The affection and love received from parents and other family members is essential for the proper development of children. The emotional bonding which close family ties give, make children feel wanted and loved. They grow up to be better adjusted adults than those who have not felt close family ties.

Education: The family is the first school of a child- where the do's and don'ts of society are learnt. Learning how to interact with others, learning to respect and obey elders, learning to be honest, etc., starts at home. The traditional skills are also learnt at home and the child is prepared for future roles and career by the family.

Financial security: The family acts as a provider for all its members. It provides the food, the shelter and the clothes that everyone needs. Other requirements of the family members are also fulfilled.

The work in the family is divided among all the members. Different members perform different tasks. Some earn, some perform the household tasks. Take a look at your own family and make a list of all the things that each person in your family does. You will notice that through this division of labour, all the work gets done, and the basic needs of everyone are fulfilled.

Recreation: Family members act as companions to one another. There is always someone to play with or talk to. Also, celebration of festivals and events in the family like birth or marriage, etc., provide recreation to members.

LIFE STYLE

Life-style related health determinants are multi-dimensional. These determinants are linked to number of major health problems. Also, some health issues share same determinants such as tobacco, alcohol, and nutrition.

Health problems linked to life-style related health determinants can be life-situation specific e.g. in childhood or in old age, but they can also be strongly linked to cultural aspects. In addition, socio-economic factors are an important reason for variations in health. Addressing these factors will be considered in all actions aimed at tackling lifestyle-related health determinant. Comprehensive health promotion in various settings e.g. schools, workplaces, families and local communities has proven to be efficient in addressing health determinants.

All these dimensions (determinants, health problems, life cycle, settings) are linked to each other. Depending on the situation, action focussed on a specific disease or on a specific determinant can be justified.

Equally population group or setting specific actions, which simultaneously address all relevant health determinants, can be the most efficient approach in many situations.

A variety of lifestyle or health related habits (behavioural factors), material factors (such as the environment and living standards), and psychosocial factors (for example, stress and risk taking) can have a major impact on a person's health. Factors often cluster together, for example, where a particular social group tend to live in close proximity within a neighbourhood, producing inequalities in ill health and inequalities in such causes of ill health. Behavioural and social issues that impact on health include smoking, diet, nutrition and alcohol (which together account for many cancer deaths), poor diet leading to obesity (reducing life expectancy) or alternatively malnutrition, lack of physical exercise, sexual behaviour (for example, leading to infection or teenage pregnancy), and problems resulting from drug taking. Consistent small area estimates of lifestyle factors are not available.

OBESITY

Being overweight can contribute or lead to a range of health conditions, such as heart disease, high blood pressure, diabetes, indigestion and some cancers. Adult and child obesity levels are becoming an increasing issue for the health service, as greater numbers of people put on extra weight, through poor diet or insufficient exercise. Obesity is measured using the Body Mass Index (BMI) formula, which is based on an individual's height and weight. A BMI of 25 to 29.9 is considered overweight; a score of 30 or above is considered obese. Synthetic estimates of obesity have limitations. Analyses of 2005 data on obesity levels indicate that poorer women are gaining weight, whilst poorer men are becoming thinner. Correlations between obesity and deprivation, apparent historically, are no longer clearcut, in particular amongst young people, where obesity rates are rapidly increasing.

ALCOHOLISM

Alcohol related problems can lead to ill health and premature death, especially through cirrhosis of the liver, and through alcohol related violence resulting in emergency admission to hospital. Whilst the focus has been on how alcohol related illnesses can affect the middle aged, binge drinking is increasingly of concern, affecting both teenagers and younger adults, and becoming an all too frequent way to spend a night out. In addition to alcohol related accidents, which can result in attendance at Accident and Emergency departments, binge drinking impacts on alcohol related crime and many social problems.

SMOKING

Smoking is a major cause of lung cancer, cardiovascular disease and chronic obstructive pulmonary disease (COPD), although it can, in addition, be a cause of, or contribute to, many other cancers and conditions, such as asthma or high blood pressure. Research indicates that smoking can reduce life expectancy by seven to eight years.

DRUGS

Drug taking, and in particular addiction, can have a devastating effect on personal health and circumstances, as well as impacting on family, friends and communities. The majority of those in contact with structured treatment services report problems resulting from the use of opiates.

MENTAL HEALTH

There is no Health without mental health. The public health approach to mental health and mental illness is based in a population-based model characterised by concern for the health of a population in its entirety and by an awareness of the linkage between health and the physical and the psychosocial environment.

HYGIENE

Hygiene is the science of health and its preservation. The term also refers to practices that are conductive to good health. Good personal hygiene usually means those measures a person takes to keep his skin and its appendages (his hair, finger nails, and toe nails) and his health & mouth clean and in good condition. Physical health is an important component of total health. The subject of physical health includes care of the skin, hair, teeth, eyes, ears, hands, feet, rest & sleep, exercise, recreation & posture. The students must know not only the anatomy of the body organs but also known how these can be maintained in a state of optimum health. The science of preserving and promoting health is known as hygiene. Hygiene has two aspects:

- Personal Hygiene
- Environmental Hygiene

The Subject of personal hygiene is physical health and how to maintain it. Preventive medicine is defined as "The Science and art of preventing decease, prolonging life & promoting physical and mental health and efficiency". Where as in preventive medicine the focus is on the individual in community health. Personal Hygiene helps in the following manner:

- To maintain a good and clean physique.
- To maintain good muscle strength.
- To maintain clean mouth and Teeth free from carries.
- To keep the eyes, ears and nose in a healthy condition and free from infection.
- To maintain a healthy skin.
- To preserve ones energy and not get tired in carrying out daily tasks.
- To maintain resistance and prevent infection.

HYGIENE PRINCIPLES

- The intact skin is the body first organ of defence against infection and injury.
- Individual differences exit in the nature of the skin and its appendages.
- Changes occur throughout the life span in the skin, mucus membrane, hair, nails and the teeth.
- The health of the skin and mucus membrane is highly dependant on adequate nourishment, fluid intake and exercise.
- A person general health affects both the status of his skin and appendages, teeth and mouth.
- Hygiene practices are learnt.
- Hygiene practices vary with cultural norms, personal values and ability to maintain good habits of cleanliness and grooming.
- Drugs and other form of therapeutic treatment affect the skin and its appendages.

NURSING

Most people think of Nursing as caring for the sick or helping the doctor in the care and treatment of patients. It is much more than this, nursing includes carrying activities in hospital and in community. Nursing includes preventing illness, disability and death. Nursing responsibility is also includes health education, research, training and supervision of health personnel and administration.

Nursing is helping a person with those things he cannot do for himself, but are necessary for him to get back to his former health and independence. In nursing we should try to do even more.

We should do, all we can to help people to live a life that is fully healthy in body, mind and spirit and social relationship. When nursing an individual we should remember his feelings and beliefs, try to understand his problems, also the needs of his family and of the community. Nursing is an important part of work of a health worker.

PERSONAL HYGIENE

Skin Care

To preserve cleanliness of skin and to keep healthy, regular baths and proper clothing are necessary. Other wise, the sebaceous glands will be locked, which in turn will interfere with the excretion process and further lead to certain skin condition such as scabies, impetigo, prickly heat and ring worm etc. Skin is the one of the most vital organ of the body. The functions of the skin are:

- It protects the body from heat, cold, humidity and entry of micro organisms.
- It acts as a sensory agent for touch.
- It converts sunlight into vitamin D.

Bathing of the skin: Skin comes in contact with the external environment and accumulates dirt. Taking daily bath with soap and water removes dirt and free us from all body odours. Soap is good surface cleaning agent. It gives a sense of freshness and well being and also prevents infection.

Bathing help not only in cleanliness, but also in maintaining good circulation of blood, tone of muscle and improves appetite. Baths may vary according to climatic conditions and be classified according to condition of the patient and temperature of the water. Main purposes of bath are:

- To remove waste products and clean the skin.
- To refresh and promote relaxation.
- To stimulate circulation.
- To maintain the condition of the skin
- The best time for the bath is either before breakfast or at least one hour after meals.

The skin must be maintain and protected by the following ways:

Regular baths: A daily bath, taken twice a day, is essential in India because of the hot climate. It keeps the skin clean and prevents infections such as boils, scabies, ringworm and itching.

Oil baths: Periodical oil baths are beneficial especially during winter months for healthy skin and prevention of dryness of the skin.

Balanced diet: A daily balanced diet and a diet including vitamin A rich foods should be taken to promote health of the skin.

Mosquito nets: The skin is a portal of entry to many communicable diseases such as malaria and filariasis through insect bites. So the people must use mosquito nets to prevent insect bites.

Protective clothing: People who are working in industries and factories, those who come in contact with acids, alkalis and other chemical and physical agents should wear protective cloths to prevent accidents and injuries.

Cosmetics: As long as there is no allergy and skin irritation, they should be no objection in using cosmetics. Overuse of cosmetics may cause more harm than benefits because this may blocks the sweat glands.

Clothing: Clothing is one of the essential needs of the man. The main purposes of clothing are:

- To protect the body from climatic factors such as extreme cold and heat, to protect from injuries and bites of animals and insects.
- To maintain the body heat.
- For personal value such as ornamentation and decoration.

Choice of clothing is important and the material for clothing should be appropriate, for example, wool is best clothing for winter season. Cotton cloths are best in summer season. So, one should wear clean cloths after bath.

Hair Care

The condition of hair often reflects the general condition of the body and its nutritional status. In children who have streaked, yellowish brown, dry hair indicates deficiency of vitamins. In kwashiorkor hair becomes thin, sparse and easily breakable. Hair breaking shows that the shafts are not receiving sufficient nourishment. Greying or loss of hair pigment is due to deficiency of diet, physical and mental diseases. Using of soaps, shampoos and soap nuts take care of the hair. Soaps are mostly made up of with animal or vegetable oil such as coconut oil, olive oil, glycerine and sandalwood.

A good shampoo is prepared from synthetic detergents and it removes the surface grease, dirt and skin debris without affecting the scalp. Soap nuts are natural products and cause no harm to hair and remove dirt thoroughly. After using these, we should wash hair thoroughly with warm water. Before and during washing, the scalp should be massaged properly with the fingertips.

The regular care of the hair is washing with shampoo, twice a week. Massaging the scalp is also useful. It is a type of positive exercise. It stimulates the blood flow and improves the nutrition of the hair. Oils are easily absorbed in the skin. So, once in a week massaging the scalp with coconut oil is very beneficial. Good scalp hygiene prevents infections like scabies, head lice, ringworm and dandruff.

Dandruff: Dandruff is due to the excessive shedding of dead skin cells from the scalp. As it is normal for skin cells to die and flake off, a small amount of flaking is normal and in fact quite common. Some people, however, either chronically or as a result of certain triggers, experience an unusually large amount of flaking, which can also be accompanied by redness and irritation. Most cases of dandruff can be easily treated with specialized shampoos. Excessive flaking can also be a symptom of seborrhoeic dermatitis, psoriasis, fungal infection or excoriation associated with infestation of head lice.

Those affected by dandruff find that it can cause social or self-esteem problems. Treatment may be important purely for psychological reasons. Regular washing with shampoo can control dandruff. Shampoo containing selenium and sulphur are available in the market to treat dandruff, but they should not be use regularly.

Pediculosis: For infestation of lice or pediculosis, one part of kerosene, one part of the pure oil may be rubbed well into the hair at night, covered with a towel or a cap, and the hair washed next morning. Warm vinegar will soften the nits and then they can be washed off the hair. The more recent treatment is 10% DDT dusting powder applied to the hair and covered with a towel for several hours. The hair can be combed with a fine toothcomb and DDT applied again a week later. In the meantime the hair should not be washed after the first dusting so that the new lice can be killed as they hatch.

Oral Hygiene

The most two common dental ailments are dental carries (tooth decay) and periodontal disease (gum diseases of pyorrhoea). Dental hygiene is an important aspect of personal health of an individual. Good oral hygiene implies sound teeth and healthy gums with health surrounding tissues. A physical act of chewing promotes saliva and gastric secretions, which helps in digestions. Teeth are not only useful for mastication but also for good appearance and clear speech. Improvement of oral hygiene improves the general health. Dental Disease in children often continues into the adult life. Some of the dental disease conditions are as follows:

Dental Caries: Dental caries is the most destructive of all dental diseases, leading to cavity formation and tooth decay. Dental caries is due to the action of acids on tooth enamel and these acids are produced certain mouth bacteria acting upon food particles lodging in the mouth. Due to bad oral hygiene dental caries develop. If the acids secrete for a prolonged period and touch the enamel, a cavity develops on the enamel surface. Once the enamel is damaged, it cannot be repaired. That means dental caries may be developed due to bad oral hygiene. A lot of research has shown that sugar consumption can increase caries, particularly when the sweat food is in a sticky form.

Periodontal disease: This disease is also called as pyorrhoea or pockets of pus around the teeth. It develops very slowly. It is a painless condition and unnoticed by the patient for a long time. It is responsible for more tooth loss than any other single factor. It also affects supporting structures surrounding the teeth which causes tooth fall. Hygiene of the mouth is essential for the control and prevention of this disease.

Halitosis: It means bad breath. It is due to poor oral hygiene, periodontal disease, sinus infection, tonsillitis, and infection of nose and throat. These conditions are quiet common in India and often start in early childhood.

The care of the teeth is explained below:

Tooth brushing: Teeth should be cleaned at least twice a day. Many people in the village use tender twigs of neem or babbul (acacia) as a toothbrush. Some use ash, charcoal and some tooth powders. The toothbrush is the best for removal of food debris and dental plaque, which accumulates around the neck of the teeth. Along with the toothpaste and powders, tooth brushing is ideal for cleaning the teeth. The bristles of the toothbrush should be soft that and should not be too sharp or too hard.

For brushing the teeth generally a vertical or circular brushing techniques are recommended. Tooth should be clean and the mouth should be rinsed soon after eating food. The tongue should be scraped or brushed and the mouth should be gargled with luke-warm water to keep the throat clean.

Use of fluorides: Where ever drinking water contains less than 0.5 mg of fluorides per litre, excessive dental caries has been observed. The optimum level of fluoride in drinking water is between 0.5 to 0.8 mg per litre. Fluorides decreases enamel solubility in acids. Deficiency of fluorine in drinking water can be rectified by applying topical fluoride on the tooth surfaces. The use of fluorides is significant means of caries prevention. Fluoride present in the drinking water acts both systemically and locally.

Regular Dental checkups: Dental check-up twice a year is recommended for early diagnosis and treatment of dental ailments. In some countries, regular dental services or check ups are provided to all school children through school dental nurses and dental hygienists.

Diet: The relation between the diet and dental disease is well known. In cities the dental disease are increased. Excessive intake of refined carbohydrates such as sugar sweets, jilebees, pastries, cakes, chocolates and biscuits promotes the dental caries.

Soft and sticky foods that adhere to the teeth causes tooth decay. Intake of fruits, vegetables like carrots, cucumber, sugarcane etc. reduces the frequency of dental caries. These foods are called natural toothbrushes and their daily intake should be promoted.

Habits: The habit of sucking sweets in the mouth causes a marked increased in tooth decay. Holding a feeding bottle with milk or sweetened juices for a long time sucking may cause dental caries. This is called by dentists "baby bottle syndrome". The habit of eating snacks frequently in between meals is also a bad habit. The habit of chewing betel leaves and tobacco is an important cause of bad oral hygiene in India. The foundation of good oral hygiene is laid in early childhood.

Care of dentures: Dentures are man-made substitutes. All dentures are potentially traumatic. These should be removed after meals and thoroughly brushed. All dentures must be removed at night because they can act as incubators of bacteria. After removing the dentures the mouth should be rinsed thoroughly with warm salt water. Don't place the dentures in boiling water. Dentures can be washed with baking soda or any washing detergent.

Care of the Hands and Nails

Hands and nails are never free from micro organisms. They pick up dirt and bacteria easily because they come in contact with many things. Therefore they should be kept clean, by thoroughly washing with soap and water, especially before taking food. After attending the toilet, hands should be washed with soap and water. The nails collect dirt, so they should be kept clean by gentle scrubbing with nailbrush. The habit of biting nails and putting fingers in the nose or ears and mouth is unhygienic habit and this should be discouraged.

Nails also require rigorous cleaning. They need to be cut short periodically. Otherwise dirt will be accumulate under long nails which is unhygienic, harbour harmful organisms of typhoid, cholera, dysentery, diarrhoea and various intestinal worms. Long nails can also be dangerous like scratching or hurting the skin of a patient while giving care, especially in cases of newborn and children.

Hand washing: In the community health nursing practice, if a nurse has to wash hands before carrying out any procedure, following technique can be followed, that is wet the hands from elbow towards fingertips and apply soap well. Rub the hands thoroughly and washed the tips of fingers and thumb in and out, then wash between fingers and arms rotating motion, a rinse from elbow to the downward this helps to remove dirt. Repeat it whenever necessary to remove adhered dirt.

Care of the Elimination

The organs of elimination are the lungs, skin, kidney and the intestine. These are involuntary acts. The elimination of faeces is a voluntary action. Lungs eliminate carbon dioxide, skin eliminates sweat, and kidneys eliminate urine.

Kidney: Proper maintenance of skin as mentioned earlier and good exercise will promote elimination of wastes thoroughly by kidneys. The kidneys excrete 3-4 pints of water per a day.

Bowel: Forming a regular habit of emptying the bowels each day at about the same time will help in avoiding constipation. Some guidance and a bit of permissiveness will help the child to establish his own schedule. Irregularity of bowel habits may cause the individual to have headaches, be impatient, low spirited, or lack of energy and will be unable to concentrate and study. The hands need to be washed well with soap and water afterwards. Open field defecation is to be avoided.

Menstrual Hygiene

The menstruating woman is considered unclean and is prevented from taking part in normal daily activities in some communities. It should be explained that menstruation is a normal physiological process. The menstrual discharge is usually controlled by means of an absorbent sanitary pad or diaper, which must be frequently changed. Alternatively an absorbent tampon may be placed in the vagina.

Intra-vaginal tampons fitted with a cord are available. Commercially they are easy to insert and remove. Intra-vaginal tampons are popular because they are comfortable and convenient. Their main disadvantage is that they cannot be used unless the hymen is torn or stretched. Vaginal douching is not only unnecessary at the end of the period or at any other time, but is positively harmful in that it washes away the natural protective discharge.

The vagina can take care of it self, and it is remarkable how it cleanses itself of all the menstrual debris in the course of a few hours. Regarding sexual intercourse during menstruation, there is no medical reason to avoid, but only objection is the obvious aesthetic one.

Eye Care

Eye often reflects the physical health. Eyes needs well maintained care. When reading books they should be held 12 to 16 inches away from the eye at an angle of 45° to 75°. Skin around eyes must be cleaned with soap and water or clear water. Vitamin A foods are used for good eyesight and prevent infractions.The conditions which may affect the eyes are:

- Infections-conjunctivitis, trachoma, sty
- Injuries-corneal ulcers
- Malnutrition-Night blindness, exophthalmia
- Errors of refraction - short sightedness, long-sightedness.
- Others- cataract, glaucoma.

There are 15 million blind people in India as of year 2007. The main causes of blindness are:

- Cataract.
- Trachoma.
- Others infections.
- Malnutrition.

- Injuries.
- Glaucoma.

Blindness is preventable through simple measures such as:

- Early diagnosis and treatment
- Good personal hygiene.
- Improvement in diet.
- Control of flies.
- Health education.

The care of the eyes consists of the following:

- Prevention and control of infections.
- Injuries.
- Eye strain
- Good diet.
- Squint
- Regular check up

Prevention and Control of Infections: Eye is a delicate and sensitive organ. Trachoma is eye infection which is common in children. It spread by using infected clothes, handkerchiefs, towels, and flies. Conjunctivitis is an acute inflammation of the outer layers of the eye which is caused by bacteria, virus or allergy. The preventive measures are:

- Early diagnosis and treatment until cure is achieved
- Health education towards of clean towels and linen, fly control, prevention and good personal hygiene.

Injuries: During working or playing, eye is exposed to injuries. In industries, eye injuries are common; workers must use protective glasses. In children eye injuries are due to firecrackers. While playing they may cause eye injury. Foreign bodies also cause eye injury. Wash the eye immediately with plenty of water, eye should not be rubbed. If foreign body does not come out, refer to doctor immediately.

Eye Strain: Reading must be done in good light to avoid eyestrain. Light should come from left and behind. Hold the book at 45 to 75 degrees from the horizontal level. Avoid reading in moving trains and buses or in lying positions. Eye must be protected from direct exposure to sun light, glare and extreme brightness. If required wear glasses.

Good diet: Many eye diseases occur due to malnutrition. Vitamin A rich foods such as green leafy vegetables, fruits, milk and butter prevent deficiency diseases like neurosis, keratomalaia, night blindness.

Squint: If there is a cross eye or squint, refer to specialist. This defect can be rectified by the use of glasses or eye exercises. In some cases, it may need operation. It should be treated early in the life.

Regular check-up: Regular check up by the eye specialist once a year until the age of 10 and there after every 3 years is must in early detection and treatment of eye diseases.

Care of the Ears

The ear is an important sense organ of the body. It is useful not only for hearing, but also for body equilibrium. The ear is liable to infection and injury. Infections of nose and throat readily spread to middle ear and cause inflammation known as otitis media. The ear problems are earache, discharge, wax and foreign bodies.

Care of the ear comprises of the following:

- Keeping the ear clean.
- Removing excessive wax carefully
- Preventing entering of water into the ear during bathing.
- Protect the ear from exposure to loud noises.
- Preventing and treating all nose and throat infections.
- If the ear canal is full of wax. it must be cleaned. For its removal, put a drop of warm boiled coconut oil, olive oil, peanut oil or glycerine into the ear.
- Teaching good habits; one should not put pencils, patches and other foreign bodies into ear. If any foreign body enter into the ear refer to a doctor.

Care of Nose and Throat

Great care should be taken in blowing the nose. If possible, have disposable tissues for nasal discharge or cough. If not, rag pieces may be used (placed in covered vessel of water after use and boiled for 10 minutes then washed and hung in the sun to dry). Sari ends or fingers should never be used. When swimming keep water as much as out of the nose and throat and be sure the water is safe, (not contaminated) by waste materials. While the face is under water, expel air slowly and continuously through the nose. Breathe in through the mouth while the head is above water. Blow the nose gently after swimming. If there is any infection of nose or throat, it may spread rapidly to ear. Treat the infection immediately.

Care of the Feet

The human foot is composed of 26 bones, connected by ligaments, muscles, blood vessels and nerves. Bones are so arranged as to balance and support the weight of the body. If the foot are allowed to stay in a wrong position for a long time, it leads to poor posture. To prevent diseases and for foot hygiene, the feet should be washed with soap and water, both at night and morning. The feet may be soaked in a dilute solution of formalin (table spoon of formalin to 250 ml. of water) for 15 minutes, then thoroughly dried and dusted with boric acid or talcum powder. Special care must be taken in selection of shoes. Shoes must be broad-toed and not too fitting. The socks should be clean and dry and they should not be too tight. Walking bare foot is unhygienic. Avoid cuts and bruises. If occurs, they should be treated with mild antiseptic cream. If there are cracks, apply milk cream or coconut oil.

ACTIVITIES OF DAILY LIVING

Activities of daily living (ADLs) are the things we normally do in daily living including any daily activity we perform for self-care (such as feeding ourselves, bathing, dressing, grooming), work, homemaking, and leisure." Health professionals routinely refer to the ability or inability to perform ADLs as a measurement of the functional status of a person. This measurement is useful for assessing the elderly, the mentally ill, those with chronic diseases, and others, in order to evaluate what type of health care services an individual may need.

RECREATION

Recreation means relaxation and amusing oneself. It relieves mental tension and fatigue and provides a feeling of well-being. Recreation may be active or passive. Physical exercise is an acute form of recreation. Passive form of recreation includes listening radio, watching T.V. going cinema, or picnic, playing cards, reading etc. There are recreation centres opened in many cities so that people can use their leisure time for improvement of their physical and mental health.

Recreation or fun is the expenditure of time in a manner designed for therapeutic refreshment of one's body or mind. While leisure is more likely a form of entertainment or rest, recreation is active for the participant but in a refreshing and diverting manner. As people in the world's wealthier regions lead increasingly sedentary life styles, the need for recreation has increased. The rise of so called active vacations exemplifies this.

A few individuals view recreation as largely non-productive, even trivial. Excessive recreation is not considered healthy, and may be labelled as escapism. However, research has shown that recreation contributes to satisfaction, and that the stress management aspects of it contribute to quality of life, health and wellness, and that the use of recreation as a diversion may have clinical applications to individuals with chronic pain and other health impairments. In some cultures and religions, recreation is encouraged on certain days and discouraged on others. For example, in Judaism, the Shabbat is a day for recreation and relaxation; some Christian churches use the Sabbath. Recreation is one kind of stress management.

REST AND SLEEP

To maintain good health, the body needs rest and sleep. We spend 1/3rd of time in sleeping every day. During sleep, the body and mind relax, repair and growth take place. Fatigue disappears. After sleep or rest we feel fresh and work better. According to the age, sex, environment, family, nature of work the amount of sleep required varies. In fact, children need 9-10 hours of sleep and adult 7-8 hours per day. The sleeping bed should be flat and should not sag in the middle and also we should not use too many pillows. Only one is sufficient. During sleeping face should not be covered, room should be dark, calm and quiet and well ventilated. Candles should not be kept in the room. One should cultivate regular sleeping habits-early to bed and early to rise. Drugs should not used to sleep.

SEXUAL LIFE

Evidence points to the many health benefits of an active sex life. Sexual activity is a form of physical exercise. Having sex three times a week burns around 7,500 calories in a year – the equivalent of jogging 75 miles. It raises the amount of oxygen in cells, helping to keep organs and tissues functioning at their peak. It increases testosterone. Testosterone is believed to help keep men's bones and muscles strong. Active sexual life can lower levels of the body's total cholesterol slightly, while positively changing the ratio of good-to-bad cholesterol. Sex can lower levels of arthritic pain, whiplash pain and headache pain. Hormones that are released during sexual excitement and orgasm can elevate pain thresholds.

DHEA (dehydroepiandrosterone), a popular supplemental hormone, is released naturally during sexual act. Researchers say prostate trouble may arise or be worsened by fluid build-up within the gland. Regular ejaculation will help wash out those fluids. Sex can be a very effective way of reducing stress levels. Affectionate touch increases levels of oxytocin. Oxytocin is a desire-enhancing chemical secreted by the pituitary. Regular oxytocin release may help encourage frequent lovemaking. Regular act can increase a woman's oestrogen level, protect her heart and keep her vaginal tissues more supple.

SPIRITUAL LIFE

Spirituality involves a dimension of human experience that psychiatrists are increasingly interested in, because of its potential benefits to health. It is not necessary to hold formal religious beliefs, or engage in religious practices, or belong to an established faith tradition, to experience the spiritual dimension.

In healthcare, spirituality is identified with experiencing a deep-seated sense of meaning and purpose in life, together with a sense of belonging. It is about acceptance, integration and wholeness.

According to one definition, "The spiritual dimension tries to be in harmony with the universe, strives for answers about the infinite, and comes especially into focus in times of emotional stress, physical and mental illness, loss, bereavement and death." This desire for wholeness of being is not an intellectual attainment, for it is no less present in people with learning disability, but lies in the essence of what it means to be human.

From the spiritual perspective, a distinction can be made between cure, or relief of symptoms, and healing of the whole person. Life is a perpetual journey of discovery and development, during which maturity is often gained through adversity. The relief of suffering remains a primary aim of health care, but it is by no means the whole story.

The last ten years have witnessed a dramatic increase in studies of spirituality, health, and well-being. This research has demonstrated robust links between spirituality and health.

Surveys of health patients have shown the need for:

- An environment for purposeful activity such as creative art, structured work and enjoying nature.
- Feeling safe and secure. Being treated with respect and dignity allows you to develop a feeling of belonging, of being valued and trusted.

- Having time to express feelings to sympathetic and concerned members of staff.
- Opportunities and encouragement to make sense of, and derive meaning from, experiences including illness.
- Permission and encouragement to develop a relationship with God or the Absolute (however the person conceives whatever is sacred).

People need a time, a place and privacy in which to pray and worship, the opportunity to explore spiritual (and sometimes religious) matters, encouragement in deepening faith, feeling universally connected and perhaps also forgiven.

Spirituality can deal with diverse problems such as lifestyle diseases, mental illness, addiction, chronic pain, marital and family problems, PTSD, and spiritual struggles among people with traditional and non-traditional spiritual identifications. Studies show that Spirituality can help to promote good health and fight disease by:

- Offering additional social supports.
- Improving coping skills through prayer and a philosophy that all things have a purpose.

EDUCATION

It is well accepted that education is positively related to health. Education can have benefits for individuals and society. Education lead to more than just better employment opportunities or higher potential income. Wolfe and Haveman (2001) list a number of possible non-market and social effects of education.

These include an association between an individual's education and:

- Higher levels of schooling of their children.
- An improved ability to make efficient choices, including consumer choices.
- Outcomes of individuals in their neighbourhood.
- The ability to plan fertility decisions.
- Their and their children's health outcomes.

FINANCIAL MANAGEMENT

Financial stress affects most people in one way or another. Some people become stressed to the point where they will self-medicate with either alcohol or some other drug, others will work to find some help and others will eat. Depression is also a common result from this kind of stress, especially in people who are at a complete loss as to what they can possibly do to deal with their financial troubles. How they choose to self-medicate or deal with their situation will often depend on the individual.

With the economy going the way it is these days, financial strife is affecting more people, and those who were suffering enough before will most likely be in worse trouble now. This means that there will be more people looking for ways to alleviate the immense stress they are feeling when finding themselves unable to pay bills, pay for enough proper food to feed their family and finding it increasingly difficult to make rent each month. As if making ends meet weren't bad enough already, it seems like just about everything from rent to food is jumping in price. For many, it can seem an impossible situation that continues to get worse with each passing day, especially if they are one of the many unfortunate victims of layoffs.

In this world today, living beyond one's means is easily accomplished, though many find it difficult to fix. How lack of money relates to a person's physical health all depends on how they handle their stress, as well as how well they are eating. For most finding themselves in financial strife, they may begin gaining more weight than is healthy for them because they have changed to a diet they believe is cheaper even if it isn't necessarily healthier. Others may find themselves losing weight because they are so focused on trying to get their bills and loans paid off that they are cutting the amount of food they are purchasing for themselves. Even children can be affected by the changes in diet their parents go through when trying to save money during tough financial times. In fact, thousands of children every day go to school hungry because their parents simply cannot afford to buy them food for breakfast.

Overeating or under eating is not the way to deal with financial stress. It will only cause health problems that may only make financial difficulties worse. Speaking with an online counsellor is probably the best place to start when looking for a real way out of a poor financial situation. Online counselling can be useful to anyone who is looking for some suggestions as to how they can improve their situation. Online therapists are available to help anyone looking for some help, or even just someone to talk to, and they can help one to find the best way to deal with their unique situation. In the end, online therapy can set one on the right track to changing their financial strife into a better situation.

INCOME

Richer, better-educated people live longer than poorer, less-educated people. Lower mortality and morbidity is associated with almost any positive indicator of socioeconomic status, a relationship that has come to be known as "the gradient."

Economists also have emphasized the negative correlation between socioeconomic status and various risky behaviours, such as smoking, binge drinking, obesity, and lack of exercise. They have also pointed to mechanisms that run from health to earnings, education, and labour force participation, and to the role of potential third factors, such as discount rates, that affect both education and health.

Epidemiologists argue that the economists' explanations at best can explain only a small part of the gradient; they argue that socioeconomic status is a fundamental cause of health. They frequently endorse measures to improve health through manipulating socioeconomic status, not only by improving education but also by increasing or redistributing incomes.

Even if income inequality has no direct effect on health, the fact that the relationship between health and income depends on the ratio of the between-to-within group components of income inequality.

REFERENCES

Edwards N, Mill J, Kothari A. Multiple Intervention Research Programs in Community Health. Can J Nurs Res. 2004;36(1): 40-55.

Emmons KM. Behavioural and Social Science Contributions to the Health of Adults in the United States. In Promoting Health: Intervention strategies from social and behavioural research. BD Smedley & SL Syme (Eds.), National Academy Press, Washington, D.C., 2000. p. 254-321.

Ensor T, Cooper S. Resource allocation and purchasing: influencing the demand side. Prepared for World Bank, Resource Allocation and Purchasing (RAP) Project. (March, 2002).

Ensor T, Cooper S. Resource allocation and purchasing: influencing the demand side. The University of York, Centre for Health Economics, Heslington, University of York.

Farquharson K. Influencing policy transnationally: Pro- and anti-tobacco global advocacy networks. Aust J Pub Admin. 2003;62(4): 80-92.

Fielen AC, Girasek DC. Integrating perspectives on the prevention of unintentional injuries, p. 203-227. In: N Schneiderman, MA Speers, JM Silva, H Tomes & JH Gentry. Integrating behavioural and social sciences with public health. United Book Press, Inc., Baltimore, 2001.

Frankish J. Study on the implementation of health goals in Canada. Institute of Health Promotion Research, UBC, 2000.

Frankish J, Kwan B, Flores J. Assessing the health of communities: Indicator projects and their impacts. Institute of Health Promotion Research, UBC, Sept 2002.

5

Epidemiology

Epidemiology is the study of how often diseases occur in different groups of people and why. Epidemiological information is used to plan and evaluate strategies to prevent illness and as a guide to the management of patients in whom disease has already developed.

The word 'epidemiology' has been used since the time when most of the infectious diseases were epidemic. Today, when infectious morbidity has considerably decreased, the concept of epidemiology includes the study of objective laws of aetiology, distribution and control of infectious diseases in a human community, and also elaboration of methods to prevent and control these diseases.

The following definition of the term 'epidemiology' was formulated at the International Symposium of Epidemiologists in Prague (1960): "Epidemiology is an independent branch of medicine studying aetiology and spreading of infectious diseases in a human community and is aimed at prevention, control, and final eradication of these diseases". General and special epidemiologies are distinguished. General epidemiology studies the laws of distribution of infectious diseases among people (characteristics of sources of infection, the mechanism of transmission, susceptibility to infection, and the like) and the general principles of prevention and control of these diseases. Special epidemiology studies epidemiologic characteristics of each particular infectious disease and the methods to prevent and control it.

HISTORY

Ancient people had their own concept of contagiosity of some diseases and took first prophylactic measures; they rejected people with infectious diseases from their community, used variolation (deliberate inoculation with smallpox virus), disinfection, etc. All these measures were empirical and their efficacy was low. At those times it was impossible to prove instrumentally that infectious diseases might be evoked by living microorganisms, but in the 14-15th centuries, aroused such suspicions in physicians.

Fracastorius, an Italian physician (1483-1553), produced a theory that proved contagiosity of these diseases. In Russia of the 11th century, they isolated people with contagious diseases and hurried the dead separately from the others. First quarantines were organized in the 16th century: patients were separated from their relatives, and funeral services over the dead were forbidden. In the 17th century, quarantine piquets were organized during epidemics out at the entrance to the city and at the houses with the diseased. When a family died, the house with the dead and the utensils was burned. According to the law, any case suspected for a contagious disease had to be reported to the officials.

In the 18th century, Edward Jenner an English physician, (1749-1823) devised a safe and effective method to prevent natural smallpox by inoculating people with cowpox vaccine. Development of industry and trade between different countries stimulated advances in medicine, including sanitary, quarantine, and anti-epidemic services. The second half of the 19th century was marked by vigorous development of physics chemistry, biology and other sciences, which all provided conditions for developing a new science microbiology. The scientific discoveries made by Pasteur, Mechnikov, Koch, Ivanovsky and many others promoted the study of aetiology, pathogenesis, course of infectious disease and also their epidemiology. The study of epidemiology of some infectious diseases and working out of prophylactic measures revealed the important role of social factors in the spread of epidemics. Inadequate labour and living conditions, poverty, and poor sanitation promoted the spread of contagious diseases.

Advances in epidemiology are infeasible without improvement of labour and living conditions, adequate health care, and planned anti-epidemic measures.

CONCEPT OF EPIDEMIC PROCESS

Micro organisms causing infectious diseases parasitize on host and persist due to continuous reproduction of new generations which change their properties in accordance with evolution of the environment conditions. Living inside its host, the micro organism persists for a definite period of time. Then the pathogenic micro organism can survive by changing its residence, i.e., by moving to another host via a corresponding transmission mechanism. This continuous chain of successive transmission of infection (patient - carrier), manifested by symptomatic or asymptomatic forms of the disease, is called an epidemic process.

The source of infectious micro organisms is an object which is the site of natural habitation and multiplication of the pathogenic micro organisms, and in which the micro organisms are accumulated. Since pathogenic micro organisms are parasites, only a living macro organism can be such an object, i.e., a human or an animal.

An epidemic focus is the residence of infection source including the surrounding territory within the boundaries of which, the source can, under given conditions, transmit a given disease through the agency of the pathogenic micro organisms. The focus of infection remains active until the pathogenic micro organisms are completely eradicated, plus the maximal incubation period in persons that were in contact with the source of infection.

The following three obligatory factors are necessary for the onset and continuous course of an epidemic process: the source of pathogenic microorganism, the mechanism of their transmission, and macroorganisms susceptible to infection. Infectious diseases are classed according to their source as anthroponoses (the source of infection is man), zoonoses (the source of infection is animal), and anthropozoonoses (both man and animal can be the source of infection). An infected macroorganism (man or animal), being the sole source of infection, can have either clinically manifest or asymptomatic form of the disease. A diseased person is the primary source from which the infection spreads.

DYNAMICS OF DISEASE TRANSMISSION

An infectious process is the interaction of a pathogenic microorganism with a macroorganism under certain environmental and social conditions. The concept 'infectious disease' means the condition manifested by a disease state of a patient and the so-called carrier state. The specific properties of infective agents, various pathogenicity and virulence of these agents, as well as the quantity of microorganisms that enter the macroorganism, resistance of the macroorganism and duration of specific immunity account for the multitude of clinical manifestations of infection. Infection can be clinically pronounced or it may be asymptomatic, which is known as the carrier state (parasite, bacterium, virus carrier state). A clinically manifest infection can run a typical or atypical course.

Patients with a typical form of infection demonstrate all symptoms specific for a given disease. One or several symptoms of a given disease are absent from the clinical picture of an atypical form, or the symptoms can be modified. A disease can be acute or run a protracted or even a chronic course.

A clinically manifest disease is usually classed as mild, moderate, and severe; according to the duration, the disease can be acute or chronic. An acute infection (smallpox, measles, plague) is characterized by a short stay of the causative agent in the body and development of specific immunity in the patient toward the given infection. A chronic infection (brucellosis, tuberculosis) can last for years. Asymptomatic infections can be subclinical and latent.

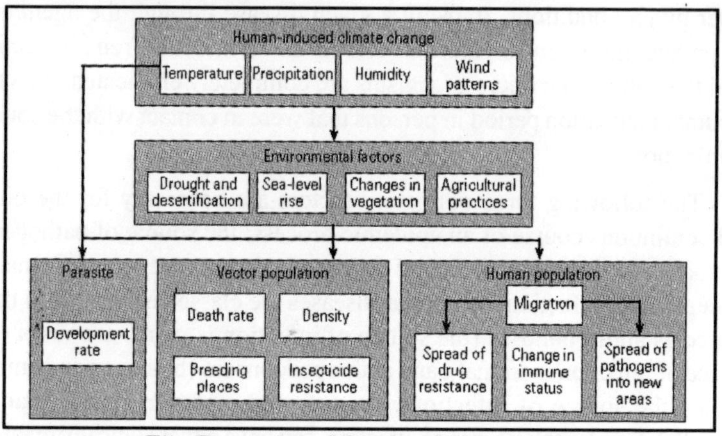

Fig. Dynamics of Disease Transmission

A person with a subclinical infection (acute and chronic) looks in full health, and the disease can only be diagnosed by detecting the causative agents, specific antibodies, and functional and morphological changes in the organs and tissues that are specific for a given disease. Such patients (or carriers) are a special danger for the surrounding people since they are the source of infection. At the same time, a repeated subclinical infection in poliomyelitis, diphtheria, influenza, and some other acute infections promotes formation of an immune group of people (herd immunity). Acute and chronic subclinical forms (carrier state) are more common in typhoid fever, paratyphoid B, salmonellosis, viral hepatitis B, etc. Latent or persistent forms of human and animal infections are a prolonged asymptomatic interaction of macroorganisms with the pathogenic agents which are present in modified ('defective') forms.

These are defective interfering particles in latent viral infections, and L forms, spheroplasts, etc. in bacterial infections. Being inside the host cell, these forms survive for long periods of time and are not released into the environment. Under the action of various provoking factors (such as thermal effects, injuries, psychic trauma, transplantation, blood transfusion, various disease states), persistent infection can be activated and become clinically manifest. The microbe regains its pathogenic properties. Persistence of virus has been studied best of all, but at the present time, persistence of other pathogenic factors has been intensively studied as well, e.g. of the L forms of streptococci, staphylococci, meningococci, cholera vibrio, typhoid fever bacilli, microbes causing diphtheria, tetanus, etc. Protozoa and rickettsia can also persist. For example, latent epidemic recrudescent typhus infection is manifested by relapses of epidemic recrudescent typhus (Brill's disease).

Mechanism of Transmission

For the epidemic to break out it is not sufficient to have a source of infection alone. The causative agent can survive only if it is transmitted from one host to another, because any given macroorganism destroys the pathogenic microorganisms by specific antibodies that are formed in it in response to the ingress of these microorganisms. Death of an individual host terminates the life of the parasitizing microorganisms. The only exception are sporeforming microbes (causative agents of anthrax, tetanus, botulism).

The combination of routes by which the pathogenic microorganisms are transmitted from an infected macroorganism to a healthy one is called the mechanism of infection transmission. Four mechanisms of infection transmission are distinguished according to the primary localization of pathogenic agents in macroorganisms: (1) faecal-oral (intestinal localization); (2) air-borne (airways localization); (3) transmissive (localization in the blood circulating system); (4) contact (transmission of infection through direct contact with another person or environmental objects).

Three phases are distinguished in the transmission of infection from one macroorganism to another: (1) excretion from an infected macroorganism; (2) presence in the environment; (3) ingress into a healthy macroorganism. The method by which microbes are excreted from an infected macroorganism (the first phase) depends on the locus of infection in the infected individual or a carrier. If pathogenic microorganisms reside on respiratory mucosa (influenza, measles, pertussis) they can be released from the patient only with expired air or with droplets of nasopharyngeal mucus. If the infection is localized in the intestine, the pathogenic microorganisms can be excreted with faeces (dysentery). The pathogenic organisms in the blood infect blood-sucking arthropods.

Epidemiological Triad

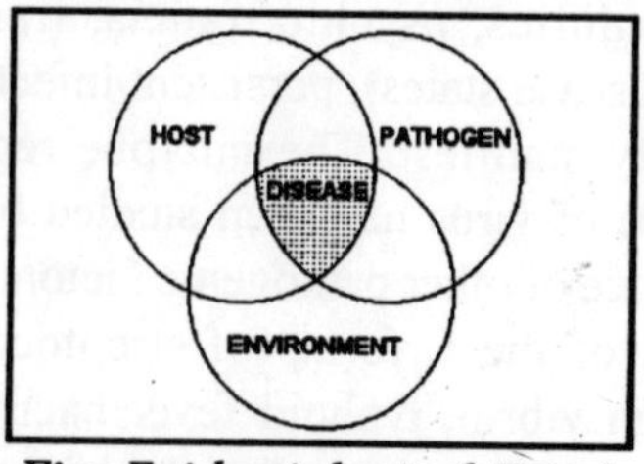

Fig. Epidemiological Triad

The traditional model of infectious disease causation. It includes three components: an external agent, a susceptible host, and an environment that brings the host and agent together, so that disease occurs.

MORBIDITY AND MORTALITY

Morbidity refers to a diseased state, disability, or poor health due to any cause.[12] The term may be used to refer to the existence of any form of disease, or to the degree that the health condition affects the patient. Among severely ill patients, the level of morbidity is often measured by ICU scoring systems. Comorbidity is the simultaneous presence of two medical conditions, such as a person with schizophrenia and substance abuse.

In epidemiology and actuarial science, the term morbidity rate can refer to either the incidence rate, or the prevalence of a disease or medical condition. This measure of sickness is contrasted with the mortality rate of a condition, which is the proportion of people dying during a given time interval.

Mortality rate is a measure of the number of deaths (in general, or due to a specific cause) in some population, scaled to the size of that population, per unit time. Mortality rate is typically expressed in units of deaths per 1000 individuals per year; thus, a mortality rate of 9.5 in a population of 100,000 would mean 950 deaths per year in that entire population. It is distinct from morbidity rate, which refers to the number of individuals in poor health during a given time period (the incidence rate) or the number who currently have that disease (the prevalence rate), scaled to the size of the population. One distinguishes:

1. The crude death rate, the total number of deaths per 1000 people. The crude death rate for the whole world is currently about 9.6 per 1000 per year (based on 62 million deaths in 2006, for a population of 6470 million).

2. The perinatal mortality rate, the sum of neonatal deaths and foetal deaths (stillbirths) per 1,000 births.
3. The maternal mortality rate, the number of maternal deaths due to childbearing per 100,000 live births.
4. The infant mortality rate, the number of deaths of children less than 1 year old per thousand live births.
5. The child mortality rate, the number of deaths of children less than 5 year old per thousand live births.
6. The standardised mortality rate (SMR)- This represents a proportional comparison to the deaths that would have been expected if the population had been of a standard composition in terms of age, gender, etc.
7. The age-specific mortality rate (ASMR) - This refers to the total number of deaths per 1000 people of a given age (e.g. 16-65 or 65+).

PREVENTION

Prevention and control of infectious diseases include the following:

- Mass-scale measures aimed at improvement of public health, prevention and spread of infectious diseases.
- Medical measures aimed at reduction of infectious morbidity and eradication of some diseases.
- Health education and involvement of population in prevention or restriction of the spread of infectious diseases.
- Prevention of import of infectious diseases from other countries.

Improvement of peoples' well-being, adequate housing, medical aid, and health education should be adequately planned and carried out. Preventive sanitary supervision is also necessary. Industrial objects, residential houses, children's and medical institutions should be constructed with strict adherence to the special sanitary requirements that are intended to improve labour and living conditions, prevention of onset and spread of infectious diseases. Preventive measures aimed to control infectious diseases taken by medical personnel are divided into preventive and anti-epidemic. Preventive measures are carried out regardless of the presence or absence of infectious diseases at a given time and locality. These measures are aimed at prevention of infectious diseases. Anti-epidemic measures are necessary when an infectious disease develops. It has already been said that the following three basic factors are necessary for development of an epidemic: the source of infection, transmission mechanism, and susceptibility of population. Exclusion of any of these factors terminates the spread of an epidemic process. Prophylactic and antiepidemic measures are therefore aimed at control of the source of infection, disruption of the route by which infection spreads, and strengthening of non-susceptibility of population.

Control of Infection Source

Patients with some infectious diseases, e. g. measles, pertussis, dysentery or cholera, liberate the pathogenic microorganisms into the environment during the last days of the incubation period or during the first day of the disease. Timely revealing of the sick is thus very important. Active detection of the sick is performed by medical personnel at hospitals, polyclinics, medical posts and the like. Health education of population by medical personnel promotes early attendance of the sick for medical aid and thus helps timely detection of infectious patients.

Examination of population in outpatient conditions (in residential districts) is helpful in this respect. An infectious disease is diagnosed on the basis of clinical findings, epidemiologic anamnesis and laboratory tests. All patients with the diagnosis of an infectious disease should be entered into a special record. The record should be made by a physician or a medical nurse.

All cases of infectious diseases or suspected cases should be entered into the record, and higher epidemiologic authorities should be informed not later than within 24 hours. In cases of plague, cholera or other disease that requires quarantine measures, local medical personnel must inform higher authorities of the health system. The infectious patients must be isolated in proper time. Patients with plague, cholera, viral hepatitis, typhoid and paratyphoid fever, diphtheria, and similar contagious diseases should be immediately hospitalized. The patients should be handled in special ambulance cars that should be disinfected after transportation of each patient.

The patient delivered to the hospital must be given appropriate sanitary treatment before placing in the appropriate ward or an isolated room, if the diagnosis is not clear, or infection is mixed by its character. Special measures should be taken in order to prevent spread of infection within the hospital. In order to remove the danger of spreading infection, the patient should be given appropriate therapy. Patients with scarlet fever, escherichiasis, dysentery and the like diseases can remain at home where they must be isolated from the other family. The family must be instructed how to prevent infection and to disinfect the household utensils. Observation of the patient by the medical personnel must be constant.

Persons cured from infectious diseases should be discharged from hospital after alleviation of all clinical symptoms, and examination for the carrier state, specific for each particular infection; for example, person who sustained diphtheria, can be discharged from hospital after a complete clinical cure and two negative bacteriological tests of the faucial and nasopharyngeal smears.

Persons who recovered from typhoid fever, paratyphoid, salmonellosis, dysentery should be observed in outpatient conditions. The term of observation depends on each particular disease. Carriers of infection should be revealed and isolated for medical examination and treatment. Since it is impossible to screen the entire population, only those who can be a danger for the surrounding people (personnel of children's institutions, food catering, and the like establishments) should be inspected. If the epidemiologic situation requires, the following groups of people should be examined for the carrier state:

- Persons who can be in contact with typhoid fever patients, patients with dysentery, paratyphoid, diphtheria, and meningococcal infection;
- Persons with a history of sustained typhoid fever, paratyphoid, and dysentery;
- Persons suspected for being a source of infection in the focus of infection.

The carriers must be immediately withdrawn from their occupation at food catering or children's institutions till they are completely cured and given multiple tests for the absence of the carrier state. Chronic carriers should be moved to other jobs that are not connected with food or children. Infection carriers must be regularly treated and observed according to special instructions. If animals are the source of infection, measures differ.

Veterinary measures should be taken with respect to domestic animals. Animals with brucellosis should be slaughtered. Horses with glanders should also be killed. Food and materials obtained from diseased animals must be given special treatment. Farms where infection is revealed, must be disinfected and quarantine established. Wild animals that are not the object of quarry must be destroyed, and measures for their isolation from man should be taken.

Disruption of Infection Transmission Pathways

The pathways by which infection can be transmitted are disrupted by acting on the transmission factors. Since intestinal infections are transmitted by the faecal-oral route, all preventive measures are aimed to preclude contact of the infected material with water, food, or hands. General sanitary measures should be taken constantly and universally, regardless of the presence or absence of infection in a given locality.

Community hygiene is very important in prevention of infection spread. Layout of settlements, housing conditions, the presence or absence of water supply and sewage systems are important factors in this respect. Permanent control of water supply system, a correct selection of water body and the site of water intake, protection of the water intake zone, purification and decontamination of water are important preventive measures. Soil protection from contamination with domestic wastes and sewage and timely cleaning of settlements are decisive measures against flies. Almost all intestinal infections can spread by ingestion of food.

METHODS OF EPIDEMIOLOGY

A complex epidemiologic method is used to study the laws of infection spread among population. The method includes epidemiologic observation and experiment. Epidemiologic observation, in turn, includes epidemiologic study of the focus of infection (incidental case) and outbursts; statistic analysis of morbidity; study and description of epidemic process on the whole within a given district or area.

Epidemiologic inspection of an infectious focus is necessary to reveal the source of infection and determine the mechanism of its transmission, to estimate the environmental factors and the living conditions that might promote the spread of the infection.Inspection includes analysis of the incidence of a given infection within its focus (residence, office, children's institution) during 2-3 previous months. In order to reveal the source of infection and the routes of its transmission, the patient and the surrounding people are inquired, and laboratory tests and experiments carried out. In accordance with the findings, concrete measures are taken to prevent further spread of the infection.

An epidemiologic examination of an outburst includes the study of morbidity before the outburst, the dynamics of morbidity during the outburst (by days and longer periods of time), the analysis of morbidity by its main signs, epidemiologic findings in separate foci, clinical course of the disease, the laboratory findings, examination of various objects, isolated strains of the causative agents, materials characterizing the sanitary and technical condition of food catering and other establishments.

This complex examination gives information about the type of infection outburst (water-borne, food infection) and causes of its development, which facilitates conduction of rational measures to eradicate the infection outburst. Analysis of morbidity on the basis of statistic findings is necessary for the study of epidemiology of infectious diseases by some indices during the course of a year, or several years. The infectious process is characterized by numerous indices. The most important of them are distribution of the incidence by age, sex, occupation, season, area, source of infection, lethality, etc.

Statistic data are usually absolute or relative figures, but they can also be presented in the form of tables, graphs, diagrams, and the like. Primary material for a statistic presentation of an epidemic process is the material collected for each particular case of the disease which is entered into a chart of epidemiologic examination.

Statistic analysis gives a summary in absolute indices, which are not, however, convenient for comparison of morbidity in various cities, areas or countries. In order to enable such comparison, absolute figures are converted into mean or relative values. Intensive and extensive indices are usually used in epidemiology.

Intensive Indices

Intensive indices characterize the distribution of a given infection. The coefficients are calculated from proportions reducing absolute figures to one base (1000, 10 000, 1 000000 of population). Intensive indices include morbidity, mortality, and lethality.

Morbidity (incidence or sick rate) is the ratio of the diseased during a given period of time (e. g. a year) to the number of residents of a given city or country during the same period. Morbidity is expressed by the following ratio:

$$\frac{\text{Sick persons}}{\text{Average population}} \times 100000$$

Mortality (death rate) is the number of dead expressed by a coefficient per 100 000 of adult population, and 10 000 of children. The death rate is expressed by the ratio:

$$\frac{\text{Number of dead}}{\text{Average population}} \times 100000$$

Lethality is the percentage of the dead due to the given infection. Lethality index is expressed by the ratio:

$$\frac{\text{Number of dead}}{\text{Number of sick persons}} \times 100$$

Lethality index is used to estimate severity of infection and efficacy of treatment.

Statistic analysis enables their comparison with the previous experience and thus to draw conclusions concerning the increase or reduction of morbidity, efficacy of therapeutic measures, and hence to plan further measures. Description of an epidemic process within a confined area makes it possible to demonstrate the effect of separate elements of social conditions on morbidity.

Experiment includes microbiologic and serologic examinations, entomologic, physical and chemical studies, experiments on humans and animals. Microbiologic and serologic methods are used to study aetiology of infectious diseases, stability of causative agents in environment, inside the macroorganism and resistance to desinfectants; experiment is also used to diagnose infectious disease, to assess treatment efficacy, to reveal acute and chronic carrier state. Microbiologic tests are used to detect pathogenic microbes in food and water.

These tests are also used to locate accurately the source of infection, its transmission routes, time during which a sick person remains dangerous to the surrounding people, and to determine the immunologic structure of population.

Entomologic studies are concerned with ecology of the arthropods, the living carriers of the pathogenic microbes, multiplication of these microbes in the macroorganism in various environmental conditions, and establish the carrier type in a particular disease. Chemical studies of water, food and other objects are necessary to solve disputable questions (e.g. in order to exclude chemical poisoning).

Single and mass-scale experiments can be carried out on animals and people. Experiments on animals are usually used for diagnostic purposes. Besides, they are used to assess harmlessness and efficacy of new vaccines, sera, immunoglobulins and therapeutic preparations. New vaccines, sera, or immunoglobulins can be used in experiments on humans only after they have been tried in laboratory (experiments on animals included).

REFERENCES

Frankish J, Veenstra G, Moulton G. Population health in Canada: Issues and challenges for policy, practice and research. Can J Public Health. 1999;90(1): S71-S75.

Glasgow RE, Vogt TM, Boles SM. Evaluating the public health impact of Health Promotion Interventions: The RE-AIM Framework. Am J Public Health. 1999;89(8): 1322-1327.

Goodman RM. Bridging the gap in effective program implementation: From concept to application. J Community Psychol. 2000;28(3): 309-321.

Gostin LO. Legal and public policy interventions to advance the population's health. In Promoting Health: Intervention strategies from social and behavioural research. BD Smedley & SL Syme (Eds.), National Academy Press, Washington, D.C., 2000, p. 390-416.

Goyer KC, Gow J. Alternatives to current HIV/AIDS policies and practices in South African prinsons. J Public Health Policy. 2002;23(3): 303-323.

Green LW, Richard L, Potvin L. Ecological foundations of health promotion. Am J Health Promot. 1996;10(4): 270-281.

Hancock T, Labonte R, Edwards R. Indicators that count: Measuring population health at the community level. Can J Public Health. 1999;90(1): S22-S26.

Hawe P. Needs assessment must become more change-focused. Aust NZ J of Public Health 1996;20(5): 473-478.

Hawe P, Noort M, King L, Jordens C. Multiplying health gains: The critical role of capacity-building within health promotion programs. Health Policy. 1997;39(1): 29-42.

Hawe P, Shiell A. Social capital and health promotion. Soc Sci Med. 2000;51(6): 871-885.

Health Systems: Improving Performance, WHO, Geneva, especially chapter 2 "How Well do Health Systems Perform" (pages 23-46).

Healthcare Management FORUM, spring. Health Canada (2002), Economic Burden of Illness in Canada, 1998, Minister of Public Works and Government Services Canada.

Integrating Behavioural and Social Sciences with Public Health, Schneiderman N, Speers MA, Silva JM, Tomes H, and Gentry JH (Eds.), p. 141-158.

The International Union for Health Promotion and Education. The Evidence of Health Promotion Effectiveness: Shaping Public Health in a New Europe. A Report for the European Commission. Part One, Core Document. 2nd Ed., Jouve Composition and Impression. Paris. 2000.

6

Epidemiology and Management of Common Communicable Diseases

A communicable disease is a clinically evident disease resulting from the presence of pathogenic microbial agents, including pathogenic viruses, pathogenic bacteria, fungi, protozoa, multicellular parasites, and aberrant proteins known as prions. These pathogens are able to cause disease in animals and/or plants. Infectious pathologies are usually qualified as contagious diseases (also called communicable diseases) due to their potentiality of transmission from one person or species to another. Transmission of an infectious disease may occur through one or more of diverse pathways including physical contact with infected individuals. These infecting agents may also be transmitted through liquids, food, body fluids, contaminated objects, airborne inhalation, or through vector-borne spread.

The term infectivity describes the ability of an organism to enter, survive and multiply in the host, while the infectiousness of a disease indicates the comparative ease with which the disease is transmitted to other hosts. An infection however, is not synonymous with an infectious disease, as an infection may not cause important clinical symptoms or impair host function.

The prevention, management and control of communicable diseases requires the active participation and cooperation of all health-care professionals. While this chapter is intended to act as a guide to the management and control of communicable diseases, professional judgment will still be required by those charged with providing health care services.

CLASSIFICATION

Among the almost infinite varieties of microorganisms, relatively few cause disease in otherwise healthy individuals. Infectious disease results from the interplay between those few pathogens and the defences of the hosts they infect. The appearance and severity of disease resulting from any pathogen depends upon the ability of that pathogen to damage the host as well as the ability of the host to resist the pathogen. Infectious micro organisms, or microbes, are therefore classified as either primary pathogens or as opportunistic pathogens according to the status of host defences.

Primary pathogens cause disease as a result of their presence or activity within the normal, healthy host, and their intrinsic virulence (the severity of the disease they cause) is, in part, a necessary consequence of their need to reproduce and spread. Many of the most common primary pathogens of humans only infect humans, however many serious diseases are caused by organisms acquired from the environment or which infect non-human hosts.

Organisms which cause an infectious disease in a host with depressed resistance are classified as opportunistic pathogens. Opportunistic disease may be caused by microbes that are ordinarily in contact with the host, such as pathogenic bacteria or fungi in the gastrointestinal or the upper respiratory tract, and they may also result from (otherwise innocuous) microbes acquired from other hosts (as in Clostridium difficile colitis) or from the environment as a result of traumatic introduction (as in surgical wound infections or compound fractures).

An opportunistic disease requires impairment of host defences, which may occur as a result of genetic defects (such as Chronic granulomatous disease), exposure to antimicrobial drugs or immunosuppressive chemicals (as might occur following poisoning or cancer chemotherapy), exposure to ionizing radiation, or as a result of an infectious disease with immunosuppressive activity (such as with measles, malaria or HIV disease). Primary pathogens may also cause more severe disease in a host with depressed resistance than would normally occur in an immuno-sufficient host.

SMALL POX

Aetiology: The disease is due to DNA-containing virus belonging to the family of Poxviridae. The virus is highly stable in the environment. In dry pustules and exudates, that contaminate cloths and fomites, it can survive for days and weeks. Moreover, it can remain viable for years in dry pustular crusts. The virus is stable to disinfectants. It can only be killed by an 8 per cent lysol, 3 per cent chloramine, or 2 per cent clarified lime chloride solutions.

Epidemiology. The source of infection is a diseased human. The patient becomes contagious from the very onset of the disease and remains so till the time when crusts fall off (6 weeks). The most dangerous period in this respect is from the 3rd to the 9th day of the disease. Patients with atypical clinical course of the disease (varioloid) are especially dangerous for the surrounding. The virus is dissipated with the respiratory secretions and skin elements.

Clinical picture. Smallpox can be mild, moderate and severe. The course of the disease can be divided into the incubation, initial period, rash, drying and falling off of the crusts and scabs. Moderately severe smallpox has an incubation period of 9-12 days, with extremes of 5-22 days. The initial period is 3-4 days. The disease begins with a shaking chill. The body temperature abruptly rises to 40 and even 41°C by the second day. Pulse and respiration rates are high. The patient develops weakness, nausea, vomiting, pain in the legs and in the lumbar region; sacral pain is also characteristic. Insomnia occurs. Delirium, loss of consciousness and cramping are possible. The face, conjunctiva and mucosa are hyperaemic.

In 2-3 days of the disease, 30-40 per cent of patients develop prodromal or toxic rash. Polymorphous rash (like that in measles or scarlet fever) can be seen mainly on the face and limbs, the lower abdomen and the inner surfaces of the thighs, and also in the region of the chest muscles and the inner surface of the upper shoulder. Rash persists from several hours to 2 days, and then subsides.

On the 3rd or 4th day, the body temperature drops substantially, and the patient feels relieved. During the early eruption period the temperature normalizes. Small pink spots develop on the face, especially on the forehead, the haired part of the head, and the hands. The spots turn copper-red and form papules. During next 2-3 (less frequently 4-5) days, firm papules (nodules the size of a pea) develop on the whole trunk and the mucosa of the soft palate and nasopharynx. Less frequently eruptions develop on the mucosa of the bronchi, conjunctiva, urethra, vagina and the rectum, which causes' severe pain. In 2-3 days the nodules turn into vesicles in the same sequence: face, haired part of the head, the upper extremities, the trunk, and the lower extremities. The vesicles are pale pink, surrounded by red rim; they contain clear fluid.

In 4-5 days the fluid turns cloudy, and by the 6th day (8-9th day of the disease) the vesicles turn into pustules (Plate III). The hyperaemic rim, oedema and infiltration around the pustules increase. Like vesicles, the pustules are multichamber, with a navel-like retraction in the centre. Formation of the pustules also begins with the face. The body temperature rises with purulation to attain 39-40°C and above, and at this level it is maintained for 3-5 days. The general condition of the patient worsens, consciousness is dimmed, pulse accelerates, dysrhythmia develops, arterial pressure drops. Pus and "saliva issue from the mouth; odour is offensive. The face changes beyond recognition: the eyelids are oedematous, the eyes are closed, the nose and the lips are swollen. The patient fails to find a posture in which the tension in the skin can be released. Swallowing is painful, skin is itching.

Diagnosis. The diagnosis is based on clinical, epidemiologic findings, and the results of laboratory studies. Cases suspected for smallpox should be tested in the laboratory because the vaccinated can develop an atypical modified smallpox. The contents of the vesicles, pustules, and also blood, crusts and scabs, can be examined in the laboratory.

Treatment. Treatment should be complex and depend on severity and the period of the disease. Specific therapy of smallpox is unknown. Early injections of immunoglobulin (1 ml/kg) are sometimes effective. Methisazone and other chemical preparations are used for therapeutic and prophylactic purposes. Antibiotics should be given parenterally for suppurative complications.

Toxaemia can be decreased by intravenous infusions of haemodez, rheopolyglucin and polyglucin, a 5 per cent glucose solution, etc. Strophanthine, corglicon, adrenaline, cocarboxylase, and other preparations should be given for cardiovascular insufficiency. Care of the smallpox patient is important. Mattresses should be convenient, inflatable cushions are recommended. Linen and cloths should be renewed frequently. A 5-10 per cent potassium permanganate solution should be used to treat vesicles and pustules. Pruritus can be relieved by applying zinc oxide or menthol ointment; warm baths are recommended.

CHICKEN POX

Aetiology: The viral agent causing this disease belongs to the genus Herpesvirus that also causes herpes zoster. The virus is unstable in the environment.

Epidemiology: The source of infection is the diseased person who becomes contagious 1-2 days before skin eruption develops and remains so 3-4 days after appearance of the last rash element. Patients with herpes zoster can also be the source of infection. Infection is transmitted by air-borne route even during a short exposure in a room where the chickenpox patient is present. Besides, the disease can spread over a significant distance (to a neighbouring room, flat, through corridors). Infants aged from 6 months to 7 years are especially susceptible to chickenpox. Susceptibility is quite high. Life-long immunity is produced in those who sustained the disease. Chickenpox is highly contagious. It occurs in epidemics, especially in large cities and in the cold season.

Pathogenesis: The portal of entry is the mucosa of the upper airways. From the mucosa, the virus enters the blood. In the epidermis the virus evokes a pathologic process with formation of spots, papules, and vesicles.

Clinical picture: The incubation period is 11-21 day, more commonly 14-17 days. The prodromal symptoms are mild, but scarlatina-like rash can develop. The body temperature rises to 38°C and higher (less frequently the temperature is normal); then circumscribed rose spots develop on various parts of the body.

In few hours, the spots turn into papules and then into vesicles filled with clear fluid. The fluid then turns cloudy. A red rim is formed around the vesicles. In 1-2 days after their appearance, the vesicles dry, rupture (or are destroyed by the child), and crusts are formed. New eruption develops within few days, and rash elements in all their stages can therefore be seen simultaneously on the skin of the patient. These eruptions are roseoles, papules, vesicles, and crusts.

Diagnosis: The diagnosis is based on clinical and epidemiologic findings. Whenever necessary, viroscopy, and complement fixation test can be conducted.

Treatment: The patient must keep bed. His skin should be treated with a week potassium permanganate solution after eruption subsides. Baths are also recommended. Patient's nails should be cut and his hands kept clean. Rash elements should be treated with a 5 >per cent potassium permanganate solution or a 1 per cent brilliant green solution. Antibiotics should be given for suppurative complications.

MEASLES

Aetiology: The disease is due to RNA-containing virus Paramyxoviridae. The virus is pathogenic to humans and monkeys. In laboratory the virus is cultivated on human and monkey kidney cells. Attenuated strains of the virus are used as live antimeasles vaccine. The virus is rapidly killed when exposed to high temperature, ultra-violet radiation, or disinfectants. In the environment it is destroyed in 30 minutes.

Epidemiology: The only source of infection is a measles patient, who becomes contagious during the last one or two days of the incubation period, during the catarrhal period, and during 3-5 days following development of rash. In the presence of complications, the period of contagiosity elongates to 10 days from the day when rash develops. The infection is transmitted by air-borne route. The virus can be carried by air to adjacent rooms and flats within a house.

All persons who have not sustained measles or were not vaccinated against measles are susceptible to this disease. Vaccination with live measles vaccine considerably decreases the morbidity. Stable (life-long) immunity develops in those who sustained the disease. Repeated infections are rare. Before active immunization has become common practice, measles epidemic occurred at 2-3 year intervals. Morbidity usually increases in the cold season.

Pathogenesis: The portal of entry is the mucosa of the upper airways, where the virus multiplies in epithelial cells to evoke inflammatory process. The virus then enters the blood to cause toxaemia and to affect various organs and tissues. The virus is contained in droplets of mucus that are dissipated from the upper airways and the nasopharynx during coughing or sneezing. As the titre of antiviral antibodies increases, the virus is eliminated from the patient. Complications are due to weakness of the patient and superimposition of secondary infection.

Clinical picture: The incubation period is usually 9-10 days but can last to 17 days; in the immunized with immunoglobulin, it can be as long as 21 day. The onset of the disease is usually gradual. Symptoms of initial catarrhal or prodromal period develop with elevation of body temperature to 38-39 °C; these are headache, rhinorrhoea, dry barking cough, conjunctivitis, and photophobia. Whitish small papules surrounded by narrow hyperaemic rims (Koplik's spots) appear on the buccal mucosa on the 2nd or 3rd day of the catarrhal period; the spots persist for 2-3 days.

Diagnosis: The diagnosis is based on clinical and epidemiologic findings.

Treatment: In uncomplicated cases, treatment includes preventive and hygienic measures. The room of the patient should be well aired. The patient requires thorough care: he should be given warm baths every other or third day; visible mucosa should be given regular sanitary treatment. The diet should be adequate, easy to assimilate and rich in vitamins; much liquid should be given to drink. Amidopyrin should be given for headache; codeine is helpful in dry cough. If measles is complicated with pneumonia, the patient should be given antibiotics, intravenous infusions of plasma, 20 per cent glucose solution, 10 per cent solution of calcium gluconate, cocarboxylase, corglucon, and ascorbic acid.

INFLUENZA

Aetiology: The disease is caused by the virus belonging to the family Orthomyxoviridae. Three serotypes of the influenza virus are distinguished: A, B, and C. Virus A is of greatest epidemiologic danger. Its antigen structure is constantly changing. Four subtypes of virus A have been established: AO, Al, A2 and A3. Virus B has a more stable antigen structure. Virus C is the most stable influenza virus. Two various antigens are contained in the outer envelope of the influenza virus: haemagglutinin (H) and neuraminidase (N). Haemagglutinin (H) has four independent subtypes: HO, HI, H2 and H3, which relate to viruses AO, Al, A2 and A3, respectively. The other antigen of the influenza virus of the envelope, neuraminidase (N), has two subtypes: Nl (common for viruses AO and Al) and N2 (common for viruses A2 and A3).

Diagnosis: It is not difficult to establish the diagnosis of influenza during an epidemic outbreak. During the interepidemic period, when the course of influenza is mild, it should be differentiated from other acute respiratory viral infections. Influenza is characterized by an acute onset, marked toxaemia, mild catarrhal phenomena, and leucopenia. A final and accurate diagnosis of influenza and other acute viral respiratory infections can be established in the laboratory by serologic, virologic and immunofluorescent methods.

The first specimen of serum is taken not later than on the third day of the disease, the second not earlier than in three weeks. A four-fold increase in the titre is considered as a decisive diagnostic evidence. Serologic reactions are used to confirm the clinical diagnosis. The influenza virus can be isolated from the pharyngeal washings obtained during the first days of the disease or when the disease is in its full swing. The filtrate of the washings is mixed in the laboratory with a 2 per cent suspension of hen or guinea pig erythrocytes. The mixture is kept on ice for 20-30 minutes and the erythrocytes are precipitated by centrifuging.

Treatment: Regardless of severity of the disease, the patient must keep bed until his body temperature normalizes and symptoms of toxaemia subside. Drinking of great amount of hot liquid (tea with lemon, jam or honey; warm milk) is recommended. Polyvitamins should be taken 3 times a day. If the nose is stuffy, a 2 per cent ephedrine (naphthyzine, or sanorine) solution should be instilled into the nose. Codeine, libexin preparations and steam inhalations are useful for cough. Analgin, amidopyrin, ascophen should be given to lessen headache and myalgia. Anti-influenza donor immunoglobulin is an effective specific preparation. It is given in severe forms of influenza, preferably during the first days of the disease. Immunoglobulin should be given to children intramuscularly, 0.15-0.2 ml/kg body weight. Adults should be given 6 ml. Influenza due to virus A should be treated with remantadine, which is effective only during the first 2 days.

Remantadine is given as follows: 2 tablets (100 mg) three times after meals during the first day, 2 tablets 2 times a day during the 2nd and 3rd day, and 2 tablets (by one intake) on the 4th day. Severe forms of influenza should be treated by repeated administrations of anti-influenza immunoglobulin, detoxicating fluids (isotonic sodium chloride solution, haemodez, polyglucin, rheopolyglucin), 800-1000 ml a day, with an obligatory administration of lasix, brinaldix (saluretics), or urea and mannitol. Development of complications is an indication for antibiotic therapy.

RUBELLA

Aetiology: The disease is due to the virus belonging to the family Togaviridae. This RNA-containing virus is cultivated on tissue cultures. It is sensitive to chemicals and is unstable to environmental changes.

Epidemiology: The source of infection is a rubella patient and a virus carrier. The patient is a danger to the surrounding people beginning with the last 1-2 days of the incubation period and remains so till the second week after the onset of the disease. Patients with latent or asymptomatic rubella, and also children with congenital rubella, in whom the virus can live for 18 months and longer, can also be the source of infection. The infection is transmitted by air-borne route. Respiratory Infections 193 Infants aged from 1 to 7 years are mostly affected. The disease also occurs in adults, especially in the pregnant, in whom it is particularly dangerous because the infection can be transmitted to the foetus and become the cause of stillbirth, congenital deafness, microcephaly and other malformations. Stable immunity is produced in those who sustained the disease. Rubella occurs as small epidemics, with the rise in morbidity during the winter and spring. Epidemics occur at 5-7 year intervals.

Diagnosis: The diagnosis is based on clinical, epidemiologic and laboratory findings (blood tests).

Treatment: Treatment is symptomatic. The patient must remain in bed for 2-3 days. If complicated with encephalitis, the disease should be treated with glucocorticosteroids.

PNEUMONIA

Aetiology: Typical pneumonia is usually acquired by bronchogenic spread of the pathogen. The organism may also manifest itself as a suprainfection in patients previously infected by an upper or lower respiratory viral infection. There is no age-specific predisposition, however the incidence of infection increases with advancing age. Most patients are adults above the fifth decade and who have some underlying chronic obstructive pulmonary disease (COPD), cardiovascular or other chronic disease.

Streptococcus pneumoniae is a bacterial pathogen that affects children and adults worldwide. It is a leading cause of illness in young children and causes illness and death among the elderly and persons who have certain underlying medical conditions. Pneumococcal infection causes an estimated 40,000 deaths annually in the United States. Approximately half of these deaths potentially could be prevented through the use of vaccine. Despite appropriate antimicrobial therapy and intensive medical care, the overall case-fatality rate for pneumococcal bacteremia is 15%-20% among adults. The organism colonizes the upper respiratory tract and can cause the following types of illnesses: a) disseminated invasive infections, including bacteremia and meningitis; b) pneumonia and other lower respiratory tract infections; and c) upper respiratory tract infections, including otitis media and sinusitis. Each year in the United States, pneumococcal disease accounts for an estimated 3,000 cases of meningitis, 50,000 cases of bacteremia, 500,000 cases of pneumonia, and 7 million cases of otitis media.

Epidemiology: Pneumonia causing organisms are air-borne and droplet infection from infected persons is responsible for the infection. The germ that causes the pneumonia can spread if the person is still infectious at the time the pneumonia develops. Most of the germs that cause pneumonia spread by direct or close contact with mouth and nose secretions and touching contaminated objects.

Pathogenesis: A microorganism enters the alveoli and proceeds to grow in the rich environment provided by the lung. Oftentimes the organism contains a capsule or is intracellular and can avoid phagocytosis for a period of time. As a result of tissue injury an inflammatory response occurs. Tissue injury can occur due to exotoxins produced by bacteria, cell lysis caused by a virus, or death of alveolar macrophages and dumping of their lysosomal contents in the alveoli due to growth of an organism in the phagocyte. Vascular permeability increases and PMNs arrive at the area attempting to contain and eliminate the organisms. Along with PMNs come many of the serum components. Meanwhile other alveolar macrophages are being recruited to the area of inflammation.

This accumulation of microorganism, immune cells, and serum components causes the alveoli to fill up and can result in spread to other alveoli in close proximity. This inflammatory response is what is described as an opacity or consolidation when viewing a roentgenograph (a X-ray film). Not only are serum components coming into the alveoli but certain products made by the microorganism are able to leave the lung and exert systemic effects. Examples include endotoxin from gram negative bacteria eventually resulting in fever and septic shock, and cell wall components of gram positive bacteria that can eventually lead to fever production and septic shock. All of the microbial products producing or indirectly resulting in systemic changes have yet to be clearly determined.

Diagnosis: The diagnosis of pneumonia is usually made from a medical history, a physical examination, and a chest X-ray. A doctor who suspects pneumonia begins by taking a thorough medical history and performing a physical examination. Bacterial pneumonias often come on suddenly; creating a cough that produces mucous that is often colored or "rusty", fever, and pain along the chest wall. Based on the medical history and physical exam, a doctor may choose to begin treatment right away without doing other tests. The need for more tests often is guided by the severity of symptoms and a person's age and state of health.

In general, the sicker a person is, the more tests may be done. This is particularly true for older adults and infants. Blood tests are generally performed when a pneumonia is suspected: a full blood count often showns neutrophilia (except in some immunocompromised and all neutropenic patients). Renal function may have deteriorated if there is sepsis. Electrolytes can show hyponatremia (low sodium levels); this is often due to secretion of antidiuretic hormone by pulmonary tissue. In nosocomial (hospital-acquired) pneumonia and the pneumonias of the immunocompromised, diagnosis can be difficult, and CT scanning of the lungs can be required to differentiate possible causes (e.g. pulmonary embolism). CT scanning is also used when the symptoms and physical examination point at possible different causes for the complaints (e.g. vasculitis, sarcoidosis, lung cancer).

Treatment: Treatment of pneumonia consists of respiratory support, including O_2 if indicated, and antibiotics, which are selected on the basis of Gram stain results. If Gram stain is not performed or does not establish a diagnosis, antibiotics are selected on the basis of probabilities according to patient age, epidemiology, host risk factors, and severity of illness.

Antibiotics are the main causal therapy for pneumonia. The antibiotics that are used depend on the nature of the pneumonia and the immune status of the patient. Amoxicillin is used as first-line therapy in the vast majority of community patients, sometimes with added clarithromycin. Clarithromycin, azithromycin, and the fluoroquinolones have displaced the penicillin-derived drugs as first line therapy. In hospitalised patients and immune deficient patients, local guidelines generally determine which combination of (generally intravenous) antibiotics is used. When in the hospital, respiratory treatments to remove secretions may be necessary. Occasionally, steroid medications may be used to reduce wheezing if there is an underlying lung disease.

MUMPS

Aetiology: The causative agent of mumps belongs to the family of Paramyxoviridae. Paramyxoviruses are characterized by high contagiosity and low stability in the environment.

Epidemiology: Human beings are the source of infection. The patient is contagious from the last days of the incubation period and remains so for 7-9 days. Patients with an obliterated form of the disease are a special danger. The infection is transmitted mainly by air-borne route. Susceptibility to mumps is high, but lower than in measles, influenza, or chickenpox.

Children aged from 5 to 15 are especially susceptible. Outbreaks of the disease among adults are also possible. Stable immunity is produced in those who sustained the disease. Seasonal variations in the infection rate are characteristic: the morbidity rises in the cold season. Epidemics of mumps occur at 4-5 year intervals.

Pathogenesis: The portal of entry is mucosa of the mouth, nose or pharynx through which the virus enters the blood that carries it to the parotid, submandibular, sublingual and other glands. Besides, it can afflict the sex glands, the pancreas and the central nervous system. The virus is excreted from the body with saliva.

Diagnosis: Typical cases are easy to diagnose. Atypical disease should be differentiated by consideration of epidemiologic anamnestic findings. Serologic tests (complement fixation test, direct haemagglutination reaction) can be used.

Treatment: Treatment is symptomatic. The patient is given liquid or semiliquid food. Dry warmth (cotton wool pad) should be applied over the involved gland. Mouth care is necessary (frequent rinsing with sodium hydrocarbonate solution). Analgin, amidopyrin and other analgesics are useful. Cold is necessary during the first 2-4 days of orchitis; immunoglobulin (9-12 ml) should be prescribed on the 4-5th day. Cerebrospinal puncture and dehydration therapy are indicated for developing symptoms of meningitis or meningoencephalitis.

DIPHTHERIA

Aetiology: This disease is produced by Corynebacterium diphtheriae, non-motile, gram-positive rod with a characteristic swelling at one end. Neisser-stained bacilli viewed microscopically by the fluorescent method demonstrate the presence of volutin grains (Babes-Erns granules) in their ends. The genus Corynebacterium diphtheriae includes toxicogenic (causative agent of diphtheria) and non-toxicogenic corynebacteriae which do not cause diseases with clinical symptoms of diphtheria. By their cultural biochemical and other properties Corynebacteria diphtheriae are classed into mitis, gravis, and intermedins groups.

Epidemiology. The source of infection is a diphtheria patient with clinically manifest symptoms or with an asymptomatic course of the disease, convalescents, and carriers of toxicogenic strains of the bacteria. The infected person can be the source of infection during the last days of the incubation period and remain contagious for the entire duration of the disease. From the epidemiologic standpoint, the greatest danger are patients with mild and obliterated forms of the disease that now prevail and can be mistaken for lacunar or catarrhal tonsillitis, rhinitis, and the like. Eradication of the agent from convalescents usually ends in 15-20 days, less frequently in 1-2 months. Healthy carriers of toxicogenic strains of the bacteria are dangerous because their number is much greater than of diphtheria patients and convalescents. The number of toxicogenic carriers depends on the morbidity; their number is much greater in the foci of diphtheria.

Diagnosis: The diagnosis is based on clinical, epidemiologic and laboratory findings. The bacteriologic method is very important in identification of diphtheria. Sterile cotton tampons are used to take materials from the tonsils and the nasal mucosa (separate tampon for each smear). The material is taken in the morning before meals or at least 2 hours after meals. When taking material for a tonsillar smear, it is necessary that the tampon should not touch the tongue, the buccal mucosa or the teeth. A spatula should therefore be used. In the presence of membranes, the material is taken at the border between the affected and healthy tissues.

Treatment: The main treatment is early administration of antidiphtheritic serum (diphtheria antitoxin). Before administering the serum, the patient should obligatory be tested for sensitivity to foreign protein (intracutaneous test). The dose of the serum depends on the clinical form of the disease, its severity, and duration. The severer the disease and the longer its duration, the greater the dose. The first single dose for faucial diphtheria is 10 000-30 000 U; if the disease is diffuse, 30 000-40 000 U; and if its form is toxic, the dose should be 50000-120000 U. Injections should be repeated at 8-12 hour intervals, and then given every day, until signs of toxaemia disappear and the fauces are cleared of the membranes.

Depending on severity of the disease, the daily dose for laryngeal diphtheria during the first day of the therapy should be from 15 000 to 30 000 U. Administration of the diphtheria antitoxin should be combined with antibiotics: the tetracyclines and erythromycin, in common doses depending on the age of the patient (for seven days). Detoxicating therapy of faucial diphtheria of the first and second degree includes haemodez and rheopolyglucin with a 10 per cent glucose solution (intravenous drip), the injection dose is 20-30 ml/kg. 182 Special Epidemiology Ascorbic acid, cocarboxylase, and insulin should be added to the solution. Diuretics should also be given.

Operative treatment (intubation and tracheostomy) is necessary in croup patients with severe stenosis, if conservative treatment fails (thermal procedures, steam inhalations, oxygen therapy, etc.), and if the second stage transforms into the third stage (asphyxia). Intubation consists in passing a tube into the lumen of the constricted larynx. In this time, diphtheritic croup is rare. After abatement of acute symptoms, patients with mild diphtheria are allowed to leave their beds. Patients with toxic diphtheria should be kept in hospital regardless of the absence or presence of complications. Patients with subtoxic forms and toxaemia of the first degree should remain in bed for at least a month, with toxic diphtheria of the second degree, 40-45 days, and of the third degree, 50-60 days.

Prevention and control: Active immunization is the main prophylactic measure against diphtheria. Epidemiologic efficacy of immunization depends on timely vaccination of the entire children's population. Primary immunization in infants (in the absence of contraindications) should be conducted at the age of 3 months, using adsorbed vaccine (combined vaccine against pertussis, diphtheria, and tetanus).

WHOOPING COUGH

Aetiology: Whooping cough is due to Bordetella pertussis that belongs to haemophilic bacteria. The bacilli are highly pathogenic to humans and unstable in the environment.

Epidemiology: The main source of infection is a pertussis patient which is especially contagious during the initial period of the disease. As the disease progresses, contagiosity decreases, and by the end of the sixth week the patient presents no danger to the surrounding people even in the presence of cough. Antibiotics accelerate elimination of the microbes from the patient. Patients with mild atypical form of whooping cough are an active source of infection spread. Carriers can also be the source of infection. The pathogenic agent is transmitted by air-borne route. Susceptibility to pertussis is high from the very first day of life. Preschool children are usually affected by the disease; only rare cases occur among adult population. Stable life-long immunity is produced in those who sustained the disease. The whooping cough morbidity has substantially decreased since active immunization has been elaborated. Seasonal variations in the infection rate are not typical of this disease.

Pathogenesis: The portal of entry are the upper airways. The pathogenic agent multiplies on the laryngeal, tracheal and bronchial mucosa. The endotoxin irritates the respiratory mucosa thus evoking cough. Besides, it acts directly on the central nervous system, irritates the nerve receptors of the respiratory mucosa and stimulates the cough reflex to provoke paroxysm of cough.

Diagnosis: The diagnosis is based on clinical, epidemiologic, anamnestic, and laboratory findings. It is difficult to differentiate between pertussis and parapertussis only by clinical signs; bacteriologic and serologic studies are therefore diagnostically decisive. Bacteriologic studies are based on isolation of the causative agent from the patient and its identification in the culture. A specimen is taken from the posterior wall of the pharynx by a sterile cotton tampon in patients or suspected persons, and the material is used for immediate inoculation of the culture medium (carbon-caseine). If the material is sent to the laboratory, it should be kept protected from cold. A preliminary answer is ready in 3 days, and the final, in 5 days. Agglutination reaction can be informative during the second or third week of the disease. The test is considered positive with titres of 1: 20 and higher. In view of mass-scale vaccination against whooping cough, the diagnosis is considered trustworthy with progressively increasing antibody titres in repeated examinations. Complement fixation test can be conducted on the second week of the disease. It is positive with titres of 1: 10 and higher. The diagnosis of whooping cough can be confirmed by an accelerated luminescent serologic method that has advantages over isolation of cultures. It is highly sensitive and the result is ready in short time.

Treatment: Bedrest is prescribed only in the presence of severe complications and fever. Fresh air is curative, and the room must therefore be well aired. In the warm season, the child must remain out-of-doors as much as possible; in winter, at least for several hours. It is necessary to organize children's leisure time in order to distract them from coughing. Highly caloric adequate diet rich in vitamins should be given. The child must eat by small portions, better soon after an attack of cough. During the catarrhal period and in the early paroxysmal period, the tetracyclines should be given to infants with a severe disease and in the presence of complications. The doses are 0.025 g/kg a day for 8-10 days. Erythromycin should be given in a dose of 0.005-0.01 g/kg to infants under five, 3-4 times a day for 10 days. Antipertussis immunoglobulin is also given: 3 ml during 3 days in succession, and then every other day several times depending on the patient's condition. Oxygen therapy, vitamins, and neuroplegics (aminazine, propazine, etc.) are widely used since they remove anxiety in children, improve sleep and appetite, and decrease the frequency and severity of paroxysms.

MENINGOCOCCAL INFECTION

Aetiology: The causative organism is Neisseria meningitidis. Several serogroups of meningococci are distinguished by their antigen structure: A, B, C, D, N, X, Y, Z. Particular groups of meningococcus prevails in certain areas. Meningococci are rapidly destroyed in the environment, especially at low temperatures and in the absence of moisture.

Epidemiology: Human beings are the only source of infection. These may be patients with apparent or obliterated forms of meningitis or carriers of the cocci. Patients with meningococcal nasopharyngitis, who dissipate the microbes into the air during sneezing and coughing are a special epidemiologic danger. Patients with meningococcal meningitis and meningococcaemia liberate the pathogenic microbes into the environment during the prodromal period, but the acute symptoms of the disease help early diagnosis and isolation of patients.

The duration of the contagious period depends on the duration of the presence of meningococcus in the nasopharynx. The carrier state in convalescents persists for three weeks. Carriers are less dangerous for the surrounding people than patients, but the number of carriers is much greater, and it is more difficult to reveal them. The carrier state can be sooner terminated by treating with antibiotics and sulpha drugs. Healthy carrier state continues for 2-3 weeks. Longer carrier state (to 6 weeks) occurs in chronic inflammation in the nasopharynx.

Meningococcal infections afflict a comparatively small percentage of population even in intensive epidemic periods (actually not more than 10-15 per cent). The main part of the infected are carriers and patients with acute nasopharyngitis. Generalized forms are rare. In the years of sporadic incidence the microbes live in the carriers whose number is around 1 per cent (from 8 to 12 per cent in the focus). During epidemics, the number of carriers in the focus of infection can exceed 40 per cent. The infection is transmitted by air-borne route during talking, sneezing and coughing. Since the agent is unstable in the environment, the infection is transmitted only during intimate and prolonged contacts of susceptibles with the source of infection. Susceptibility to meningococcus can be considered universal, but the pronounced clinical picture of the disease can be seen only in few of the exposed.

Diagnosis: Meningitis is diagnosed on the basis of clinical and epidemiologic findings. Isolation of meningococcus is diagnostically decisive. The cerebrospinal fluid, blood and mucus (from the nasopharynx) should therefore be examined. The cerebrospinal fluid is taken into two sterile test tubes. The first specimen (1 ml) is sent to the laboratory for liquor test, while the second (2-5 ml) is immediately examined microbiologically. Two or three drops of the cerebrospinal fluid are used to inoculate serum agar (direct inoculation) and for preparing two smears (for bacterioscopy).

The remaining fluid is kept under a layer of semiliquid agar (for enrichment). The blood (5-10 ml) is immediately used to inoculate 50 ml of broth containing 0.1 per cent of glucose. The vial is kept in a thermostat for seven days: serum agar in Petri dishes is inoculated every day. The nasopharyngeal mucus is taken on fast stomach or at least in 3-4 hours after meal from the posterior wall of the nasopharynx using a sterile cotton tampon on a soft wire (2-3 mm in diameter). The root of the tongue is retracted using a spatula.

The mucus is immediately seeded on solid nutrient medium (serum agar or lincomycin medium that inhibits the growth of gram-positive cocci). During transportation to the laboratory, the materials should be protected from cold. Direct haemagglutination reaction, latex test, counter electrophoresis and radioimmune methods are important, since antibodies and the specific antigens can be detected in the blood serum and the cerebrospinal fluid of the patient during the very first days of the disease.

Treatment: Acute nasopharyngitis of moderate severity should be treated with sulpha drugs in a dose of 4-6 g a day for adults and 0.3 g/kg for children in the course of 3-5 days. Prolonged action sulpha drugs (sulphapyridazine or sulphadimethoxin) can be given to adults in a dose of 2 g during the first day and 1 g during subsequent 4 days. Meningitis and meningococcaemia patients are treated with antibiotics. Penicillin should be given in daily doses of 300 000 U/kg for 5-8 days for adults and 300000-400000 U/kg for infants under 3 months of age. The daily dose is given intramuscularly at a 4-hour 208 Special Epidemiology interval maximum, and to infants under 2 months, at 3-hour intervals.

Treatment should be continued for 5-8 days (until the cerebrospinal fluid normalizes). Chloramphenicol sodium succinate given in a dose of 0.05-0.1 g/kg for 6-8 days is highly effective. Ampicillin (0.15-0.2 g/kg a day) and other antibiotics can also be prescribed. Aetiotropic therapy is given simultaneously with pathogenetic treatment which depends on severity of the disease and the presence of complications. Toxaemia can be controlled by administering a sufficient amount of fluid containing the necessary amounts of salts to maintain the electrolyte balance. The liquid can be given per os or intravenously (polyion solutions, glucose, haemodez, plasma). Dehydration is attained by diuretics.

TUBERCULOSIS

Aetiology: Tuberculosis is a common and often deadly infectious disease caused by mycobacteria, mainly Mycobacterium tuberculosis. Tuberculosis usually attacks the lungs (as pulmonary TB) but can also affect the central nervous system, the lymphatic system, the circulatory system, the genitourinary system, the gastrointestinal system, bones, joints, and even the skin. Other mycobacteria such as Mycobacterium bovis, Mycobacterium africanum, Mycobacterium canetti, and Mycobacterium microti also cause tuberculosis, but these species are less common.

Epidemiology: When people suffering from active pulmonary TB cough, sneeze, speak, or spit, they expel infectious aerosol droplets 0.5 to 5 μm in diameter. A single sneeze can release up to 40,000 droplets. Each one of these droplets may transmit the disease, since the infectious dose of tuberculosis is very low and the inhalation of just a single bacterium can cause a new infection.

People with prolonged, frequent, or intense contact are at particularly high risk of becoming infected, with an estimated 22% infection rate. A person with active but untreated tuberculosis can infect 10-15 other people per year. Others at risk include people in areas where TB is common, people who inject drugs using unsanitary needles, residents and employees of high-risk congregate settings, medically under-served and low-income populations, high-risk racial or ethnic minority populations, children exposed to adults in high-risk categories, patients immunocompromised by conditions such as HIV/AIDS, people who take immunosuppressant drugs, and health care workers serving these high-risk clients.

Diagnosis: Tuberculosis is diagnosed definitively by identifying the causative organism (Mycobacterium tuberculosis) in a clinical sample (for example, sputum or pus). When this is not possible, a probable diagnosis may be made using imaging (X-rays or scans) and/or a tuberculin skin test.

The main problem with tuberculosis diagnosis is the difficulty in culturing this slow-growing organism in the laboratory (it may take 4 to 12 weeks for blood or sputum culture). A complete medical evaluation for TB must include a medical history, a physical examination, a chest X-ray, microbiological smears and cultures. It may also include a tuberculin skin test, a serological test. The interpretation of the tuberculin skin test depends upon the person's risk factors for infection and progression to TB disease, such as exposure to other cases of TB or immunosuppression.

Treatment: Treatment for TB uses antibiotics to kill the bacteria. The two antibiotics most commonly used are rifampicin and isoniazid. However, instead of the short course of antibiotics typically used to cure other bacterial infections, TB requires much longer periods of treatment (around 6 to 12 months) to entirely eliminate mycobacteria from the body. Latent TB treatment usually uses a single antibiotic, while active TB disease is best treated with combinations of several antibiotics, to reduce the risk of the bacteria developing antibiotic resistance. People with latent infections are treated to prevent them from progressing to active TB disease later in life. However, treatment using Rifampicin and Pyrazinamide is not risk-free. The Centers for Disease Control and Prevention (CDC) notified healthcare professionals of revised recommendations against the use of rifampin plus pyrazinamide for treatment of latent tuberculosis infection, due to high rates of hospitalization and death from liver injury associated with the combined use of these drugs.

SARS

Aetiology: SARS (Severe acute respiratory syndrome) is a respiratory disease in humans which is caused by the SARS coronavirus (SARS-CoV). There has been one near pandemic to date, between November 2002 and July 2003, with 8,096 known infected cases and 774 deaths (a case-fatality rate of 9.6%) worldwide being listed in the World Health Organization's (WHO) 21 April 2004 concluding report. Within a matter of weeks in early 2003, SARS spread from the Guangdong province of China to rapidly infect individuals in some 37 countries around the world.

Epidemiology: The primary way that SARS appears to spread is by close person-to-person contact. SARS-CoV is thought to be transmitted most readily by respiratory droplets (droplet spread) produced when an infected person coughs or sneezes. Droplet spread can happen when droplets from the cough or sneeze of an infected person are propelled a short distance (generally up to 3 feet) through the air and deposited on the mucous membranes of the mouth, nose, or eyes of persons who are nearby.

The virus also can spread when a person touches a surface or object contaminated with infectious droplets and then touches his or her mouth, nose, or eye(s). In addition, it is possible that SARS-CoV might be spread more broadly through the air (airborne spread) or by other ways that are not now known.

Pathogenesis: Available information suggests that persons with SARS are most likely to be contagious only when they have symptoms, such as fever or cough. Patients are most contagious during the second week of illness. However, as a precaution against spreading the disease, CDC recommends that persons with SARS limit their interactions outside the home (for example, by not going to work or to school) until 10 days after their fever has gone away and their respiratory (breathing) symptoms have gotten better.

Diagnosis: The chest X-ray (CXR) appearance of SARS is variable. There is no pathognomonic appearance of SARS but is commonly felt to be abnormal with patchy infiltrates in any part of the lungs. The initial CXR may be clear. White blood cell and platelet counts are often high. Early reports indicated a tendency to relative neutrophilia and a relative lymphopenia - relative because the total number of white blood cells tends to be low. Other laboratory tests suggest raised lactate dehydrogenase and slightly raised creatine kinase and C-Reactive protein levels.

With the identification and sequencing of the RNA of the coronavirus responsible for SARS in 2008, several diagnostic test kits have been produced and are now being tested for their suitability for use. Three possible diagnostic tests have emerged, each with drawbacks. The first, an ELISA (enzyme-linked immunosorbent assay) test detects antibodies to SARS reliably but only 21 days after the onset of symptoms. The second, an immunofluorescence assay, can detect antibodies 10 days after the onset of the disease but is a labour and time intensive test, requiring an immunofluorescence microscope and an experienced operator. The last test is a polymerase chain reaction (PCR) test that can detect genetic material of the SARS virus in specimens ranging from blood, sputum, tissue samples and stools. The PCR tests so far have proven to be very specific but not very sensitive. This means that while a positive PCR test result is strongly indicative that the patient is infected with SARS, a negative test result does not mean that the patient does not have SARS.

Prevention and control: Infection control precautions should be continued for SARS patients for 10 days after respiratory symptoms and fever are gone. SARS patients should limit interactions outside the home and should not go to work, school, out-of-home day care, or other public areas during the 10-day period.

During this 10-day period, all members of the household with a SARS patient should carefully follow recommendations for hand hygiene, such as frequent hand washing or the use of alcohol-based hand rubs.

Each patient with SARS should cover his or her mouth and nose with a tissue before sneezing or coughing. If possible, a person recovering from SARS should wear a surgical mask during close contact with uninfected persons. If the patient is unable to wear a surgical mask, other people in the home should wear one when in close contact with the patient.

Disposable gloves should be considered for any contact with body fluids from a SARS patient. However, immediately after activities involving contact with body fluids, gloves should be removed and discarded, and hands should be washed. Gloves should not be washed or reused, and are not intended to replace proper hand hygiene.

SARS patients should avoid sharing eating utensils, towels, and bedding with other members of the household, although these items can be used by others after routine cleaning, such as washing or laundering with soap and hot water.

Common household cleaners are sufficient for disinfecting toilets, sinks, and other surfaces touched by patients with SARS, but the cleaners must be used frequently.

Other members of the household need not restrict their outside activities unless they develop symptoms of SARS, such as a fever or respiratory illness.

INTESTINAL INFECTIONS

POLIO

Aetiology: Poliomyelitis (Gr. polios gray and myelos marrow) is caused by a virus belonging to the family of Picornaviridae, the genus Enterovirus; coxsackievirus and echovirus also belong to this group. Three separate serotypes of the poliovirus are distinguished: I, II, and III. The poliovirus is sufficiently stable in the environment: it withstands absence of moisture and cold; in water it can survive for 100 days and in milk to three months; in faeces it remains viable for 6 months; the virus is sensitive to disinfectants. The virus is also pathogenic for monkeys. Albino mice and cotton rats are sensitive to some strains of type I virus.

Epidemiology: Humans are the source of poliovirus; these can be patients with manifest clinical symptoms and also persons with asymptomatic forms of the disease. According to some authors, the ratio of clinically manifest cases to asymptomatic cases can (before prophylactic vaccination) be from 1: 100 to 1: 1000. Patients in the acute period of the disease are of greatest danger for the surrounding people.

The virus is eradicated from the convalescent in 15-20 days after recovery. This period is sometimes longer: 30-40 days or even 4-5 months. The infection is transmitted by the faecal-oral route. Infected dishes, toys and other objects in common use are the transmitting factors. The causative agent can be transmitted with food (milk, etc.), thus accounting for the epidemic spread of the disease. Water-borne epidemics have also been reported. Poliomyelitis can be transmitted by droplets borne in air. Children aged under 5-7 years are mostly susceptible to the infection. Older children and adults are less susceptible, which is explained by the fact that they might have already sustained this disease (or carrier state) in an abortive form.

Pathogenesis: The portal of infection is the mucosa of the mouth, alimentary tract and the upper airways. From mucosa the virus passes to the regional lymph nodes where it multiplies and is carried with the lymph to the blood to cause virusaemia. Blood carries the virus to the cells of cornua of the spinal cord. The cervical and the sacrolumbar enlargements are mostly involved. About one fourth or third of the nerve cells in the enlargements are destroyed to cause paresis. A complete paralysis occurs in cases where three thirds of the cells die. The virus also damages the cells of the macrophagic system, respiratory mucosa, lung, gastrointestinal tract, etc.

Treatment: Specific therapy of poliomyelitis is unknown. Immunoglobulin (0.3-0.5 ml per kg body weight) is given intramuscularly during the preparalytic period. In order to lessen oedema of the brain and its meninges, 20-40 ml of a 40 per cent glucose solution are given intravenously. Vitamins (vitamin C, B, B12) should be given. Anaesthetic and amino acids are also used. An apparatus for artificial respiration should be used in patients with respiratory failure. The patient must remain in bed for 2-3 weeks. When paralysis develops, it is necessary to see that the paralyzed extremities are in normal position; this helps prevent deformation, contractures, etc. Medical exercises, massage, physio- and stimulation therapy are prescribed in the restorative period. The orthopaedist should observe the patient. Sanatorial treatment is recommended in the stage of residual phenomena.

VIRAL HEPATITIS

Several forms of hepatitis are designated by the collective term 'viral hepatitis'. The main forms are viral hepatitis A and hepatitis B. A group of viral hepatitides that are clinically similar to hepatitis A and B have been recently separated and given a conventional name of non-A, non-B hepatitis. The epidemic characteristics of non-A, non-B hepatitis are similar to those of hepatitis B.

Aetiology: Hepatitis A virus (HAV) contains RNA and is similar to enterovirus by its physicochemical properties. It is completely destroyed at a temperature of 100 °C for 5 minutes; it is also sensitive to U-V radiation. Hepatitis B virus (HBV) contains two-spiral DNA. In addition to Dane particles (mature viral particles), the blood serum of a hepatitis patient contains also other viral particles: small oval (or spherical) and tubular (subviral) forms that are the main antigen carriers.

Three antigens are distinguished: surface antigen HBsAg (it is also known as Australia antigen); it appears in liver cells, biological fluids, in the faeces of hepatitis patients and HBV carriers in 2-6 weeks following the infection, and persists over the entire period of the disease or the carrier state); antigen E, designated HBeAg (it is present not only in the Dane particle but is also found to circulate in the blood; in the free form or bound with immunoglobulin; persistence of HBeAg over 3 weeks indicated transition of the disease into its chronic form (infectivity antigen); and antigen C, or core antigen, designated HBeAg; it is contained inside Dane particles.

Pathogenesis: As virus A is ingested, it multiplies in the gastrointestinal mucosa and then in the regional lymph nodes (incubation period). During the pre-icteric period, the virus invades the blood (virusaemia), and is carried to the parenchymatous organs, mainly to the liver, where it multiplies in the macrophage and liver cells to destroy them. Growing immunity promotes eradication of the virus from the patient by the end of the second or third week of the icteric period. Transition of the disease into its chronic and protracted form is more frequent in hepatitis B than hepatitis A.

When infection is transmitted parenterally, virus B gets into the blood and is rapidly eradicated from the body (short-lasting virus carrier state), provided immunity is sufficiently active. If the virus is retained in the body, it is carried to the liver and other organs. Ingress of the virus into the macrophage and liver cells evokes the cytolysis, cholestasis and mesenchymal inflammatory syndromes.

The virus alters the antigen composition of the hepatocyte plasma membranes, arouses the immune response to the hepatocytes containing the virus, and causes their subsequent cytolysis. Secondary and subsequent invasions of the virus in the blood accounts for the unduiant course of the disease, its exacerbations, and transition into the chronic form. Increasing specific immunity eradicates the virus from the patient. The cholestatic syndrome is associated with disturbed liver architecture, upset production of bile and its excretion.

Intralobular cholestasis, dilatation of the bile capillaries with cholestasis and formation of thrombi dominate other disorders. Gall pigments and acids are carried with blood to account for the yellow colour of the skin and mucosa, and, in some cases, itching. Hyperbilirubinaemia, choiuria, hypercholesterolaemia and increased transaminase activity in the blood are noted. The mesenchymal inflammatory syndrome is manifested by infiltration of and damage to the stroma and cells of the macrophagic system, their proliferation, hypoproteinaemia, low albumin and high globulin levels.

Treatment: Specific therapy is unknown. Mild viral hepatitides in their acute phase should be treated by adequate regimen, diet, and sparing conditions for the liver. During the first 7-10 days of clinical jaundice, the patient must remain in bed but later he can occasionally leave his bed. The diet should be sparing but adequate. The daily ration must include at least 100 g of protein, to 30-40 g of butter, and carbohydrates. Fried, smoked or pickled food, and also alcohol should be excluded.

Food must be rich in vitamins. Taking much liquid (2-3 litres a day) as stewed fruits, tea with lemon, fruit juices, and the like, is recommended. Daily evacuation of the bowels is necessary. Patients with moderate disease attended with signs of toxaemia, who are unable to drink great quantity of liquid because of nausea, should be given detoxicating therapy. A 5-10 per cent glucose solution, Ringer-Locke solution (250-500 ml each) with an addition of 10 ml of a 5 per cent ascorbic acid solution should be given by drip infusion. Nicotinic acid (60 mg), thiamine (6 mg), riboflavin and pyridoxine should also be given. If necessary, haemodez or rheopolyglucin (200-400 ml), plasma (100-150 ml) or the like should be administered.

CHOLERA

Aetiology: The disease is caused by Vibrio cholerae. The bacillus has a single polar flagellum due to which it becomes motile. The vibrio is divided into two subspecies: the classic one and El Tor vibrio. Each biotype is in turn subdivided into three serotypes: Inaba, Ogawa and Hikojema. Non-agglutinating (NAG) vibrios, that can produce cholera-like diseases, are sometimes isolated from water and humans. Cholera vibrio is sufficiently stable in the environment.

It can survive for 150 days in faeces in the absence of light, for 60 days in soil, for several days in milk, for 20-30 days in butter, and from 3 to 10 days on fruits and vegetables. Cholera vibrio withstands low temperature. Under equal conditions, El Tor vibrio survives in the environment longer than the classic biotype. Vibrios are sensitive to the absence of moisture; they are killed immediately on boiling. Even weak hydrochloric and sulphuric acids (1: 10000) kill them in few seconds.

Epidemiology: The only source of infection is a diseased human or a carrier. Humans with the disease in full swing are especially dangerous for the surrounding: they liberate from 7 to 30 litres of liquid daily with stools and voinitus that contain large amounts of the vibrio. The degree of danger depends on the clinical form of cholera. If the disease runs a severe course, the patient attends for medical aid immediately and the spread of the infection is usually confined to a family.

Patients with atypical and obliterated course are a great danger. They continue performing their routine duties and diffuse the infection among their coworkers and mates thus promoting the infection spread over a large area. Convalescents, chronic and healthy carriers can also be the source of infection. Convalescents usually stop being carriers during the first 1-2 weeks after recovery; healthy carriers, in few days. Chronic carrier state is rare in cholera; the state persists from several months to years. Especially it concerns El Tor cholera. It can also run an asymptomatic course; healthy carrier state is possible too. Like other intestinal infections, cholera is mainly transmitted by the faecal-oral mechanism. The vibrios are ingested with infected food or water. Infection is also possible through direct contact with the patient: the vibrios are then carried into the mouth with soiled hands.

Pathogenesis: The microorganisms are ingested. Since the cholera vibrio is highly sensitive to dilute hydrochloric acid, it can survive only in an empty stomach in the absence of gastric secretion, inside a food lump, or when ingested with ample water, or else if gastric secretion is inhibited. The vibrio multiplies in an alkaline medium intensively, mainly on the surface of the intestinal mucosa and in the intestinal lumen. As die vibrio multiplies, its great quantities are accumulated and a great amount of cholera toxins (endo- and exotoxins) is found inside the small intestine.

The clinical symptoms of cholera develop due to the general effect of the cholera toxins. The symptoms depend on the lesion of the central and vegetative nervous system, gastrointestinal tract, and the parenchymal organs (kidneys, adrenal glands, liver, etc.). Due to the effect of exotoxin (choleragen), large amounts of water and electrolyte, especially of sodium and potassium chlorides are released through the membranes of epithelial cells of the small intestine. Water is not absorbed in the large intestine and excess liquid in the intestine stimulates peristalsis to cause profuse diarrhoea, which is attended by vomiting. In severe cases (dehydration of degrees III and IV), a considerable amount of liquid and salts is lost.

As a result, exsiccosis develops along with salt depletion. Blood thickens, the activity of the cardiovascular system becomes deranged, hypothermia develops (the body temperature drops below 36°C); the condition is also attended by acidosis, hypoxaemia and deranged gas metabolism (to asphyxia). The liver function is also upset: the mucosa and the skin become icteric; renal function is deranged with subsequent development of oliguria and possibly anuria. Acidosis and saline depletion cause muscular cramps.

Treatment: Treatment depends on the pathogenesis of the disease and includes restoration of the lost fluid and electrolyte. Patients with a severe form of cholera are examined for determination of heart and respiration rate, arterial pressure, body weight, body temperature, and also the physicochemical indices (plasma density, concentration of electrolytes in the plasma and in the red blood cells, degree of acidosis, and the haematocrit). This done, treatment can begin. To replenish the lost water and electrolyte, polyion solutions (sterilized and warmed to a temperature of 38-40°C) are usually infused intravenously at a rate of 40-48 ml per minute in the II degree dehydration, and 80-120 ml per minute for III and IV degrees of dehydration.

After administration of 2-4 litres of solution, the rate of subsequent infusion should be gradually slowed to 10 ml/min. The volumes of stools and vomitus are measured at 4-hour interval; the physicochemical properties of blood are also determined. After termination of vomiting and recovery of the patient from the dehydration state (III and IV degree), the polyion solution should be continued per os. Depending on the amount of lost liquid, 120-200 ml/kg (to 1000 ml/h) should be given during the first 6-8 hours and then the intake should be decreased to 15 ml/kg per hour until diarrhoea has stopped. Patients with I degree dehydration and also patients with II degree dehydration (depending on their condition) can be given the polyion solutions per os from the very beginning of rehydration therapy (primary rehydration).

After vomiting discontinues, tetracycline (0.3 g 4 times a day for 5 days) should be given per os; the preparation shortens the duration of diarrhoea and eradicates the pathogenic microorganisms from the patient. The diet should be sparing during the first days of the disease, but beginning with the 3-5th day, dietary restrictions are unnecessary. The patient should be given a thorough care. Hot water bottles should be placed to keep him warm. The ambient temperature in the room must be adequate. Rehydration should be performed in an intensive care unit or in a special ward provided with the necessary equipment: a special bed with an aperture to collect faeces, volumetric receptacles for excrements, etc.

The patient should be discharged from hospital after clinical recovery (usually in 10-11 days) and three negative bacteriologic tests that are carried out not earlier than in 24-36 hours after suspension of antibiotics. The tests should be performed during three successive days. The duodenal contents should be examined only once. Faeces should be collected after administration of a laxative salt. Vibrio carriers are given tetracycline for 3-5 days. If the vibrio is detected repeatedly, chloramphenicol should be given.

DYSENTERY

Aetiology: The disease is due to Enterobacteriaceae, the genus Shigella, that includes more than 100 types. According to the international classification, 4 groups of shigellae are distinguished: A, B, C and D. Group A includes 10 serotypes of Shigella dysenteriae among which are S. shigae, S. schmitzii; group B includes S. flexneri (6 serotypes); group C includes S. boydii (15 serotypes); group D includes S. sonnet Shigellae are released from the patient or carrier with the excrements. The microorganisms can survive in soil for 3 months, on soiled utensils, dishes, moist linen for weeks or even months, for several days on food (bread, meat); in milk they persist for 30 days and longer; in running water they can survive from several hours to 5-9 days.

Epidemiology: The source of infection are humans, either patients with acute or chronic dysentery, or carriers. The patient is contagious from the very first day of the disease till complete recovery. Patients with mild forms of the disease are especially dangerous because they often remain out of hospital. Clinical recovery of patients does not always coincide in time with bacteriologic convalescence. If a convalescent carrier continues excreting shigellae for more than 3' months, he (or she) is considered a chronic carrier (for 2 years).

Chronic dysentery patients are the habitat for the pathogenic microorganisms and they excrete them (either constantly or periodically) into the environment. Like other intestinal infections, dysentery is transmitted by the faecal-oral route. The main transmitting factors are food, water, soiled hands, linen, toys, dishes and the like articles. Depending on the transmitting factor, the conditions for infection spread are different. The number of infected people is the decisive factor.

Food that is not cooked before eating (milk and dairy products, salads, stewed fruits, berries, etc.), in which the bacteria multiply and accumulate, is an important factor in dysentery due to S. sonnei. Ingestion of infected food is often responsible for group morbidity. Outbreaks of food-borne dysentery can be due to negligence of sanitary and technical requirements in food and milk industries, at food catering and similar establishments. If the shigellae multiply and accumulate in food, food-borne epidemic toxicoinfections occur. This is especially characteristic of dysentery due to S. sonnei. Food-borne outbreaks can occur during the whole year but their incidence is more common in the warm season.

Water-borne dysentery is explained by the fact that water is easily contaminated with the microorganisms that persist in it for long periods of time. Water in open bodies is polluted by surface effluents (run-off), untreated sewage, faecal sewage included (ship sewage), by leakage of faecal sewage into the open water bodies from lavatories and other sites of refuse accumulation. Tap water can be contaminated during breakdown in the sewage system, through maintenance wells, etc. The character of morbidity with water-borne infection can be different.

Diagnosis: The diagnosis is based on the clinical, epidemiologic, instrumental and laboratory findings. Whether or not a particular patient should be taken to hospital should be decided on the basis of the clinical and epidemiologic picture. If any diagnostic doubt arises, the patient must be examined in the diagnostic department of the hospital. The epidemiologic anamnesis helps reveal contacts with the diseased or persons suspected for dysentery, carriers in the family, house, or at a children's institution. Laboratory diagnosis includes bacteriologic, serologic and immunofluorescence studies. Freshly taken mucus, pus and other pathological admixtures (not blood) obtained by natural defaecation or by tampons are used for cultures.

Best results are obtained with cultures of fresh excrements taken directly at patient's bedside. If this is infeasible, the material is placed in a sterile tube containing a preservative (glycerol mixture, or the like) and delivered to the bacteriologic laboratory not later than in 2 hours. If the material cannot be delivered to the laboratory within this time, the test tube should be kept in a refrigerator (not longer than 12 hours). Cultures are more informative if the material is taken during the early stage of the disease, before treatment is started. A preliminary result is ready in two days, while the final result, in 4 days. Indirect haemagglutination reaction is additionally performed using an erythrocytic dysentery diagnosticum beginning with the 5th day of the disease. The minimum diagnostic titre of indirect haemagglutination test is 1: 160. The immunofluorescent technique is used for rapid diagnosis. The diagnosis can also be established rapidly by adding a suspension of native faeces to a mixture of carbon and serum containing shigella antibodies. If the test is positive, large dark flakes precipitate in few minutes (agglomeration). The test is performed on glass.

Coprologic analysis (microscopy of the patient's faeces aimed to detect the pathologic admixtures such as mucus, leucocytes, or erythrocytes) is used as an additional diagnostic method. Another additional method is rectoromanoscopy by which the mucosa of the large intestine can be observed to a distance of 25-30 cm from the anus. This method helps follow the changes in the pathology inside the intestine. Rectoromanoscopy is contraindicated to pregnant, infants under 1 year, and in the presence of acute processes in the intestine.

Treatment: This should be complex and begin as early as possible. Patients with mild and moderate forms of dysentery attended by marked symptoms of colitis should be treated with nitrofurans (furazolidone, furazolin, etc.), 0.1-0.15 g 4 times a day after meals for 3-5 days. Derivative of 8-oxyquinoline can be given: mexase, mexaform, 2 tablets 4 times a day after meals for 3-5 days. Nitrofurans and 8-oxyquinolines act aetiotropically on shigellae and do not kill the normal intestinal flora.

Aged patients with moderate shigellosis superimposed upon other diseases, and also patients with severe forms of shigellosis should be treated with antibiotics: ampicillin 0.5 g 4 times a day after meals for 2-3 days. If this treatment fails, neomycin sulphate should be given in 0.1-0.2 g doses 2-4 times a day, or kanamycin 0.5 g 4 times a day for 3-5 days. Prolonged-action sulpha drugs can also be given: sulphadimethoxine, sulphapyridazine, phthazin. Sulphadimethoxine should be given per os: 2 g in a single dose on the first day, and then 1 g a day for the following two days; colibacterin, lactobacterin, bificol, bifidumbacterin should be given 5-6 times a day for 3-4 weeks to prevent intestinal disbacteriosis. If toxaemia is marked and the signs of dehydration are obvious, isotonic salt solutions should be given intravenously (1-2 litres). If the disease is severe (in the absence of dehydration), colloid solutions are also indicated: haemodez, rheopolyglucin, or polyglucin to 400- 800 ml a day. In addition to vitamin C (500-600 mg/day), nicotinic acid (40-60 mg/day), thiamine and riboflavin (9 mg/day) are also prescribed. Symptoms of cardiovascular pathology and collapse should be managed with subcutaneous injection of cordiamine, caffeine, etc.

TYPHOID FEVER

Aetiology: Typhoid fever is caused by Enterobacteriaceae, genus Salmonella. The microorganism is motile, it is pathogenic only toward man. It is stable in the environment: in running water it persists for 5-10 days and in stagnant water for a few months. It can survive over winter in ice. In fruits and vegetables it lives for 5-10 days, in other foods from 2 to 8 weeks. On some objects of the environment it persists from several hours to a month and even longer. When dried in direct sun rays the pathogenic microorganism is rapidly destroyed. Boiling kills it instantaneously. A 3 per cent solution of lysol and a 3 per cent chloramine solution kill the bacteria within 2-3 minutes.

Epidemiology: The source of infection is a typhoid patient or a carrier. Patients with mild or abortive forms of the disease are especially dangerous because they often continue performing their routine duties and thus promote the infection spread. Patients with typhoid fever are contagious for the surrounding people beginning with the first week of the disease, but they are the greatest danger during the second and third week of the disease, when the maximum amount of pathogenic microorganisms are excreted with the urine and stools. Chronic carrier state is a chronic form of typhoid infection. The microorganism persists in the cells of the macrophague system in the L form.

Under certain conditions, it can be reactivated into the initial pathogenic form and cause bacteraemia with development of secondary foci in the absence of clinical symptoms. Beginning with the first week of the disease, specific immunity develops in most patients. It helps the patient to free from the pathogenic microorganisms and to terminate toxaemia. The leading role in the spread of infection belongs to chronic carriers, especially if they are engaged occupationally in handling of food that is not cooked before use. Chronic carriers are dangerous not only as the source of infection, which cause disease in other persons and epidemic outbreaks, but also as depots of typhoid infection. The epidemiologic importance of healthy (transitory) carriers, compared with chronic carriers, is not great because they release the microbes only for a short period of time and in small amount.

Pathogenesis: The pathogenic microorganisms enter a human through the mouth. If the defensive function of the stomach is adequate, the microorganism is killed in the stomach and the person does not develop the disease. If the defense function is impaired and the number of microorganisms that enter the stomach is great, they can reach the lower portions of the small intestine where they get into the aggregations of lymphatic follicles (Peyer's plaques) and solitary follicles, and into the nearest mesenteric lymph nodes, where they multiply.

At the end of the incubation period, the pathogenic microorganisms are released from the mesenteric nodes into the blood to cause bacteraemia.

The pathogenic microorganisms are thus carried throughout the entire body and precipitate in the spleen, bone marrow, lymph nodes and the liver. As the microbes die, they release endotoxin that poisons the human body. The endotoxin acts on the central nervous system to induce status typhosus, which is characterized by dimmed consciousness, inhibition, sleepiness alternated by insomnia, headache. The rate of bacteria removal from the patient depends largely on the function of the excretory organs and systems (the liver, the intestinal glands, the intestine, the kidneys) and formation of specific antibodies.

From the liver, the microbes are released with bile into the intestine and are partly excreted from the patient. The remaining microbes precipitate in aggregated and single lymphatic follicles, primarily sensitized by the microbes, in the lower portion of the small intestine. The re-entrance of the microbes into the presensitized aggregated and solitary lymphatic follicles causes an allergic inflammation with ulceration and necrosis of tissues (Plate I). Involvement of the sympathetic nervous system induces meteorism (inflation of the intestine), diarrhoea, bradycardia, and hypotension. Endotoxin affects also bone marrow and induces leucopenia.

Diagnosis: The diagnosis of typhoid fever is based on the clinical picture of the disease, epidemiologic anamnesis, and the laboratory findings. The main method of laboratory diagnosis is bacteriologic study. The blood, urine, faeces and bile (duodenal contents) are examined in the laboratory.

The blood culture method is rapid and accurate for early diagnosis. A sterile syringe is used to take 10-15 ml of blood from the patient's ulnar vein. The blood specimen is placed into a vial containing Rappoport medium or 10-20 per cent bile culture medium (1: 10). The flask is kept in a thermostat at 37°C and then Endo agar and Ploskirev medium are inoculated in 1, 2 and 7 days. Blood cultures are mostly positive during the first days of the disease, before antibiotic therapy is started. The immunofluorescence method is also used for early diagnosis of typhoid fever. It reveals the typhoid bacillus in 10-12 hours after inoculation, but this does not exclude confirmation of the diagnosis by the classical blood culture method. Stool and urine cultures are less important because they are positive only beginning with the second week of the disease. Cultures are inoculated from the first day of the disease. In order to take a specimen of faeces, a disinfected pan is used; 3-5 g specimen is transferred into a test tube containing a 30 per cent glycerol mixture.

The test tube is handled to the laboratory where the taken material is used to inoculate Endo or Ploskirev medium and an enriched culture medium. A urine specimen shtmld be better taken by a sterile catheter. If a catheter is not available, the outer orifice of the urethra should be washed with an isotonic sodium chloride solution, the first portion of the urine discarded, and then a 20-50 ml specimen taken into a sterile flask. In the laboratory, the urine is centrifuged or settled, and the sediment is used to inoculate the medium. In order to reveal carriers, the duodenal contents should be examined not earlier than 5-10 days following the fall of temperature. Bile is taken from a fasting patient using a duodenal tube. A, B and C biles are taken in separate sterile test tubes. Serologic studies are used to confirm the diagnosis.

Widal's test is used along with passive (indirect) haemagglutination test with erythrocytic diagnosticum (O, H and Vi antigens). Widal's test is performed with 2-3 ml of blood taken from the ulnar vein of the patient on the 8-9th day of the disease. Indirect haemagglutination reactions with H, O and Vi antigens are more specific than the Widal reaction, and they are used to reveal antibodies from the 4th or 6th day of the disease. The reaction is positive with the titre of 1: 200 and over. In order to differentiate acute carriers from chronic ones, and also vaccinated persons from carriers, indirect haemagglutination tests with cysteine are used. Of the known immunoglobulins of five classes (IgA, IgM, IgG, IgD and IgE), immunoglobulins IgG (cysteine-resistant antibodies), which are not destroyed by cysteine, are of greatest diagnostic importance.

Treatment: Chloramphenicol is used to treat typhoid fever. It is given in doses from 0.5 to 0.75 g four times a day until the body temperature normalizes, and then for another 8-10 days (0.5 g three times a day). Chloramphenicol is given per os, 20-30 minutes before meals. If vomiting develops, chloramphenicol sodium succinate should be given intramuscularly or intravenously, 1.0 g three times a day. Ampicillin in doses of 1 g four times a day (for 14 days) is also effective. Bactrim (biseptol), 2-3 tablets two times a day (for 3-4 weeks), or nitrofurane preparations in doses of 0.15-0.2 g four times a day are given to patients with antibiotic-resistant bacilli. Antibiotics combined with vaccines decrease the incidence of relapses and prevent carrier state.

Treatment with Vi antigen is more effective. It is given subcutaneously twice in 1 g doses at 8-10 day interval during any stage of the disease. In order to lessen toxaemia in severe course of the disease, a 5 per cent glucose solution (500-800 ml) is given by intravenous drip or haemodez (400 ml) in combination with cocarboxylase and ascorbic acid. Furosemide is given per os, 0.04 g in the morning, for 1-2 days; vitamins BBu B6B, B12 and rutin are also given. Cardiovascular preparations are given in cases of medium severity. An immediate surgical operation is necessary in intestinal perforation. Patients with intestinal haemorrhage must remain in bed, and an ice bag should be placed on the abdomen. Blood of the appropriate group should be transfused in haemostatic doses (75-100 ml). Vikasol should be given in a dose of 0.01 g twice a day. A 10 per cent solution of calcium chloride should be given intravenously in a dose of 5-10 ml. In profuse bleeding, 1-2 litres of blood, polyionic and colloid solutions (polyglucin, gelatinol) should be transfused.

During the first 10-12 hours the patient is allowed only to drink tea or water. Thin (5 per cent) milk semolina and fruit jellies can be given later until stools normalize. Patients must remain in bed regardless of severity of the disease. The patient is allowed to assume a sitting position only in 7 or 8 days after normalization of body temperature. The patient is allowed to leave the bed and walk only in 10-11 days (provided there are no contraindications). In 21 day after normalization of body temperature the patient can be discharged from hospital, provided his condition permits. If the patient did not receive antibiotics, he can be discharged from hospital in 14 days after normalization of temperature. Care of typhoid patients is important. Sanitation of the mouth, ears, nose and skin is of great significance.

If the disease runs a severe course, the patient's tongue should be treated with a piece of gauze wetted with a 2 per cent boric acid solution; dry lips can be treated with vaseline oil. In order to prevent congestion in the lungs and bedsores, a critical patient should be helped to turn from one side to another. Cleansing enema is necessary in constipation. If the abdomen is inflated, a tube should be passed into the intestine to release gases. Careful attitude to the patient and his complaints, control of his pulse, etc. help timely reveal possible complications. Food must be easily assimilable, rich in vitamins and caloric. It is recommended that food should be cooked by steam and contain no solid ingredients (thin porridges, broth, minced meat, omelette, puree, fresh fruits, rubbed through a sieve, and juice. Food that might evoke meteorism should be avoided.

BOTULISM

Aetiology: Botulism (from Latin botulus sausage) is caused by spore-forming Clostridia (Clostridium botulinum). Seven serologic types of these motile anaerobes are distinguished by the structure of the antigen and exotoxin: A, B, C, D, E, F, and G types. Types A, B and E are commonly found in soil; these are responsible for the onset of botulism in humans. Clostridial spores withstand boiling for 5-6 hours; if treated in an autoclave, the Clostridia are killed in 10-20 minutes. As the vegetative forms of the microbes propagate in anaerobic conditions in food, they produce exotoxin, it is destroyed completely by boiling for 5-15 minutes.

Epidemiology: Botulism microbes are widely distributed as they are stable in the environment because they can form spores that are distributed with air-borne dust and water, and also by humans and animals. The intestinal contents of healthy people and animals are not suitable for multiplication of the microbes and formation of toxins. The spores are therefore released from the macroorganism with faeces and contaminated soil. From soil, the spores get on vegetables, mushrooms or other plant materials that are used for canning.

Accumulation of the causative agents and their toxins in food occurs in anaerobic conditions at a temperature not below 4-10°C (depending on the type of the microbe). The optimum temperature for production of toxins is 28-37°C. The disease develops after ingestion of food contaminated with the toxin and live microbes, which multiply and intensify toxaemia. A form of the disease known as wound botulism is also known. The disease is caused by infection of a wound. The disease is usually associated with ingestion of pickled or salted mushrooms, or home-canned vegetables, home-smoked meat, and other foods infected with botulism spores. Industrially canned food is safe because it is treated in autoclaves in which the spores are quickly killed. Botulism microorganisms and their toxins propagate in separate foci rather than in the whole bulk of smoked meat, fish or sausage.

This explains the fact that only few people may be infected, v/hile others, who took the same food, may remain healthy. Botulism occurs sporadically; group morbidity is less frequent. Pathogenesis. Clostridium botulinum and its toxin are ingested with food. In the gastrointestinal tract, the toxin is rapidly absorbed and is carried by blood throughout the whole body to affect, in the first instance, the nervous system. Motoneurons of the medulla oblongata and the bone marrow are more sensitive to the toxin. This explains development of bulbar paralysis.

The toxin inhibits the release of acetylcholine in the nerve synapses thus interfering with normal transmission of the impulses from the nerve to the muscle. Specific paralysis of the chest musculature, dysphagia, and vision disorders develop as a result. The toxin constricts the blood vessels, increases their permeability, and causes their paresis and ruptures. Humans are more sensitive to toxins of serotypes A, B and E. Simultaneous effects of several serotypes are additive by their character.

Treatment: The stomach of the patient should be lavaged as soon as possible with a 5 per cent sodium bicarbonate solution; the patient should also be clysterized (siphon). The specific treatment includes early administration of antitoxic vaccine after determination of sensitivity to equine protein (skin test). If the causative microbe has not been identified, a polyvalent vaccine containing A, B, C and E antitoxins is used. The vaccine is given intramuscularly or intravenously (10000 U of types A, C and E and 5000 U of type B). Patients with moderately severe botulism are given a single dose of the vaccine once a day for 3-4 days. In severe cases, or if the treatment begins late after the onset of the disease, the vaccine is administered at 6-8 hour intervals for 2-3 days, and then 2 times a day.

The course of serotherapy should not exceed 4-6 days. After identification of the causative microorganism, monovalent vaccine should be used. Chloramphenicol (0.5 g 4 times a day), and the tetracyclines (0.3 g 4 times a day) should be additionally given for 7-8 days. Antitoxin types A, B, C and E are used to produce active immunity. The preparations are given as follows: 0.5 ml of each type for the first injection, 1 ml of each type for the 2nd and 3rd injections. (The second and third injections should be separated by a 5-7 day interval.)

Monovalent antitoxin should be used after identification of a particular type of the causative agent. In order to lessen toxaemia in moderate and severe forms of the disease, neocompensan or haemodez should be given intravenously; 2000 or 3000 ml of a 5 per cent glucose solution with an equal amount of sodium chloride solution should be infused. Vitamins B and ascorbic acid, cocarboxylase, ATP, cardiacs (cordiamine, camphor, cardiac glycosides) and hormone preparations are indicated. Patients with severe respiratory distress should be taken to an intensive care unit and artificial respiration given.

AMOEBIASIS

Aetiology: Amoebiasis is caused by Entamoeba histolytica that exists in the form of the motile trophozoite and the cyst. The former is subdivided into forma magna, or the tissue form which is found in the ulcers of the intestinal wall (it can phagocytize erythrocytes), and forma minuta that inhabits the lumen of the upper portions of the large intestine. Cysts are formed from the forma minuta in the lower portions of the large intestine; they contain from 1 to 4 nuclei.

The disease is produced only by a mature cyst containing 4 nuclei. The tissue form is found in faeces of patients during the acute period and during exacerbation; the forma minuta can be found in convalescents and in cyst carriers. Outside a human body the trophozoites are rapidly destroyed. The cyst is encased in a dense coat that protects it from the environmental changes. The cyst can survive in water for 8 months, in moist faeces-to a month; it readily withstands low temperature, but is rapidly killed at a temperature of 85°C and above. The cyst is more stable against chlorine preparations; it is sensitive to lysol and phenol solutions.

Epidemiology: The source of infection is man, either an amoebiasis patient or a carrier. Cyst carrier state in epidemic areas can last from several months to years. The transmission mechanism is the same as in shigellosis (faecal-oral). The main route of amoeba transmission is by water (by drinking infected water from open sources such as a river) and by contact (soiled hands or domestic objects). If the sanitary conditions at food catering or children's establishments are below standards the infection can be transmitted with food contaminated by soiled hands of patients or carriers. Foods served without preliminary cooking (vegetables, fruits) are of special importance in transmission of amoebiasis. The highest incidence is during the warm season. The disease is common for countries with hot climate.

Pathogenesis: The cyst of Entamoeba histolytica is ingested with food or water. In the lower portion of the small or in the upper portion of the large intestine the cyst is dissolved and the trophozoite is released into the lumen, where it multiplies, descends to the lower portion of the large intestine in the form of cysts, and is released into the environment.

In the patient, the trophozoite is embedded into the submucous layer of the upper portion of the large intestine; it increases in size and converts into the pathogenic form. As the microorganisms multiply in the submucous membrane, they form abscesses which rupture into the intestinal lumen and form ulcers. The caecum and the ascending colon are usually involved. Ulcers can be deep and reach the serous coat which may result in perforation of the intestinal wall. Blood can carry amoeba to the liver, lungs, brain, kidneys and other organs, where abscesses can be formed.

Diagnosis: The diagnosis is based on laboratory studies. From 4 to 6 smears of fresh warm faeces or material taken during rectoromanoscopy are examined to reveal amoeba. The discovery of the trophozoite with ingested erythrocytes (haematophagous trophozoites) indicates an active disease in the intestine. The enzyme-linked immunosorbent method is also used. Serologic tests (indirect haemagglutination test, immunofluorescent antibody test) are used for the diagnosis of amoebic abscess of the liver and abscesses of other organs. Rectoromanoscopy is an additional diagnostic technique by which specific deep ulcers can be revealed in the lower portion of the intestine.

Treatment: Specific treatment of patients with intestinal and extra-intestinal forms of amoebiasis includes metronidazole (trichopol, flagil), 0.6-0.8 g 3 times a day for 5-10 days. The trophozoites are more readily killed by entamizole, the preparation that includes metronidazole and diloxanide. Two tablets of the preparation are given three times a day for 5-7 days. Acute amoebiasis can be treated with emetine hydrochloride (1 per cent solution, 1.5-2 ml intramuscularly) 2 times a day for 5-7 days. The course is repeated in a week.

Dihydroemetine is less toxic than emetine. The preparation is given as 1-2 per cent solution intramuscularly (1-1.5 mg per kg body weight) for 5 days; the maximum dose is 90 mg/day. Chingamin (delagil, chlorochin) 0.25 g three times a day, quiniofon (yatren) 0.5 g three times a day and antibiotics (tetracyclines, monomycin) should be given in the intervals of the emetine therapy. After the specific treatment, the patient should be given colibacterin, bificol or other preparations for 20-30 days. In the presence of vast abscess of the liver, surgical treatment is indicated in addition to medication with metronidazole in combination with tetracycline and monomycin. General envigorating therapy (vitamins, repeated transfusions of blood or dry plasma) is indicated.

HOOKWORM INFECTION

Aetiology: Hookworm is an infection of one of two different 7 to 13 mm long roundworms (either Ancylostoma duodenale or Necator americanus). If not treated, Hookworm infection can lead to abdominal pain and iron-deficiency. Approximately one-quarter of the world's population is infected with Hookworm.

Epidemiology: Hookworm eggs are passed in stool and infection results when a person comes in contact with the eggs from the contaminated soil or stool. The larvae enter through the skin and travel to the lungs through the blood. They climb up the lungs through the bronchi and trachea and then are swallowed. As the larvae pass into the digestive tract, they attach themselves to the wall of the small intestine. Here they mature into adult worms, mate and feed on the blood of the host. Adult hookworms may live up to ten years.

Pathogenesis: Most of the time a Hookworm infection does not show any symptoms. However, the lifecycle of Hookworm takes it from the skin to the blood, to the lungs and then, eventually, to the intestines; thus, there may be symptoms from the infection in any of these places. There may be a local irritation of the skin where the worm penetrated or even an itchy rash. In the lungs, there may be asthma-like symptoms or pneumonia.

The most common symptoms of Hookworm infection, however, are from their residence in the intestine. Here, Hookworm can lead to abdominal pain, diarrhea, weight loss, loss of appetite and excessive gases. In chronic infections, the patient may become anemic as the worms feed on the individual's blood. The loss of blood leads to a loss of iron and protein; causing difficulty in breathing, pale complexion, tiredness and weakness, fast heartbeat, generalized swelling or bloating and impotence. If the infection lasts a very long time or is very severe, there may be a slow growth, heart problems or even heart failure.

Diagnosis: Looking for the eggs in a stool sample directly, with a microscope, can identify hookworm infection. A blood sample will also indicate if there is an iron or protein deficiency from the infection. It will also indicate how serious the infection has affected on the patient.

Treatment: Hookworm is generally treated with the drug mebendazole. This drug cures more than 99 percent of all cases of hookworm if given twice per day for three days. It kills both the worms and the eggs. This drug is contraindicated during pregnancy. Other drugs that may be given are albendazole and pyrantel, which are given once per day for three days. Since iron deficient anemia is a major problem with a Hookworm infection, taking iron supplements and eating a high protein diet can improve the person's recovery.

ASCARIASIS

Aetiology: Ascariasis is a human disease caused by the parasitic roundworm Ascaris lumbricoides. Perhaps as many as one quarter of the world's people are infected, and ascariasis is particularly prevalent in tropical regions and in areas of poor hygiene. Other species of the genus Ascaris are parasitic and can cause disease in domestic animals.

Epidemiology: Infection occurs through ingestion of food contaminated with feces containing Ascaris eggs. The larvae hatch, burrow through the intestine, reach the lungs, and finally migrate up the respiratory tract. From there they are then reswallowed and mature in the intestine, growing up to 30 cm (12 in.) in length and anchoring themselves to the intestinal wall. Infections are usually asymptomatic, especially if the number of worms is small. They may however be accompanied by inflammation, fever, and diarrhea, and serious problems may develop if the worms migrate to other parts of the body.

The source of transmission is from soil and vegetation on which fecal matter containing eggs has been deposited. Ingestion of infective eggs from soil contaminated with human feces or transmission and contaminated vegetables and water is the primary route of infection. Intimate contact with pets which have been in contact with contaminated soil may result in infection, while pets which are infested themselves by a different type of roundworm can cause infection with that type of worm (Toxocara canis, etc) as occasionally occurs with groomers.

Transmission also comes through municipal recycling of wastewater into crop fields. This is quite common in emerging industrial economies, and poses serious risks for not only local crop sales but also exports of contaminated vegetables. Transmission from human to human by direct contact is impossible.

Pathogenesis: First appearance of eggs in stools is 60-70 days. In larval ascariasis, symptoms occur 4-16 days after infection. The final symptoms are gastrointestinal discomfort, colic and vomiting, fever; observation of live worms in stools. Some patients may have pulmonary symptoms or neurological disorders during migration of the larvae. However there are generally few or no symptoms. A bolus of worms may obstruct the intestine; migrating larvae may cause pneumonitis and eosinophilia.

Patients can remain asymptomatic for very long periods of time. As larval stages travel through the body, they may cause visceral damage, peritonitis and inflammation, enlargement of the liver or spleen, toxicity, and pneumonia. A heavy worm infestation may cause nutritional deficiency; other complications, sometimes fatal, include obstruction of the bowel by a bolus of worms (observed particularly in children) and obstruction of the bile or pancreatic duct. More than 796 Ascaris lumbricoides worms weighing 550 g [19 ounces] were recovered at autopsy from a 2-year-old South African girl. The worms had caused torsion and gangrene of the ileum, which was interpreted as the cause of death.

Ascaris takes most of its nutrients from the partially digested host food in the intestine. There is limited evidence that it can also pierce the intestinal mucous membrane and feed on blood, but this is not its usual source of nutrition. As a result, Ascaris infection does not produce the anemia associated with some other roundworm infections.

Diagnosis: The diagnosis is usually incidental when the host passes a worm in the stool or vomit. Stool samples for ova and parasites will demonstrate Ascaris eggs. Larvae may be found in gastric or respiratory secretions in pulmonary disease. Blood counts may demonstrate peripheral eosinophilia. On X-ray, 15-35 cm long filling defects, sometimes with whirled appearance (bolus of worms).

Treatment: Pharmaceutical treatments include:

Mebendazole (Vermox) ($C_{16}H_{13}N_3O_2$). Causes slow immobilization and death of the worms by selectively and irreversibly blocking uptake of glucose and other nutrients in susceptible adult intestine where helminths dwell. Oral dosage is 100 mg 12 hourly for 3 days.

Piperazine ($C_4H_{10}N_2.C_6H_{10}O_4$). A flaccid paralyzing agent that causes a blocking response of ascaris muscle to acetylcholine. The narcotizing effect immobilizes the worm, which prevents migration when treatment is accomplished with weak drugs such as thiabendazole. If used by itself it causes the worm to be passed out in the feces. Dosage is 75 mg/kg (max 3.5 g) as a single oral dose.

ARTHROPOD INFECTIONS

MALARIA

The disease is caused by protozoa of the genus Plasmodium (class Sporozoa). More than 100 types of malarial plasmodia are known. Four of them are parasitic in man: P. vivax, the causative organism of tertian malaria (the Plasmodium has two variants: the Northern and Southern strains with long and short incubation periods respectively); P. malariae, the causative agent of quartan malaria; P. falciparum, the agent of falciparum malaria; and P. ovale, the causative agent of ovale malaria, a mild variant of tertian malaria. There are several variants of P. falciparum: Indian, Italian, Nigerian, etc.

The Italian strain causes the most severe malaria. Humans are susceptible to some types of agents that cause malaria of monkeys. The life cycle of malarial plasmodia includes two hosts: the final host - male mosquito of the genus Anopheles, in which the sexual phase of growth occurs (known as sporogony); and the intermediate host, which is a human or a vertebrate (in which the asexual multiplication occurs, known as schizogony)

Epidemiology: The source of infection are infected humans, whose blood contains gametocytes, patients with primary or relapsing form of malaria, and carriers. Humans can infect mosquitoes during the very first days of malaria induced by P. vivax, P. ovale, and P. malariae, and remain so until the parasites are contained in the blood. Malaria falciparum patients become contagious only in 10-12 days after development of the first malarial attacks, because gametocytes are formed in the capillaries of the internal organs during 9-11 days.

The life of plasmodia in a human body varies depending on the type of the parasite: P. falciparum survives for 18 months, some African species can live to 3 years; P. vivax can live to 3 years, P. ovale to 41/2 yearsf while P. malariae can survive for decades without inducing apparent clinical symptoms and the disease is only revealed occasionally after transfusion of blood from such infected donors. Only erythrocytic schizogony occurs in such persons. The transmitters of plasmodia are about 80 types of mosquitoes of the genus Anopheles. In Africa the parasites are transmitted by A. gambiae and A. funestus, in Asia by A. minimus, A. culicifacies, A. fluviatilis, A. sundaicus, A. superpictus, etc., in Europe and North America by A. maculipennis, A. superpictus, in Central and South America by A. aquasalis, A. pseudopunctipennis, A. darlingi and A. albimanus, in New Guinea and Australia by A. punctulatus. The mosquitoes of various geographic zones have different susceptibility to plasmodia. After sucking blood, a mosquito female deposits 100-500 mature eggs on the surface of well insolated water surface (ponds and the like).

The larvae undergo their development from 2 to 7 days, depending on the ambient temperature (15-30°C). If the temperature of water is below 10°C the larvae do not grow. In temperate climate, the larvae give imagoes during 2-5 months, while in subtropic countries this period is as long as 5-8 months. In tropic countries mosquitoes appear during the whole year (except during the season of rainfalls). The time of malaria transmission is therefore only 2-5 months in temperate climate, 5-8 months in subtropic countries, and 8-10 months in the torrid zone. Malarial plasmodia can be transmitted from an infected mother to the foetus through the placenta, during labour or blood transfusion, through syringes and needles, etc. Susceptibility to malaria is high, especially in children, who make the prevalent incidence in endemic areas. Strictly specific immunity to a given species and strain is induced in persons who sustained malaria. The immunity persists only on the condition of repeated infections. Immunity can be lost if a person leaves the endemic area.

Depending on the intensity of plasmodia transmission and the infection rate of population, four types of malaria are distinguished (according to WHO classification). 1. Hypoendemic malaria-the spleen index (the percentage of population having enlarged spleens) in children aged from 2 to 9 years is about 10 per cent. 2. Mesoendemic malaria-the spleen index in children aged from 2 to 9 is from 11 to 50 per cent. 3. Hyperendemic malaria-the spleen index in children aged from 2 to 9 is constantly above 50 per cent; the index is also high in adults.

In the holoendemic areas, natives sustain an acute form of malaria during early childhood, the death rate being high. Adults acquire immunity and do not develop acute malaria during their later lives. In meso- and hypoendemic areas, acute malaria occurs in children and adults but the overall morbidity is not high. Malaria is common in almost all countries of Africa, Asia and Oceania. The most common form is tertian malaria. Its causative agent (P. vivax) is well adapted to both temperate and torrid climate. Tropic malaria caused by P. falciparum occurs in the torrid zone on both sides of the equator (45° N. lat.-20° S. lat). Quartan malaria occurs in about the same areas. Ovale malaria occurs in West and East equatorial Africa.

Pathogenesis: Paroxysms of malaria are associated with the response of the thermoregulating centres to the release into blood of a great number of merozoites and other proteins that are formed during division of schizonts and decay of red blood cells. Foreign proteins cause a toxic allergic response in the patient. This response is characterized by oedema of tissues and proliferation of immunocompetent cells (lymphocytes, monocytes, stellar reticuloendotheliocytes, etc.). Destruction of erythrocytes by the parasites and autoantibodies, inhibition of physiologic regeneration of red blood cells in the bone marrow due to splenic hyperfunction cause progressive anaemia, leucopenia, and thrombocytopenia.

Anaemia evokes dystrophic changes in the myocardium, central nervous system, liver and other parenchymatous organs. Malarial plasmodia and their metabolites, the malarial pigment, and the products of protein degradation evoke anaphylaxis: hyperadrenalinaemia, hyperglycaemia, hypercholesterolaemia, hyperkalemia, and relative hyponatraemia. Hyperadrenalinaemia provokes hypertension, tachycardia, spasm of the peripheral vessels and upsets microcirculation in the internal organs. Increased immunoglobulins (IgM, IgG), activated phagocytosis of invaded erythrocytes, and decay of the parasites in macrophages stop the first series of paroxysms after the second or third attack. The disease passes into its next phase, secondary occult period, or early (short) interparoxysmal period.

Due to imperfect initial immune reactions, the blood fails to be completely freed from the parasites. Decreased immune reactions promote an increase in the number of malarial plasmodia and development of a new wave of attacks-early relapses. They follow in 2 weeks to 3 months after termination of the first series of paroxysms. During early relapses, the developed immunity becomes sufficiently strong to suppress schizogony and to promote clinical recovery. In quartan malaria, an equilibrium between the immune system of the macroorganism and the parasites is attained; it can persist for decades. When this equilibrium is upset, the parasites retained in the erythrocytes begin propagating and attain a certain level (paroxysm) at which erythrocytic relapses become possible.

Late relapses also develop in tertian malaria, but they are due to exoerythrocytic forms of the parasites that develop from the persisting forms. Thus, unlike in other forms of malaria, true relapses of the disease and parasitaemia occur in tertian malaria. The malarial agent of vivax (tertian) malaria persists in the macroorganism for 2-4 years, of ovale malaria for 3-6 years, of falciparum malaria for 1-1 i/2 years and of quartan malaria from 2-3 years to decades. Unstable type-specific (non-sterile) immunity develops after the sustained disease.

Diagnosis: Diagnosis is established on the basis of clinical, epidemiologic and laboratory findings. The laboratory methods include microscopy of thin and thick blood smears in which plasmodia are detected. The number of malarial plasmodia is not great during the first attacks. Blood should therefore be studied up to 3 times a day during 2-3 days. Blood specimens should be taken at the height of fever as well as during apyrexia.

Specific diagnosis of malaria is possible with serologic studies: indirect immunofluorescent test, indirect haemagglutination and enzyme-labelled antibody tests. These methods are used to examine blood donors (to reveal carriers of P. malariae), to reveal malaria in persons who took antimalarial preparations before attendance for medical aid, and to establish the absence of disease transmission in endemic areas.

Treatment: Treatment of malaria patients is aimed at termination of acute paroxysms, prevention of relapses and elimination of gamonts. All antimalarial preparations are divided into four groups:

- Gametoschizotropic drugs, preventing development of erythrocytic schizoites: quinine, mepacrine, proguanil, derivatives of 4- aminoquinoline: chloroquine (chloroquine diphosphate), nivaquine (chloroquine sulphate), plaquenil, amodiaquine, pyrimethamine.

- Histoschizotropic preparations preventing development of trophozoites: proguanil, 8-aminoquinoline derivatives (primaquine, quinocide), pyrimethamine.
- Gametocides destroying gamonts: pyrimethamine, 8-aminoquinoline derivatives.
- Sporontocides preventing maturation and growth of gamonts in the mosquito stomach: proguanil, pyrimethamine, and 8-aminoquinoline derivatives.

DENGUE HAEMORRHAGIC FEVER

The disease is also known as Philippine haemorrhagic fever, Southeast haemorrhagic fever, and Thai haemorrhagic fever.

Aetiology: The causative agent is the dengue virus of the genus Flavivirus, the family Togaviridae, which is similar to the other group B arboviruses causing yellow fever and tick-borne encephalitis. At least four serotypes of the dengue virus are known (dengue types 1, 2, 3, 4). The virus survives for several years in the dry state in the blood serum at 5°C and in the frozen (- 70°C) state.

Epidemiology: The source of infection in the urban foci are human patients and in the sylvan foci, monkeys. The source of infection is dangerous during the first 5 days of the disease (viraemia). The infection is transmitted by female mosquitoes of the genus Aedes (A. aegypti, A. albopictus, and others) that become contagious in 8-12 days after sucking blood of an infected subject. Contagiosity persists for the entire life (3-4 months). Children and travellers are mostly affected by the disease in endemic foci. The disease occurs in the zone between 42°N. lat. and 40°S. lat. Foci of infection occur in the countries of Southeast Asia, Oceania, and in West Africa.

Pathogenesis: The virus is inoculated into the human being by the bite of an infected mosquito. The virus multiplies in the cells of mononuclear phagocytic system for 5-16 days and is then carried by the bloodstream to the central nervous system, kidneys, liver, muscles, and other organs and tissues, where the virus propagates and is again carried by the blood to cause secondary wave of fever. Since the vessels are involved, the haemorrhagic syndrome develops. Hypovolaemia develops (up to hypovolaemic shock).

Diagnosis: The diagnosis is established on the basis of clinical, epidemiologic and laboratory findings. The virus can be detected during the first 2-3 days of the disease. To this end, suckling albino mice are infected into the brain. Serologic tests (inhibition of haemagglutination, complement fixation test, neutralization test) with paired serums are used on the 5-6th day and later.

Treatment: Treatment is symptomatic and pathogenetic.

FILARIASIS

Filiariasis is the name for a group of tropical diseases caused by various thread-like parasitic round worms (nematodes) and their larvae. The larvae transmit the disease to humans through a mosquito bite. Filariasis is characterized by fever, chills, headache, and skin lesions in the early stages and, if untreated, can progress to include gross enlargement of the limbs and genitalia in a condition called elephantiasis.

Symptoms vary, depending on what type of parasitic worm has caused the infection, but all infections usually begin with chills, headache, and fever between three months and one year after the insect bite. There may also be swelling, redness, and pain in the arms, legs, or scrotum. Areas of pus (abscesses) may appear as a result of dying worms or a secondary bacterial infection.

Diagnosis: The disease is diagnosed by taking a patient history, performing a physical examination, and by screening blood specimens for specific proteins produced by the immune system in response to this infection (antibodies). Early diagnosis may be difficult because, in the first stages, the disease mimics other bacterial skin infections.

To make an accurate diagnosis, the physician looks for a pattern of inflammation and signs of lymphatic obstruction, together with the patient's possible exposure to filariasis in an area where filariasis is common. The larvae (microfilariae) can also be found in the blood, but because mosquitos, which spread the disease, are active at night, the larvae are usually only found in the blood between about 10 pm and 2 am.

Treatment: Either ivermectin, albendazole, or diethylcarbamazine is used to treat a filariasis infection by eliminating the larvae, impairing the adult worms' ability to reproduce, and by actually killing adult worms. Unfortunately, much of the tissue damage may not be reversible. The medication is started at low doses to prevent reactions caused by large numbers of dying parasites.

While effective, the medications can cause severe side effects in up to 70% of patients as a result either of the drug itself or the massive death of parasites in the blood. Diethylcarbamazine, for example, can cause severe allergic reactions and the formation of pus-filled sores (abscesses). These side effects can be controlled using antihistamines and anti-inflammatory drugs (corticosteroids). Rarely, treatment with diethylcarbamazine in someone with very high levels of parasite infection may lead to a fatal inflammation of the brain (encephalitis). In this case, the fever is followed by headache and confusion, then stupor and coma caused when massive numbers of larvae and parasites die. Other common drug reactions include dizziness, weakness, and nausea.

Symptoms caused by the death of the parasites include fever, headache, muscle pain, abdominal pain, nausea and vomiting, weakness, dizziness, lethargy, and asthma. Reactions usually begin within two days of starting treatment and may last between two and four days.

No treatment can reverse elephantiasis. Surgery may be used to remove surplus tissue and provide a way to drain the fluid around the damaged lymphatic vessels. Surgery may also be used to ease massive enlargement of the scrotum. Elephantiasis of the legs can also be helped by elevating the legs and providing support with elastic bandages.

VIRAL INFECTIONS

RABIES (HYDROPHOBIA)

Aetiology: The disease is caused by the RNA containing virus of the family Rhabdoviridae. The virus parasitizes on the central nervous system of humans and animals. The brain of the dead contains specific cytoplasmic inclusions, the Negri bodies. The virus can be cultivated in rabbits, hamsters, albino mice and some other mammals. Two types of the rabies virus are distinguished: street and fixed {fixe) viruses. As contrast to the street virus, the fixed virus cannot penetrate the central nervous system after its subcutaneous administration, nor is it present in the saliva of infected animals. Special strains of the fixed virus are used for the manufacture of rabies vaccine.

Epidemiology: The source of infection are animals. The main reservoir are foxes, wolves, jackals and polar foxes which infect domestic animals such as dogs or cats. Cattle, goats and sheep, horses, swine, cats, mice, rats and some other animals develop rabies. The contagious period begins 7-10 days before the clinical signs of the disease develop, and persists till the death of the animal. The incubation period in dogs is 14-30 days. Humans are usually infected by dogs, cats and foxes.

The infection is transmitted with the saliva through the bite of an infected animal or when the saliva gets on an injured skin. Humans are highly susceptible to the virus. The duration of the incubation period depends on the character of bite, the location of the wound, its area and depth, amount of saliva that contaminates the skin, etc.

Entrance of the virus through the skin of the head, neck or fingers, is especially dangerous. The disease occurs as sporadic cases among persons who did not attend for medical aid in due time (i.e., who were not given postexposure prophylactic treatment). Rabies occurs during the whole year but the incidence increases in the warm season. Dogs become infected more frequently during this period and hence the incidence among people increases too.

Pathogenesis: The virus contained in the saliva of a rabid animal enters a human being through an injured skin or mucosa and passes to the perineural space of the nervous trunks and finally to the brain and spinal cord. As the disease progresses, the virus moves from the central nervous system and the spinal cord to the periphery. It appears in the salivary glands and is excreted with the saliva. The disease is fatal.

Diagnosis: The diagnosis is not difficult if the history of exposure is known. Laboratory tests confirm the diagnosis only after the death of the patient or animal by isolation of the Negri bodies and by inoculation of experimental animals. Specimens of brain (hippocampus) and medulla oblongata in alcohol or sterile glycerol or the whole dead animal should be delivered to the laboratory. Fluorescent antibody method is used for rapid identification of the rabies virus in the brain and salivary glands.

Treatment: Effective treatment is unknown. As a rule, treatment is aimed at decreasing the psychomotor excitement and at lessening the patient's sufferings. Salt solutions, glucose and vitamins should be infused parenterally to supply the patient with the necessary nutrients and to replenish the liquid loss. Chloral hydrate (2 g in 100 g of starch solution), morphine, aminazine, dimedrol and cardiacs are indicated. Curare-like preparations and intensive respiratory support can prolong the life of the patient for 2-3 days. The patient should be placed in an isolated shaded room.

YELLOW FEVER

Aetiology: The disease is caused by Flavivirus febris of the genus Flavivirus, the family Togaviridae. The virus is unstable in the environment.

It resists drying and can survive in the frozen state for a year; in a sealed vial with nitrogen, the virus remains viable for 12 years.

Epidemiology: Two epidemiologically different types of foci are distinguished: sylvan (rain forest) and urban. The reservoir of the virus in the sylvan form are monkeys, possibly rodents, hedgehogs and other animals. The vector of transmission in South America are mosquitoes Haemagogus, Sperazzini and other insects; in tropic Africa these are mosquitoes Aedes simpsoni, A. africanus, A. aegypti and other species of Aedes. Sylvan yellow fever is also called endemic because it usually occurs in the form of endemic foci and less frequently as epidemics.

Transmission of the virus from epidemic foci to towns and villages, where mosquitoes Aedes aegypti occur, can cause an epidemic outbreak. The source of infection in urban foci of yellow fever are human patients; the vector is mosquito Aedes aegypti. The mosquito becomes contagious in 6-18 days after sucking blood of a human patient, this period depending on the ambient temperature: 18 days for ambient temperatures under 21°C, and 6 days at 31°C.

Once infected the vector remains infectious for its entire life (1-2 months). Susceptibility to yellow fever is universal, but part of the indigenous population in endemic areas sustains the disease in the mild or asymptomatic form. Life-long immunity is produced in people who sustained the disease. Sporadic cases and local group incidences are reported from subtropic and tropic zones of Africa, South and Central America. During summer, the disease can occur in other subtropic regions where the transmitters of the virus are available. According to the international rules, yellow fever is the infection that requires establishment of quarantine and should be reported to WHO.

Pathogenesis: As the virus is inoculated into a human by the bite of an infected mosquito, it multiplies during 3-6 days in the regional lymph nodes, in the cells of mononuclear phagocytic system, and enters the blood to cause viraemia. The blood carries the virus to the liver, bone marrow, kidneys, spleen, and brain to involve the vascular apparatus and to cause dystrophy and necrosis of their cells.

Diagnosis: Yellow fever is diagnosed on the basis of clinical and laboratory findings. Virus is isolated in the laboratory from a blood specimen taken during the first 4 days of the disease. Discovery of antibodies to the virus, using the complement fixation test and inhibition of indirect haemagglutination, is diagnostically important too: four-fold increase in the antibody titres in paired serums is diagnostically trustworthy. The virus neutralization reaction is also used. Serologic studies can confirm the diagnosis retrospectively because the antibodies to the virus can be revealed only on the second week of the disease.

Treatment: Specific therapy is unknown. Moderately severe forms are treated symptomatically: vitamin C, vicasol, vitamin P, cardiovascular preparations. Severe and fulminant forms should be treated by intensive therapy; resuscitation measures may be necessary: correction of haemostasis, complex antishock and detoxicating treatment.

JAPANESE ENCEPHALITIS

Japanese encephalitis was identified as an independent nosologic entity in 1924 after an outbreak of the disease in Japan. The mortality rate was high.

Aetiology: The disease is caused by arbovirus of the antigen group B; the virus is unstable outside the macroorganism. It can be detected in the hosts-warm-blooded animals, and infection transmitters - mosquitoes. The virus grows in tissue cultures and chick embryos.

Epidemiology: The source of infection are animals, birds (sparrows) and humans during viraemia. Mosquitoes Culex and Aedes are the transmitters. They usually inhabit wild nature where there are many lakes, swamps and sufficient sunlight. In this connection the disease is mostly endemic. At ambient temperatures below 20°C, the virus inside the mosquito propagates slowly. Natural nidi of Japanese encephalitis are reported from Japan, China, India, Korea, Vietnam, USSR, and African countries. In addition to the natural nidi, there are nidi of infection in populated places where the mosquitoes miltiply in small ponds and feed on domestic animals.

Humans get infected during work in field conditions, during hunting, fishing, road construction, etc. Men working in areas with natural nidi of Japanese encephalitis are mostly afflicted by the disease. The disease occurs in the end of summer and in early autumn. In Japan the disease occurs already in June. Stable immunity develops in persons who sustained the disease.

Pathogenesis: The virus circulates with blood and afflicts, in the first instance, capillary endothelium of the brain and internal organs. Haemorrhages, oedema of the meninges, adrenal glands, kidneys, liver, lungs and the intestine occur. Propagation of the virus in the brain tissue causes death of the neurons. The greatest changes occur in the grey and white substance of the brain, subcortical ganglia, in the hypothalamus and the mesencephalon.

Diagnosis: The diagnosis is based on clinical, epidemiologic and laboratory findings. During the first 7 days of the disease, blood, cerebrospinal fluid, urine and mucus from the upper airways are examined in the laboratory. The material is administered to albino mice intracerebrally. Complement fixation test, haemagglutination inhibition and neutralization tests are performed during the 1st and 3rd weeks of the disease. Intracutaneous test with the antigen prepared from the brain suspension of infected mice can also be performed.

Treatment: Specific immunoglobulin (3-6 ml) is given intramuscularly 3 times a day for 3-4 first days. In order to decrease oedema and brain swelling, dehydration therapy is indicated: 20 per cent solution of placental albumin, 15 per cent mannitol solution, and diuretics. Cardiac preparations and vitamins are indicated. During the recovery phase, a 0.05 per cent proserin solution and caloric diet are prescribed.

KYASANUR FOREST DISEASE

Aetiology: The disease is caused by the virus which is similar to that causing spring-summer tick-borne encephalitis.

Epidemiology: The source of infection are monkeys and possibly other animals and birds. The virus is transmitted by the bite of ticks Haemophysalis spinigera, H. turanicus, gamasoidea ticks, and fleas. The reservoir of virus are birds migrating from Omsk and Novosibirsk regions to India and back. Kyasanur forest disease occurs in India.

Clinical picture: The incubation period lasts from 3 to 8 days. The onset is acute: the body temperature rises to 39-39.4°C during the first day of the disease. The patient complains of headache and myalgia. On the 3rd or 4th day the condition worsens; the patient develops vomiting, diarrhoea, delirium, nasal, gastrointestinal, and gingival bleeding. Generalized maculopapulous rash, bradycardia and hypotension are characteristic. Fever lasts 7-14 days. Haematologic changes: leucopenia, thrombocytopenia, aneosinophilia, then neutrophilic leucocytosis. The urine is characterized by moderate albuminuria and haematuria. The recovery period lasts 1-2 months.

Complications: Encephalitis and pneumonia are the complications.

Diagnosis: Diagnosis is established on the basis of clinical, epidemiologic and laboratory findings. The virus is isolated from the blood by agglutination reaction. Blood should be tested from the first to the fifth day. Suckling mice, chick embryos and cell cultures are inoculated with the patient's blood. Complement fixation test, haemagglutination inhibition test and diffuse precipitation in agar are used for the purpose.

Treatment: Treatment is the same as in other haemorrhagic fevers.

Prevention and control: Measures include extermination of the transmitting vector and protection of people from ticks.

BACTERIAL INFECTIONS

BRUCELLOSIS

Aetiology: This infection is caused by microorganisms of six species. Human brucellosis is due to the following three species: B. melitensis (goats), B. suis (hogs) and B. abortus (cattle). The microorganisms were discovered by the English physician David Bruce in 1886 in preparations of human cadaveric spleen. (Hence the names of the pathogenic microorganism, Brucella, and the disease due to these causative agents, brucellosis.)

The causative agent of brucellosis in goats, B. melitensis, is the most pathogenic to humans. Brucella is sufficiently stable in the environment. In soil it survives for 3 months, in milk for 10 days, in sheep cheese to 45 days, and in wool to 3 months. It is sensitive to high temperature and boiling kills it instantaneously; heating to 60°C for 30 minutes is also detrimental. The microorganisms are sensitive to disinfectants (3 per cent lysol solution, 5 per cent solution of lime chloride).

Epidemiology: Brucellosis is a typical zoonosis because the reservoir of infection are domestic animals. It has already been said that goats and sheep are the commonest source of infection in man. Cattle and swine are less important. If healthy and diseased animals of various species are raised together, brucella migrates from goats to cattle and other animals. Outbreaks of the disease in man thus become possible. Cats, dogs, camels, deer, horses are a secondary reservoir of the infection. A diseased man presents no danger to the surrounding people.

Diseased animals shed the pathogenic microorganisms with amniotic fluid, abortus, urine, dung, and milk. Besides, the organisms are contained in the blood and flesh of the animals. The infection is usually transmitted by direct contact with the animal excrements and objects infected by these excrements. Humans get infected when taking care of the animals, during milking, shearing, etc. Another route of infection transmission is through infected foods, such as raw milk, curds, sheep cheese prepared from raw milk, and also through meat of the diseased animal. There is still another, although rare, route of infection transmission: by air-borne droplets. Humans get infected during processing wool of the diseased animals. Since brucella survives for a long time in water, water-borne infection should not be excluded either. Brucellosis is an occupational disease of animal breeders and farm workers.

Immunity, that is produced in those who sustained the disease, is unstable. The highest incidence of the disease is during the spring and summer. The first wave of morbidity is seen in the early spring. It is associated with bearing the young and miscarriages. The infection is spread by direct contact due to intensive liberation of the organisms with miscarriages, placenta, amniotic fluid, and the like. Another wave of seasonal morbidity occurs during maximum lactation in domestic animals; the main mechanism is alimentary. The incidence of brucellosis among the workers of slaughterhouses and meat processing plants coincides with the time of mass-scale slaughter of cattle.

Pathogenesis: When the pathogenic organism gets inside a human through a damaged skin or mucosa, it passes with the lymph to regional lymph nodes where it multiplies during the entire incubation period. By the moment when the disease becomes clinically manifest, brucella enters the blood and is carried to various organs and systems: the liver, spleen, bone marrow, and the lymph nodes.

Secondary foci of infection thus develop. In a considerable number of persons the acquired immunity does not ensure elimination of the causative agent. Retention and multiplication of brucella in the infection focus, repeated release of the organisms into the blood, and endotoxaemia account for the sensitization of the person to various allergens. If untreated, the disease converts into its chronic form with periodic exacerbation and remissions. Allergic changes are manifested by systemic lesion of the vessels, inflammation in the organs, arthritis, fibrositis, etc.

Clinical picture: The incubation period lasts for 2-3 weeks, with variation from one week to two months. The clinical manifestations of brucellosis are varied. The disease is sometimes asymptomatic and can only be diagnosed in the laboratory. Acute brucellosis (lasting to 3 months from the onset of the disease), subacute (from 3 to 6 months), chronic brucellosis (longer than 6 months) and residual phenomena following clinical recovery are distinguished. According to severity, the disease is classed as mild, moderate and severe. An acute form of brucellosis often begins with a prodromal period. The patient complains of malaise, lassitude, depression, deranged sleep, lumbar pain, myalgia and arthralgia, chills.

The prodromal period lasts from several days to a few weeks. The period of precursors is followed by a manifest clinical picture of brucellosis. The body temperature suddenly rises to hyperpyrexia. The elevation of temperature is attended by chills. The fever then lessens and sweating is profuse. Despite fever, the patient's general condition remains normal and his working capacity is preserved.

The patient then complains of rapid fatigue, headache, irritability, transient pain in some large joints. Fever can be undulant, remittent, intermittent, or, less frequently, continuous. Lymph nodes, usually submandibular and cervical, less frequently axillary and inguinal lymph nodes are enlarged in some patients. The spleen and liver are enlarged from the first days of fever; the condition persists for a long time. These organs become firm.

Among permanent symptoms of brucellosis in man is pain. By the end of the second week of the disease the patient develops pain in some large joints. Pain comes in attacks (undulant). It is due to arthritis and periarthritis, periostitis, bursitis, myositis, fibrositis, cellusitis, etc. Headache and pallor are due to the lesion of the central nervous system. Excitability and whining are characteristic.

Leucopenia (3 x 109/1) with relative lymphocytosis, aneosinophilia, neutropenia, thrombocytopenia and high ESR are seen. Late treatment of patients with weak reactivity facilitates the transition of the disease to its subacute and chronic forms. Subacute brucellosis, in addition to the mentioned symptoms, is also characterized by focal allergic lesions in the form of arthritis, neuritis, plexitis, etc.

Subacute brucellosis can gradually transform into chronic brucellosis which is characterized by a further reconstruction of allergic response with involvement of other organs and systems. The body temperature is usually subfebrile or normal during weeks and months (remissions). The chronic form of the disease is usually characterized by stable changes in the locomotorium (arthritis, bursitis, tendovaginitis, periostitis, perichondritis) and in the nervous system (radiculitis, ischioradiculitis, plexitis, neuralgia). The genital system is also involved: orchitis (inflammation of the testes), orchiepididymitis (inflammation of the testes and the epididymis) in males and oophoritis (inflammation of the ovaries and the tubes), endometritis, and abnormal menstrual cycle in women.

Chronic brucellosis proceeds with relapses and remissions and can last 2-3 years. After the patient recovers, residual phenomena are possible: pain in the joints and muscles, headache, irritability, organic changes in the locomotorium with deformation of the joints, etc. The clinical picture of the disease has lately somewhat changed. Severe forms of brucellosis are rare.

Complications: The commonest complications are orchitis and epididymitis, salpingitis and oophoritis, bursitis, pneumonia, acute and subacute endocarditis, plexitis and neuritis of the peripheral nerves, etc.

Diagnosis: The high variability of the symptoms complicates the diagnosis of brucellosis. A properly collected epidemiologic anamnesis and laboratory studies help establish a correct diagnosis. Isolation of brucella from the blood, bone marrow, urine, and the lymph nodes is diagnostically decisive although these studies take much time. Blood cultures are inoculated with 5-10 ml blood specimens taken from the ulnar vein of patients before the antibiotic therapy is started. It is recommended to cultivate specimens of blood, bone marrow and lymph nodes of patients with chronic brucellosis during exacerbation before treatment begins (test for the presence of the L forms of Brucella). The result is ready only in 5-10 days, and sometimes in 29-30 days.

Serologic tests, the immunofluorescent method, Coombs' test, direct haemagglutination test, and intracutaneous allergic test are used for serologic diagnosis of brucellosis. Wright and Huddleson tests are positive beginning with the 8-9th day of the disease, while the Burnet test in 7-8 days and later. A specimen of blood taken from the finger or the vein (1-2 ml) is tested (Wright's reaction) and result is considered positive with serum dilution of 1: 200 and more.

The Huddleson test can be carried out at patient's bedside (1 ml of blood). But this reaction is qualitative and the agglutination titres remain unknown. The test is suitable for screening of population before prophylactic vaccination. The reaction of direct haemagglutination is more specific. It is positive with the dilution of 1: 100. The Burnet intracutaneous test is performed after the 10th day of the disease. Brucellin is injected into the skin on the palmar surface of the middle third of the forearm. A painful oedema develops in 24-48 hours (positive test).

The size of the oedema is measured: if the oedema is from 1 to 3 cm in diameter, the reaction is weakly positive, if 4-6 cm-positive, and greater than 6 cm-highly positive. Coombs' test is used in chronic forms of infection. The reaction is based on the detection of incomplete antibodies using antiglobulin serum. The luminescent serologic test consists in applying a fixed smear of labelled serum in the working dilution. The smear is examined in a luminescent microscope.

Treatment: Patients with acute brucellosis and exacerbated chronic brucellosis should be taken to hospital. Antibiotics are given to patients with acute, subacute and exacerbated chronic brucellosis with signs of marked toxaemia and high fever. The tetracyclines and terramycin are most efficacious. They are given in a dose of 0.3 g 4 times a day. Chloramphenicol (0.5 g 4 times a day) and other antibiotics are also useful. The mentioned preparations are given per os for 5-7 days.

The course is repeated at a 5-day interval. Vaccine therapy is indicated after 2-3 courses. The vaccine should preferably be given intravenously. In the presence of contraindications it can be given intracutaneously. The dose of the vaccine depends on the patient's condition, the route of administration, allergization of the patient (the result of the Burnet test), and on the response to the previous vaccination. In order to lessen the response, the vaccine is administered intravenously in two steps. The daily dose of the vaccine is administered not by a single injection but in two portions at a 90-120 minute interval. From 7 to 10 administrations are necessary at 3-5 day intervals between the injections. The sensitivity is determined by administering 1-2 million microbes at 2-3 day intervals, and then subsequently 5, 10,25, 75, 100 and 125 million microbes. In 2-3 hours following the administration, the patient develops chill, arthralgia intensifies, and the body temperature rises to 38-40°C in 6-8 hours.

The temperature normalizes in 1-2 days, the patient sweats profusely, the liver and the spleen are enlarged. Subsequent administration of the vaccine is attended by desensitization of the body, lessening of pain, fall of body temperature, and improvement of the patient's condition. Especially severe cases of brucellosis with involvement of the joints, the central and peripheral nervous system, orchitis, etc., are treated with prednisolone and prednisone (in addition to antibiotics), given in a dose of 20-30 mg for 4-6 days. The corticosteroid therapy is combined with butadione and other anti-inflammatory preparations.

Symptomatic treatment should also be given: invigorating measures, preparations improving appetite, vitamins B and ascorbic acid, cardiacs and analgesics. To release arthralgia, 3, 5 or 10 ml of a 0.25 per cent novocaine solution are injected intravenously. Physiotherapy is widely used in brucellosis. Residual phenomena should be corrected by medical exercises and massage. Health-resort therapy is indicated in 6 months after recovery.

Prevention and control: Measures to prevent brucellosis in humans should be directed at eradication of the infection among agricultural animals and decontamination of environmental objects, foods and raw materials of animal origin, and protection of people against contamination. The intracutaneous Burnet test and serologic reactions should be performed in areas where brucellosis cases are reported in order to reveal timely the diseased animals. People should be protected by taking general sanitary measures and also by using means of individual protection.

These include observation of disinfection requirements at animal farms and in industry where animal materials are processed; observation of sanitary requirements during slaughtering the diseased animals with subsequent disinfection of enclosures, equipment, etc.; observation of rules for handling animals, and provision of means for individual protection of the personnel (overalls, rubber gloves, special footware, aprons, etc.). The workers must be provided with detergents, disinfectants, hot water, and the like. Materials obtained from diseased animals should be decontaminated: milk should be boiled or pasteurized, dairy products should be prepared only from pasteurized or boiled milk. Meat should be treated thermally. Sheep cheese should be cured for 60 days. Prophylactic vaccination is necessary in endemic areas. Quarantines are also necessary to prevent the infection spread.

In order to prevent brucellosis in humans, planned vaccinations (revaccinations) should be performed in people who are exposed occupationally to the risk of infection with goat brucellosis. Single epicutaneous vaccination, and revaccination in 8-12 months (also epicutaneously) should be carried out. Vaccinated and revaccinated are people with negative serologic and allergic tests for brucellosis at the age over 18 years, and also people to whom vaccination is not contraindicated. Dry live vaccine (B. abortus) is used. Vaccination and revaccination are performed 1-2 months before hiring for jobs associated with possible danger of infection, before intensive seasonal work begins (sheep shearing, mass-scale slaughtering, etc.). Persons exposed to the danger of brucellosis infection (animal breeders, slaughterhouse workers, etc.) should be observed regularly in outpatient conditions. The observation includes inspection by the general therapist and laboratory testing. Health education of population is necessary in areas where brucellosis cases are reported.

Patients with acute brucellosis are not dangerous for the surrounding but they should nevertheless be treated in hospital. Those who sustained brucellosis should be regularly examined in outpatient conditions for 2 years after recovery.

PLAGUE

Aetiology: The disease is due to Yersinia pestis, the bacillus of the genus Yersinia, the family Enterobacteriaceae. It is a barrel-shaped gram-negative nonmotile bacillus. Its pathogenicity toward humans and animals is very high. The bacillus remains viable outside the macroorganism for a long time. In dead rodents, Yersinia pestis can live 5 months (at 0°C); in dead (frozen) humans the bacillus can survive from 7 to 12 months. In the sputum the bacillus remains viable from several days to 5 months, in pus, to 40 days, and in water, to 3 months. Its stability toward disinfectants is low. At 100°C the plague agent is killed in few seconds.

Epidemiology: Plague is a typical disease of rodents which are the primary source of the disease among humans. Rodents such as marmots, sousliks, hamsters, field mice and voles, brown and grey rats, house mice, etc. are highly susceptible to plague. The primary reservoir of plague infection are sousliks, voles, marmots and rats. Rodents usually develop an acute form of plague and die. But some of them (hibernating sousliks, marmots) develop the latent disease which remains in them till next year. Other animals are also involved in the epizootics. Spontaneous infection with plague has been observed in 300 species of rodents and 29 species of other animals (camels, monkeys, jackals, hedgehogs, etc.).

Ectoparasites, such as fleas are involved in the spread of plague and its maintenance in nature. Fleas are the main vector of infection. They leave dead animals and attack another host. Fleas can survive in burrows of the dead for a year until the hole is occupied by a new animal. Epizootics in natural nidi are explained by circulation of plague microbes in the system rodent-flea-rodent. Natural nidi of sylvatic (steppe) and murine plague are distinguished. Natural nidi of sylvatic plague have been formed independently of the humans and their activities. The main nidus is found in the vast deserts of Middle Asia. Lybian and southern jirds are the main reservoir of the infection. Siberian marmots maintain the infection in the steppes of East Asia.

Natural nidi are known in Africa, North and South America, and on other continents, from which plague cases among people are reported annually. Grey, Alexandrian and black rats, and house mice are the main sources and reservoirs of infection. In these animals plague can proceed as a long-standing condition or as asymptomatic carrier state. The main sources of murine plague are found in South and East Asia. Humans are a great danger to the surrounding as a source of infection. These are patients with primary and secondary pneumonic types of the disease and the septicaemic form. Patients with uncomplicated bubonic forms are practically not dangerous.

The main route of infection transmission from an infected rodent to a human being is through a bite of an infected flea. The flea is infected through ingestion of blood of a bacteraemic animal. As the bacillus multiplies in the intestinal tract of the flea, a jel is formed at the entrance to the stomach that prevents the passage of subsequent meals. As a result the bacilli are regurgitated when the infected flea attempts to ingest another blood meal. The flea remains hungry and its activity increases. In the absence of rats, the flea attacks humans to infect them. If a human being hunts in the focus of plague he may get contaminated by direct contacts with marmots, hares or other infected animals, either dead or captured. If an individual damages the skin when removing the pelt, or touches the mucosa with the contaminated hands, he gets infected.

People also get infected during funeral ceremonies because the fluid issuing from the mouth or nose of the dead contains the plague agent. Ingestion of contaminated food also leads to penetration of the plague bacillus into the gastrointestinal mucosa. Susceptibility of humans to plague is extremely high. When infected from an animal, the patient usually develops the bubonic form. Bubonic plague is characterized by slowly increasing incidence. In primary or secondary pneumonic plague the infection is transmitted from person to person by air-borne route which is a great epidemiologic danger because the disease can spread widely within a short period of time. Pulmonic plague usually follows the bubonic form and very soon it becomes the main clinical form. The immunity developed in the plague patient is rather stable and repeated infections are rare.

Pathogenesis: The pathogenesis depends on the route by which the plague agent penetrates the body. If the infection gains entrance through the skin, the bacillus is carried to the regional lymph nodes where the microbes propagate to cause various inflammations with haemorrhagic infiltration. The whole group of the lymph nodes and the adjacent subcutaneous fat are involved in the inflammation. A primary bubo is thus formed. From the bubo, the microbes enter the blood stream to cause bacteraemia. The microbes enter the internal organs and lymph nodes that are remote from the portal of entry; secondary buboes are thus formed.

Secondary plague pneumonia is especially dangerous. Less frequently, a papule or vesicle (that transforms later into a pustule, filled with sanguinopurulent exudate) is formed at the portal of entry of the infection. The pustule turns into an ulcer with raised margins. The regional lymph nodes are also involved in the process. If a person is infected by the air-borne route, haemorrhagic pneumonia and sepsis occur (primary pulmonic and secondary septicaemic forms).

In alimentary infection, the disease is manifested by haemorrhagic enteritis and sepsis (intestinal and secondary septicaemic forms). In primary septicaemia, the lymphatic barrier is weak (usually due to incomplete phagocytosis of the plague agent and due to the massive dose of infection and low body reactivity).

Carried by the blood stream, the plague agent therefore generalizes the process. The plague microbe forms exo- and endotoxins which cause toxaemia. The cardiovascular and the nervous systems are first of all involved: the pulse changes, arterial pressure falls, the patient is excited and delirious. Vascular changes are manifested by necrosis, infiltration and serous impregnation of the vascular walls.

Clinical picture: The incubation period lasts from 2 to 6 days. It is shorter in the pulmonic form while in the vaccinated it can be as long as 8-10 days. Plague begins suddenly with a severe chill and rapid elevation of temperature to 39°C and higher. Toxaemia rapidly develops in all clinical forms. It is manifested by severe headache and vertigo, insomnia, myalgia, weakness, nausea and vomiting. The patient is first excited. His face and conjunctiva are hyperaemic, the tongue is white and swollen, speech becomes inarticulate.

All these symptoms (unsteady gait included) resemble those of alcoholic intoxication. Circulatory disorder is marked; tachycardia develops (120-160 beats per minute); arterial pressure falls; arrhythmia occurs in severe cases. Severe cases are also characterized by cyanosis, pointedness of the features (expression of fright on the face of some patients), delirium and hallucinations. Neutrophilic leucocytosis with a shift to the left and accelerated ESR are seen in the blood. The diuresis decreases; the urine contains protein, granular and hyaline casts and red blood cells. In addition to the symptoms that are common for all forms of plague, each particular form is also characterized by its specific symptoms.

Depending on the route of infection transmission, the patient may develop either a localized form of plague, such as cutaneous, bubonic, cutaneous-bubonic, or tonsillar (pharyngeal), or a generalized form, such as primary septicaemic, secondary septicaemic, primary pulmonic, secondary pulmonic or intestinal plague. In the cutaneous-bubonic form, a spot is first seen at the portal of entry, which is then converted into a papule, a vesicle, a pustule, and an ulcer.

The ulcer is surrounded by a zone of red, later it becomes covered with a dark crust and does not heal for a long time. As distinct from anthrax, a plague carbuncle is painful. The regional lymph nodes are almost always involved. Lymphadenitis (plague bubo) develops on the first or second day of the bubonic form. The bubo is tender not only during movement but also at rest.

The patient is therefore motionless. Pain makes him assume a forced position. If the bubo is the inguinal area, the patient flexes his leg. In the presence of an axillary bubo, the patient lies on his back with the arm set apart from the trunk. The bubo fuses with the subcutaneous cellular tissue; the overlying skin is tense and cyanotic. The bubo either resolves spontaneously or purulates and scleroses. Cutaneous-bubonic forms can be complicated by secondary buboes, secondary pulmonic and secondary septicaemic plague. The tonsillar (pharyngeal) plague lasts 2-3 days.

The toxaemia is weak, the body temperature rises to 38°C, the submandibular and neck lymph nodes are enlarged. The primary septicaemic form is characterized by delirious hyperactivity or complete adynamia, dyspnoea, rapid and weak pulse, Haemorrhagic rash and haemorrhages into the skin and mucosa develop, haematemesis and bleeding can be seen. Untreated patient dies during first days of the disease. The intestinal form is characterized by high body temperature, extreme weakness, loss of appetite, nausea, recurrent vomiting, ample liquid stools with streaks of blood and mucus, severe abdominal pain during the defaecation. Primary pulmonic plague is characterized by a fulminating course.

Primary axillary bubo and secondary inguinal bubo (after Mohry) with dyspnoea (40-60 breaths a minute), severe chest pain, cough with liberation of liquid blood-stained foaming sputum. Cardiovascular failure develops on the very first days of the disease. In the pre-antibiotic era, pulmonic plague transformed into its secondary septicaemic form in 1-2 days and the patient died. The prognosis is more favourable today.

Diagnosis: The diagnosis is based on clinical, epidemiologic and laboratory findings. Special precautions must be observed when taking infected material, its transportation and further handling in the laboratory. The following specimens are taken: bubo contents, spontaneously draining exudate from ruptured buboes, vesicles, pustules, carbuncles and ulcers; sputum is taken from patients with the pulmonic form; if sputum is absent, faucial mucus is taken.

Faeces should be taken from patients with intestinal lesions. Blood specimens of patients with all forms of the disease are studied. The dead should be autopsied and pieces of the buboes, cutaneous lesions, lymph nodes and the parenchymatous organs (spleen, liver, lung), as well as blood from the heart or large vessels should be examined in the laboratory. Exudates from buboes, vesicles, or pustules should be taken by a sterile syringe. Since the amount of the material is small, about 0.5 ml of a sterile broth is taken in the same syringe and the contents are transferred to a test tube. Sputum should be collected into wide-mouth bottles with ground-in stoppers. Blood (10 ml) is taken from the cubital vein.

Several smears (4-5) are prepared at the patient's bedside. A 5-ml portion of blood is inoculated in a vial containing 50 ml of broth, while the remaining blood is placed in a sterile test tube. If the laboratory is remote, the blood is placed in two 5-ml test tubes and examined in the laboratory not later than 5-6 hours (in the absence of a refrigerator). In the laboratory, the smears are stained with Gram's stain and methylene blue (Loeffler). The serologic luminescence analysis should be conducted if a luminescent microscope is available.

Hottinger's or Martin's culture media containing sodium sulphite and gentian violet are inoculated. The remaining material is used for infection of guinea pigs and albino mice. The serologic method is used for retrospective diagnosis in those who sustained a suspected plague, in patients to whom antibiotics were given, and in studies on the material taken from decaying corpses. Indirect haemagglutination and indirect agglutination inhibition tests are commonly used.

The latter test with an antigen diagnosticum is used to control specificity of the positive indirect haemagglutination test. Serologic reactions should be conducted on the 5th day of the disease and then at 5-day intervals till the patient is discharged from hospital. The reaction of fluorescent antibodies can be used to detect the plague agent within 2 hours. Fleas and rodents, and also dead animals, especially camels, should be examined bacteriologically in the focus of infection.

Treatment: Treatment of the patient must be complex. Specific treatment includes the tetracyclines (tetracycline, doxycycline, oxycycline, methacycline) 0.2 g 6 times a day. In order to prevent complications due to the antibiotics, dimedrol, 0.03 g 2-3 times a day, and vitamins (B1; B6, B12, C, K) should be given. A 40 per cent glucose solution should be infused to patients with marked toxaemia.

It should be given in the amount of 20-40 ml. A 5 per cent glucose should be given in the amount of 500-1000 ml. Isotonic sodium chloride solution or sodium hydrocarbonate should be given in marked acidosis. Haemodez, rheopolyglucin and plasma can also be given. Lasix, furosemide and other diuretics should be given if liquid is retained in the patient.

Cordiamine, camphor, caffeine, ephedrine, adrenaline and strophanthin should be used to correct cardiovascular disorders.

Prevention and control: Quarantine is necessary. The presence of natural nidi in various countries and reports of plague cases in them indicate possible export of the disease to other countries. The anti-plague measures should be taken in airports, sea ports, and railway border posts in accordance with the international requirements. Persons with plague should be detected and isolated. Those suspected for plague should also be isolated and observed. All persons who had contacts with plague patients should be observed. Objects suspected for contamination should be examined bacteriologically. Vaccination is necessary.

Current and final disinfection, disinsection, deratization and quarantine measures are necessary. Special anti-plague institutions should be involved in prevention and anti-epidemic measures in natural nidi of plague. The complex to antiplague preventive measures includes the following: (1) epidemiologic surveillance; (2) rodent control (deratization) and destruction of the flea vector (disinsection); (3) vaccination of population against plague; (4) health education of population. Eradication of natural nidi located mostly in remote locations is an expensive measure. In this connection the species structure and populations of rodents and their ectoparasites should be systematically controlled in enzootic areas.

Laboratory examinations are necessary for timely detection of epizootics, extermination of rodents and ectoparasites in populated places and the surrounding areas. Deratization and disinsection measures should be taken on the territories of the epizootic zone. Dry live vaccine is used for specific immunization of people. Vaccination should be done for epidemiologic indications. Dry live vaccine induces a 6-month long immunity in the vaccinated. The vaccine is given by cutireaction.

If plague is detected or suspected, measures should be taken to localize and eliminate the focus. These measures include: (1) revealing and hospitalization of patients, revealing and isolation of persons who had contacts with patients, the dead, or with infected materials; (2) revealing and burying the dead; (3) carrying out disinfection, disinsection and deratization in the focus, in populated places and in the field; (4) observation of population in the focus; provisional hospitalization of all patients with fever, lymphadenitis, tonsillitis, and pharyngitis; (5) establishing quarantines or restriction in migration of population; (6) epizootiologic examination of the focus and the adjacent areas; (7) vaccination of population for indications. The epidemiologic studies should be conducted by a special group into which personnel of the anti-plague institutions should be included. Plague patients and people suspected for plague are placed in Tularaemia 28 i special hospitals.

Any room is suitable for preliminary isolation. All people must be removed from the room where the patient was present. The plague case should immediately be reported to higher medical authorities. Each hospitalized patient must be placed in a separate room or at least screened from the other patients in the room. The hospital must be guarded. The personnel must wear special anti-plague overalls. Persons who had contacts with plague patients should be isolated for 6 days. Persons who had contacts with pulmonic plague patients should be isolated in individual rooms. All persons who had contacts with patients or the dead (with pediculosis) must have their body temperature measured at least twice a day and must be given. Preventive treatment for 5 days with doxycycline (0.2 g once a day\= intramuscularly) or tetracycline (0.5 g three times a day). The dead must be buried in coffins (or without coffins) to a depth of 1.5-2 metres. Dry chlorinated lime should be placed on the bottom of the grave.

The dead can be burned. If hospitalization of all contacts is impossible in view of their multitude, observation is especially important. People should be observed at home with obligatory thermometry. Patients with fever should be examined by the physician (who must establish the preliminary diagnosis) and sent to the corresponding hospital. Whenever necessary, observation should be combined with vaccination and health education of population. Current disinfection in the focus should be conducted when taking care of patients, during evacuation of patients and persons who had contacts with them. Final disinfection should be conducted in residential houses after evacuation of the patients and contacts, and also after burying the dead. Disinsection and deratization should also be conducted.

SALMONELLOSIS

Aetiology: The disease is caused by a large group of microorganisms -Salmonellae, counting about 2000 serotypes. Salmonellae include two antigen complexes; O (somatic) and H (flagellar) antigens. The international classification of Salmonellae is based on the antigen structure. About 700 serotypes have been isolated in man. Most common of them are S. typhimurium, S. Heidelberg, S. london, S. cholerae-suis, S. derbi, S. enteritidis, S. anatum. Salmonellae are stable to low temperatures, and survive over winter in field conditions in animal faeces. They withstand absence of moisture and survive in dry dung for 90 days, in home dust for 80 days, in dry animal faeces for 4 years. A 0.5 per cent chloramine solution kills salmonellae in one hour; a 3 per cent solution, in 30 minutes.

Epidemiology: The source of infection is man and animal. The main epidemiologic role belongs to animals in which the disease is clinically manifest or is characterized by the carrier state. From an infected animal the microorganisms are released with faeces, urine, milk, saliva, and nasal discharge. Infected cattle and pigs are the greatest danger. Horses, sheep, cats, dogs and rodents (mice and rats) can also be the source of infection. Birds, especially waterfowl, in which the salmonellae can be found not only in flesh but in the eggs as well, are also important epidemiologically.

Examination of animals and their meat reveals salmonellae in cattle (from 1 to 5 per cent), in pigs (from 5 to 15 per cent), in sheep (from 4 to 30 per cent), and in ducks and geese (to 50 per cent). Mice and rats are carriers in about 40 per cent of cases, and about 10 per cent of cats and dogs are carriers too. Human patients and carriers are also the source of infection. People working at kindergartens, food catering and the like establishments are a special danger for the surrounding people. The transmission factors are foods in which salmonellae not only survive but also multiply. Man is usually infected by ingestion of meat, milk, fish, etc. heavily infested with salmonellae as a result of inadequate handling, cooking, and storage.

Meat can be infected during slaughter of the diseased animals, as a result of neglected sanitary rules at slaughterhouses (intestinal contents of the diseased animals can get on meat of slaughtered healthy animals), during transportation, improper cooking and processing, and storage. Contact infection is possible during intimate association with a patient or a carrier, less frequently with animals. Infants are mostly infected by contact. Nosocomial (intrahospital) outbreaks of salmonellosis are possible in children, who are weakened by coexisting diseases, especially premature infants, neonates, infants under two years of age, asthenic persons, patients with other diseases and the aged. Since salmonellae are stable in the environment, they can be distributed with water and dust. People are quite sensitive toward toxins produced by salmonellae, and outbreaks of the disease are therefore possible among people who ingest food infected with salmonellae and their toxins.

The incidence of salmonellosis is higher during the warm (especially hot) season since the conditions for multiplication of salmonellae are most favourable during this seasons, and besides, the incidence of the disease among cattle is also the highest in summer.

Pathogenesis: An infectious process can begin only after living salmonellae (not only their toxins) reach the gastrointestinal tract. Part of the microorganisms are killed in the stomach, while the surviving salmonellae enter the small intestine and multiply in tissues (localized form). By the end of the incubation period, the macroorganisms are poisoned by endotoxins that are released from the dead salmonellae. The local response to the endotoxins is enteritis and gastrointestinal disorder.

In the generalized form of the disease, salmonellae pass through the lymphatic system of the intestine into the blood of the patients (typhoid form) and are carried to various organs (liver, spleen, kidneys) to form secondary foci (septic form). Endotoxins first of all acts on the vascular and nervous apparatus. This is manifested by increased permeability and decreased tone of the vessels, upset thermal regulation, vomiting and diarrhoea. In severe forms of the disease, much liquid and electrolytes are lost to upset the water-salt metabolism, to decrease the circulating blood volume and arterial pressure, and to cause hypovolaemic shock.

A septic shock can develop. Shock of mixed character (with signs of hypovolaemic and septic shock) are more common in severe salmonellosis. Oliguria and azotaemia develop in severe cases as a result of renal involvement due to hypoxia and toxaemia.

Clinical picture: The incubation period varies depending on the mechanism of infection and lasts from 6 to 24 hours, when salmonellae are ingested, and for 2 and more days if infection is transmitted by contact. The following forms of salmonellosis are distinguished: (1) gastrointestinal (localized), that runs a course similar to that of acute gastritis, gastroenteritis, or gastroenterocolitis; (2) generalized form, that runs a typhoid and septic course; (3) carrier state (acute, chronic, transient).

The gastrointestinal form: The onset is acute. The body temperature rises; weakness, headache, chill, nausea, vomiting develop; the appetite impairs, and the patient complains of epigastric pain. When the disease is at its height in 1-2 days, diarrhoea begins. Stools are usually ample, with admixtures of mucus, or watery, without pathological admixtures. The duration of the disease and its symptoms depend on severity of the disease. In mild forms the body temperature is normal or subfebrile, vomiting occurs only once, abdominal pain is not severe, stools are watery, five times a day. The patient recovers in 2-3 days. The liquid loss does not exceed 3 per cent of the body weight. The onset of salmonellosis of moderate severity is acute, the body temperature rises to 38-39°C and persists for 4 days; vomiting is repeated, stools are ample and fetid, to 10 times a day, cramps in the limbs are common.

The gastroenterocolitic form is characterized by mucous stools, sometimes with streaks of blood. Diarrhoea persists for 7 days. Tachycardia and dehydration of the first and second degree (liquid loss to 6 per cent) are possible. In severe cases, the symptoms manifest to their maximum extent already during the first hours of the disease. The temperature rises to 39°C, the patient develops chill, repeated vomiting, that rapidly becomes incoercible, and frequent (10-20 times a day) ample, fetid, watery stools. Diarrhoea lasts 6-7 days and more. If water-salt metabolism is upset (dehydration of the second or third degree), the patient develops cramps, pallor with a cyanotic hue, skin dryness, and hoarse voice that transforms into aphopia. The loss of moisture is from 7 to 10 per cent of body weight. The amount of urine excreted decreases; pathological admixtures appear, such as protein, erythrocytes and casts. Arterial pressure falls, tachycardia develops.

The generalized form: The disease can begin with gastroenteritis or fever without signs of this disease, whose clinical manifestations are similar to those of typhoid and paratyphoid fever. The septic form, which usually occurs in infants, is characterized by acyclic character, prolonged and severe course, remittent fever, chills and profuse sweats, tachycardia, spleno- and hepatomegaly. Secondary septicopyemic foci of various localization (pneumonia, pleurisy, osteomyelitis, arthritis, tonsillitis, cervical purulent lymphadenitis, meningitis) are formed.

Carrier state: Acute and chronic carrier state occur in convalescents. Acute carrier state probably lasts to 3 months, chronic over three months. A transient carrier state is characterized by the absence of clinical symptoms of the disease, the bacillus is isolated only once or twice at 1 day interval with subsequent negative cultures and reactions of indirect haemagglutination with salmonellous diagnosticum.

Complications: Pancreatitis, cholecystitis, cholangitis, chronic colitis, abscesses of the brain, liver or kidneys are among possible complications. Localized forms can be complicated by septic shock, acute heart failure, and renal failure.

Diagnosis: The diagnosis is based on clinical findings, a thoroughly collected epidemiologic anamnesis and laboratory findings. Bacteriologic studies should be performed as early as possible (before commencement of treatment). Blood taken from the ulnar vein in sterile conditions in quantity of 5-10 ml is cultivated in 50-100 ml of bile culture medium or Rappoport medium. Vomitus (50-100 g) and gastric washing water (100-200 ml) are taken in sterile flasks; excretions (4-5 g) are taken into a sterile test tube containing a glycerol mixture; urine (20-50 ml) is taken in a sterile bottle or a test tube; pus (in septic form of the disease) is taken from secondary foci. Suspected food (in the quantity of 50-60 g from various portions, taken in a sterile bottle) should also be delivered to the laboratory.

A preliminary result is ready in 2 days and the final result in 4 days. Direct and indirect haemagglutination reactions can be performed in a week (1 ml of blood). The result of the indirect haemagglutination reaction is ready in 4-6 days of the disease. The test is positive if the serum dilution is 1: 160 and over. Immunofluorescence test is used for rapid diagnosis.

Treatment: Mild forms of the disease can be treated at home. For detoxication, it is necessary to perform gastric lavage with ample warm water (2-3 litres) or a 2-3 per cent sodium hydrocarbonate solution. If salmonellosis is of mild or moderate severity, and vomiting or marked toxaemia are absent, the patient is given salt solutions per os. The amount of liquid given must comply with the amount of liquid lost. If toxaemia is marked while dehydration is mild, these solutions must be given by intravenous drip (40-60 drops per minute). If the course of the disease is severe (dehydration of the 3rd or 4th degree) a polyionic solution should be given at a rate of 80-120 ml/min.

The volume of the solution that is given to replenish the liquid lost, depends on the degree of dehydration (4-8 litres and over). After haemodynamic stabilization, termination of vomiting, and restoration of the excretory function of the kidneys, the patient can be given liquid per os. If adrenal insufficiency develops, the patient should be given prednisolone (60-90 mg) or hydrocortizone (125-250 mg) intravenously; later (in 4-6 hours) these preparations can be given by intravenous drip. Desoxycorticosterone acetate should be given intramuscularly (5-10 mg at 12-hour intervals). In order to restore the gastrointestinal function, the patient can be given festal, panzynorm, cholenzyme, etc., and also preparations restoring the intestinal microflora (bifidumbacterin, colibacterin, lactobacterin, etc.).

Antacids, e.g. white clay, bismuth preparations, should also be given. In typhoid forms of salmonellosis the patient should be given (in addition to detoxicating, rehydrating and desensitizing therapy) chloramphenicol sodium succinate (30-50 mg per kg of body mass a day) or chloramphenicol (0.5 g 4 times a day for 10-12 days), and ampicillin (1 g 4-6 times a day for 8-10 days).

Septic forms should be treated with ampicillin in combination with surgery of purulent foci. It is important to prescribe a proper diet to the patient. Vitamins are also necessary. The patient is recommended to eat oat and rice porridges (without milk), boiled fish, steam-cooked minced meat, fruit jellies, curds and sweet cheese during the first days of the disease.

Prevention and control: Prevention of salmonellosis includes veterinary and medical measures with respect to the source of infection and ways of infection transmission. Veterinary service acts to improve the condition of animals by timely isolation of the diseased animals and their treatment, decontamination of milk and other animal materials obtained from the diseased animals. It is prohibited to the affected animals slaughter (in case of emergency) together with healthy animals.

Healthy cattle should be slaughtered immediately after delivery to the slaughterhouse. Meat obtained from diseased cattle can be utilized only after a prolonged thermal treatment. Veterinary inspection must be effective at all stages of handling of animal materials, beginning with the slaughterhouse, transportation, thermal and other treatment, and storage of cooked food at low temperatures. Roddent control is another requisite condition. In order to locate the source of infection, all persons with acute intestinal diseases of unknown aetiology should be examined for carrier state. Those who develop intestinal dysfunction during their stay in hospital, all infants under two years of age that are admitted to somatic hospitals, should also be tested for carrier state.

All persons who are hired for work in food catering and similar establishments, and also children who are prepared for admission to children's institutions should be tested for carrier state as well. Salmonellosis patients may be isolated at home conditions or taken to hospital. Persons working at food catering and the like establishments, children visiting kindergartens, and infants under two years, who may or may not attend preschool children's institutions, should be hospitalized. Convalescent persons who work in food catering and the like establishments should be discharged from hospital after a complete clinical recovery and three successive negative stool cultures. (The first test should be performed in 3 days after completion of the specific therapy, the other two tests follow at 1-day intervals).

If cultures are positive, the person may not be admitted to perform his routine duties for 15 days after discharge from hospital. Meanwhile they are employed at jobs that do not present epidemiologic danger. Their faeces are tested three times. If a new examination reveals carrier state again, the tests should be repeated at 15-day intervals. If carrier state persists for more than 3 months, the person is considered a chronic carrier and must change his occupation for a year.

Three stool cultures and one bile culture (1-2 days later) should be cultivated a year later. If the cultures are positive again, the person should be dismissed from food catering and similar establishments. Children-carriers of antibiotic-resistant salmonellae should not be admitted to kindergartens. Schoolchildren can be allowed to attend school, but they are not allowed to help their mates in canteens.

Current disinfection should be performed at home before the patient is hospitalized or if the patient remains at home till recovery. After hospitalization or recovery of the patient, his apartment should undergo final disinfection. Persons who took care of the patient must be observed for 7 days. Persons who had contacts with the patient, or persons who work at food catering and similar establishments, and also children attending kindergartens and schools should be tested (once) for carrier state. If a group of persons are all taken ill, they are given medical aid and epidemiologic studies are undertaken to reveal the particular food that caused the disease outbreak. Circumstances under which this was contaminated should be established. Preventive measures against salmonellosis should be performed by epidemiologists and sanitary physicians.

ANTHRAX

Aetiology: The disease is caused by Bacillus anthracis. It is an aerobic spore-forming bacillus that is rapidly destroyed in the absence of air, when heated to 75-80°C, or when acted upon with disinfectants. In the presence of oxygen, the bacillus forms spores that are highly stable in the environment. Under beneficial conditions it can survive for years. These conditions include uncultivated soils in dry climates protected from direct sunlight and also underlying soil layers. In surface layers of soil, the spores pass into the prevegetative stage and are partly killed. Spores resist drying and high temperature (boiling kills them in 60 minutes); the spores also resist the action of disinfectants.

Epidemiology: The source of the anthrax bacillus are animals with acute disease (septicaemia type). Domesticated animals, such as cattle, goats and sheep, horses, deer, pigs and camels, are of primary epidemiologic importance. A diseased human is not infectious. An individual is infected during slaughtering or skinning cattle, processing infected meat, and when attending diseased animals. The transmission mechanism depends on the form of the anthrax agent.

The vegetative form is transmitted by contact; the infection can be transmitted by the bite of blood sucking insects, or by ingestion of infected meat. Spores can be inhaled by humans with dusty air. Occupational (industrial and agricultural) and non-occupational anthrax are distinguished. Industrial anthrax occurs due to inhalation of the spores during processing of infected animal materials (hides, wool, hair, etc.). In rural areas humans get infected during slaughtering, skinning, dissecting infected carcasses, preparing food from infected meat, and when attending the diseased animals.

Non-occupational anthrax develops due to accidental infection, usually with the spores. The incidence of anthrax among people depends directly on the incidence of the disease in domestic animals and efficiency of preventive measures. Sporadic cases are more common. Group incidence of the disease (usually infected from one source) are less frequent. Humans are highly susceptible to anthrax. Adults are usually afflicted. Stable immunity is produced in those who sustained the disease. Seasonal variations in the morbidity are associated with increasing incidence of the disease among animals and increasing populations of blood-sucking insects.

Pathogenesis: The portal of entry are injured skin and mucosa. Two clinical forms of the disease occur in humans: cutaneous and septicaemic anthrax. The septicaemic form can be both primary and secondary (complicated cutaneous form of the disease). The cutaneous form is more common than septicaemic anthrax. The skin of the arms, head or other exposed parts of the body are involved.

A pustule develops at the portal of the anthrax agent entrance. It is a serous-haemorrhagic inflammation of the skin and subcutaneous fat with subsequent necrosis, oedema, and regional lymphadenitis. If the body resistance is low, the agent enters the blood and multiplies to cause primary septicaemia. Involvement of the regional lymphatics is attended by severe oedema and necrosis. General infection develops, which is manifested by increasing bacteraemia and toxaemia. Toxaemia is attended by sudden rises in the body temperature, cardiovascular disorders, and shock, which is the cause of death.

Clinical picture: The incubation period lasts from 2 to 14 days in the cutaneous form and from several hours to 6-8 days in septicaemic anthrax. Cutaneous anthrax. The disease begins with development of a Skin Infections 289 pruritic spot at the portal of infection entrance. The erythematous spot rapidly develops to a copper-red papule and then a vesicle (pustule) containing cloudy sanguinous fluid. Because of severe itching, the patient scratches the pustule; sometimes the pustule ruptures spontaneously, and a black eschar forms and grows in size.

The eschar looks like coal (hence the name, anthrax, which means in Greek coal or carbuncle). Secondary pustules develop around the eschar and undergo the same stages of development. Infiltration develops under the crust. It rises above the intact skin level in the form of a brown-red ridge. The carbuncle is surrounded by a massive oedema of the skin and subcutaneous fat. The oedema is especially marked on the skin with underlying loose connective tissue. Lymphadenitis is common. Only one lymph node is usually enlarged. It becomes firm, mobile and painless.

During the first hours of the disease the patient complains of headache, lassitude and malaise. In 2-3 days, the body temperature rises to 39-40°C. Signs of toxicosis develop: headache intensifies, weakness and lassitude become more pronounced, the cardiovascular system becomes involved (the pulse is fast, small and sometimes arrhythmic; arterial pressure is low). The liver and the spleen are enlarged. The general symptoms are less pronounced in cutaneous anthrax and the patient can continue performing his routine duties. The condition improves in 5-8 days. The body temperature decreases, oedema gradually subsides. By the end of the 2nd or 4th week, the crust falls off and the ulcer rapidly heals to leave a scar. Cutaneous anthrax can be complicated by septicaemia.

Septicaemic anthrax: The disease begins suddenly with elevation of temperature to 39°C, chill, weakness, headache, non-productive cough, and dyspnoea. Diffuse abdominal pain is possible. Numerous haemorrhages develop. The temperature rises to 40-41°C. Severe toxaemia damages the vessels and thus evokes the haemor: rhagic syndrome in many organs and tissues (the lungs and intestine included). In view of this, pulmonary (inhalation) and intestinal variants of septicaemic anthrax are distinguished. Inhalation anthrax is characterized by pneumonia with oedema of the lungs and haemorrhagic pleurisy.

Cough intensifies, sputum is first seromucous and then rusty (haemoptysis). The intestinal form of anthrax is manifested by severe stabbing pain in the abdomen, vomiting with bile and blood, and bloody diarrhoea. Symptoms of intestinal obstruction develop later due to paresis of the intestine. Septicaemic anthrax is characterized by euphoria, delirium, convulsions and the meningeal syndrome. Pulse is fast and weak (thready); arterial pressure falls. The patient dies of septic shock during the first day (less frequently on the second day) of the disease. Haematologic studies show high leucocyte count (to 20-25 x 109/1) and neutrophilia with the shift to the left.

Diagnosis: The diagnosis of anthrax in human is based on epizootologic, epidemiologic, clinical and laboratory findings. Cutaneous anthrax should be differentiated from furunculosis, carbunculosis, erysipelas, insect bites, ulceroglandular tularaemia, bubonic plague, and glanders. Excretions and blood should be examined in the laboratory (preferably before treatment begins). Contents of vesicles, carbuncles and ulcers are taken with a syringe, pipette or a sterile tampon. The skin around the carbuncle should be carefully cleaned with alcohol. Blood specimen (1 ml) should preferably be taken during the fever period.

Venous blood (1-2 drops) are inoculated into a nutrient medium (agar or Hottinger's broth); two thin smears are also made on glass slides. Samples of animal material, such as pieces of hide, wool, hairs (20-30 g) should be sent to the laboratory whenever necessary. Soil (200 g) and water (at least 1 litre) should also be examined. Materials taken from the patient and animal specimens should be placed into sterile boxes, bottles, or other laboratory glassware. Dry smears are placed in Petri dishes and wrapped in dense paper. The pack must be labelled: "smear is not fixed". The lable must also contain information on the place and time of taking the sample, the name of the material, and the presumptive diagnosis. The name of the patient must be written on the label too. The specimens should be placed in a special sealed box. The box should be handled with care and not overthrown. The luminescent method, thermoprecipitation, and detection of capsule formation are used in the laboratory.

The tests are preliminary, and negative results do not exclude anthrax. Bacterioscopy and cultures help isolate and identify the anthrax agent. Inoculation of albino mice, guinea pigs or rabbits (biologic tests) is performed simultaneously with inoculation of cultures. The experimental animals are observed for 10 days. Smears are prepared from blood and organs of the dead animals; corresponding cultures are also grown. Preliminary conclusion can be formulated in 3-5 hours and the final is ready in 4 days. The final diagnosis is established only on the basis of the complex studies. A skin allergic test with dilute immunoglobulin can be conducted on the first day of the disease. It is positive by the end of the first week in almost all patients.

Treatment: Patients with mild cutaneous anthrax should be given antibiotics alone, better penicillin: 500000-1000000 units intramuscularly 6-8 times a day for 5-7 days. Next come the tetracyclines (tetracycline, oxytetracycline). They are given per os, 0.3 g 4 times a day for 5-7 days. In patients with moderate and severe diseases intravenous perfusion of fluids should be given in the volume sufficient to replenish the volume of circulating blood, to abate dyspnoea, cyanosis, and thirst (2-5 litres daily). Polyglucin, rheopolyglucin or haemodez should be added (400 ml). From 90 to 120 mg of prednisolone, cardiac glycosides (0.25-0.5 ml of a 0.05 per cent strophanthin or 0.5-1.0 ml of a 0.06 per cent corglycon solution), and 1 000 000 units of penicillin should be included into the perfusion system.

The remaining penicillin (from 7000000 to 12000000 U) should be given intramuscularly during a day. Specific anti-anthrax immunoglobulin is given in the absence of increased sensitivity of the patient to immunoglobulin (40-50 ml, in a single intramuscular injection). If the skin test with dilute immunoglobulin is positive or if an anaphylactic reaction develops to subcutaneous administration of immunoglobulin, the anti-anthrax immunoglobulin should be administered only after premedication with 90-120 mg of prednisolone.

Prevention and control: Control of anthrax among domestic animals includes veterinary sanitation. It also includes timely revealing, isolation and treatment of diseased animals, their protection from insect bites, and decontamination of faeces. Diseased animals should be killed by a bloodless method in order to prevent formation of spores. Killed animals should be burned. Utilization of killed animals or their burying is prohibited. Herds of animals where anthrax cases were registered should be observed. It is prohibited to pasture cattle on meadows suspected for infection with anthrax.

Cattle may not be allowed to drink water from suspected ponds or other water bodies. Pastures should be given sanation treatment. Animals should be vaccinated with a live attenuated vaccines. Prophylaxis of the disease among humans includes adherence to safety requirements when attending diseased cattle, slaughtering cattle, and when performing jobs such as skinning, processing of hides and wool, etc. Hides should be pickled (treated with a 2.5 per cent hydrochloric acid and a 15 per cent sodium chloride solution at a temperature of 30°C for 40 hours).

Wool should be treated with steam at 100-110°C or with a steam-formaldehyde mixture at 62-65°C for 2 1/2 hours. Furs should be given similar treatment. Current and final disinfection are required. Preventive disinfection should be conducted at least twice a year at animal farms, slaughterhouses, at plants processing animal materials, in storehouses, and in vehicles used for transportation of cattle and animal products. Workers should wear protective overalls, they should be provided with disinfectant solutions and means of individual protection: goggles, masks, etc. If a given batch of animal material is suspected for anthrax, its specimens should be sent to the laboratory for Ascoli's thermoprecipitation test.

Specimens of wool, fur, hide, etc. (20-30 g) should be handled in sterile test tubes. The specific prophylaxis of anthrax among population should be conducted with special live vaccine. Only people exposed to the danger of contamination should be vaccinated. Vaccine is given in a single dose, either subcutaneously or by scarification. Revaccinations should be repeated each year. For epidemic indications, the vaccine should preferably be given subcutaneously by jet injections. Contraindications are the same as for other vaccinations.

The patient should be hospitalized. Cutaneous anthrax convalescents should be discharged from hospital after cicatrization of the ulcer and falling off of the crust. Septicaemic anthrax patients can be discharged from hospital after abatement of clinical symptoms. Final disinfection should be done in the focus of infection. Epizootologic and epidemiologic studies are necessary. Contacts should be disjoined but they require medical observation during 8 days. The same measure is necessary in those who had contacts with diseased animals, pathologic materials, and in those who used infected meat as food.

Anti-anthrax immunoglobulin is recommended for prophylactic purpose. The immunoglobulin is given to persons attending the diseased animals, engaged in burying the dead, in processing meat of diseased animals, or to those who took this meat as food. Rapid prophylaxis can be done with antibiotics and anti-anthrax immunoglobulin. Phenoxymethylpenicillin should be given in a dose of 1 g twice a day for 5 days, or tetracycline 0.5 g twice a day for 5 days.

Other antibiotics can also be given: ampicillin (1 g twice a day) or oxacillin (1 g twice a day). Adults should be given 20-25 ml of immunoglobulin for prophylactic purposes. Adolescents should be given doses less than 12 ml; children should be given from 5 to 8 ml.

Immunoglobulin should be warmed before intramuscular injections. Individual sensitivity to horse protein should first be tested by intracutaneous test. Immunoglobulin is useless if more than 10 days have passed since the day of contact or more than 5 days after ingestion of infected meat.

LEPTOSPIROSIS

Aetiology: The causative agents of leptospirosis belong to the family of Spirochetaceae, the genus Leptospira. Leptospira contains two complexes: interrogans and biflexa. Each complex has antigenic variations, serovars. Serotypes with common antigens are arranged in serogroups: Icterohaemorrhagiae, Autumnalis, Canicola, Australis, Pyrogenes, Javanica, Pomona, Ballum, Cynopteri, Celledoni, Semaranga, Andamana. Leptospiras survive in moist environment. In water bodies they remain viable for 30 days and more, in soil for 3 months, on foods for several days. Leptospiras withstand low temperatures but are sensitive to high temperature and absence of moisture. Boiling kills them instantaneously.

Epidemiology: The main reservoir of the infection are roddents: common rats, voles, harvest mice, etc. Another source of infection are leptospirosis cattle, swines, horses, sheep, goats, dogs, and also clinically recovered animals. Human patients are practically safe for the surrounding people. Natural, anthropurgic, and mixed foci of infection are distinguished. Natural foci of leptospirosis usually occur in the vicinity of rivers, lakes, swamps and moist soils.

The infection is transmitted from roddents (which are chronic carriers of the infection) to humans by direct contact and through water or food during agricultural work, fishing, picking mushrooms, drinking water from occasional open sources of water, bathing, walking barefoot, or eating food contaminated with the leptospiras. Leptospirosis incidence rises in the end of summer and early autumn. Cattle, hogs, dogs, and rats are the reservoir of infection in the anthropurgic foci. Poultry and wild birds can also be involved in epizootics.

Leptospirosis usually runs a severe course in cattle, especially in calves. In swines, leptospirosis is usually characterized by mild clinical symptoms. The animals shed leptospiras in their urine. Leptospira carrier state can persist from a month to a year and longer. The main factor transmitting the infection from the diseased animals to man is water. Humans (especially persons with an empty stomach) get infected by drinking contaminated water, or when bathing in an open water body infected with the animal excrements. Leptospira penetrates through the mucosa of the mouth, eyes, nose, and through abraded skin during bathing, when working barefoot on rice plantation, etc. Less frequently man is infected by drinking milk of diseased animals or by ingesting food contaminated with the infected urine.

Man is also infected by contact with the infected objects, when taking care of diseased animals, during slaughtering diseased animals, and processing their tissues. Common brown rats are the source of infection in large cities, especially in sea ports. Deratizators and sanitary workers are especially exposed to the danger of infection. Outbreaks and sporadic infection cases are possible among stevedores and miners. In anthropurgic foci, leptospirosis occurs during the whole year in the form of sporadic cases.

Pathogenesis: Motility of leptospiras helps them overcome the defense barriers and enter the blood circulating system. Blood carries them to various organs, mainly to the liver, kidneys, spleen, lungs, etc. This process is actually the incubation period. The onset of the disease is characterized by re-entry of the decayed leptospira and their metabolites into the blood which carries them to various organs and tissues, especially to the kidneys, the adrenal glands, the liver, and the meninges.

Beginning with the second week of the disease, in connection with marked toxaemia, the capillaries are damaged, their permeability increases to cause the haemorrhagic syndrome (bleeding into the internal organs and the skin). Lesion of the liver cells and, to a lesser degree, red cell haemolysis due to the effect of leptospiral haemolysins, evoke jaundice. Complications in the kidneys, the nervous system and the eyes can develop during this period. Leptospiras are liberated into the environment with urine for several weeks. They can be detected also in the liquor. Recovery begins with the production of immunity to the specific serotype.

Clinical picture: The incubation period varies from 6 to 20 days (usually from 7 to 12 days). Anicteric and icteric forms of leptospirosis are differentiated. The onset of the disease is sudden and acute. The patient complains of chill, his temperature quickly rises to 38-40°C. The common symptoms are weakness, lassitude, persistent headache, insomnia, myalgia (especially in the calves and the neck). The face is hyperaemic, the scleral vessels injected, with haemorrhage into the sclera, the tongue is coated and dry. Scarlatina-like and measles-like rash develops in 4-5 days. Roseolas and petechiae are less frequent (usually in severe cases). Rash appears instantaneously on the chest, abdomen and the limbs.

The liver is enlarged and tender to palpation. Some patients develop the haemorrhagic syndrome at the beginning of the second week: petechiae on the skin, ecchymosis at the sites of injection, nasal, gastric, intestinal, and uterine haemorrhages, blood spitting, haemorrhage in the brain, myocardium and other organs. The platelet count is low. Symptoms of nephritis can develop. In mild cases, the urine of patients contains small amounts of protein, single red cells, white cells, and hyaline casts. In anicteric cases, jaundice is either absent or mild.

Severe disease is characterized by high body temperature that persists for 6-10 days. In the icteric form of the disease, the sclera and then the skin turn yellow in 3-5 days of the disease. The urine is also dark. The conjugated bilirubin of blood is high. After jaundice develops, the body temperature decreases critically or by an accelerated lysis. The patient's condition improves. Oliguria develops from the very first days of the disease, and becomes especially marked in 7-10 days. The protein level in the urine is high; the quantity of red and white cells, of hyaline and granular casts is also increased. Rest nitrogen of blood increases too.

If the disease runs a benign course and treatment begins in due time, oliguria is superseded by polyuria in the end of the second week; the pathological changes in the urine gradually subside. If the course of the disease is unfavourable, death is possible due to renal failure and uraemia. Haematologic changes include hypochromic anaemia, low haemoglobin (to 64-80 g/L), thrombocytopenia, leucocytosis (10-12 x 109/L), neutrophilosis with a shift to the left, aneosinophilia, and lymphopenia; ESR accelerates to 50-60 mm/h. In 5-6 days after normalization of body temperature, some patients develop an exacerbation. Fever during the relapse lasts from 3 to 9 days.

Complications: Severe leptospirosis can be complicated by renal failure, acute hepatorenal failure, acute cardiovascular failure, haemorrhage, myocarditis, meningitis, encephalitis, pneumonia, otitis, and diseases of the eye.

Diagnosis: The diagnosis is based on clinical and epidemiologic findings. It is necessary to examine blood taken from the ulnar vein during the first 4-5 days of the disease; 2 ml should be used for microscopy, and 4 ml for cultivating a blood culture on a water-serum medium (distilled water and rabbit serum). Nutrient medium (5 ml) should preferably be inoculated with the patient's blood straight at the bedside.

From 5 to 10 drops of the material should be added to each test tube. A 4-ml specimen of blood is defibrinated and injected to guinea pigs and 2-3 week-old rabbits (0.5-2 ml). Cerebrospinal fluid is examined in the presence of indications. The urine is taken in sterile conditions (0.5-1 ml) on the second week of the disease and later. Nutrient media are inoculated with the urine in 3-4 test tubes.

Blood (2 ml) is tested in the laboratory on the 7-8th day: microscopic agglutination and lysis reactions are carried out with live leptospira cultures; the complement fixation test is also performed. Paired serums should be tested because the specific antibodies persist in convalescents from few months to several years. Direct haemagglutination test and the immunofluorescent method are also used.

Treatment: Treatment should be early and complex. Mild forms can be treated symptomatically and by proper diet and vitamins. Mild and moderate diseases should be treated with penicillin (3 000000-4000000 U daily intramuscularly until body temperature normalizes and then for 2-3 days more). Detoxication therapy is also necessary. Severe forms should be treated with penicillin in doses to 10-16 million U daily.

Polyvalent leptospiral immunoglobulin containing antibodies to common leptospiras, that are pathogenic to man, should also be administered. Immunoglobulin is first tested for tolerance by the patient and then administered intramuscularly in doses of 3 ml for children from 8 to 13 years of age, and 5-10 ml for older children and adults. Treatment continues for 3 days. In the presence of symptoms of cardiovascular insufficiency, cardiotonics and glucocorticoids are prescribed.

In cases with acute renal failure and oliguria, a 20 per cent mannitol solution (300 ml), a 20 per cent glucose solution (500 ml), and a 4 per cent sodium bicarbonate solution (150-200 ml) should be administered by drip infusion in two sessions. The anuria stage of acute renal failure should be treated with haemodialysis (artificial kidney apparatus).

Prevention and control: Prophylactic measures should be taken against all epidemic factors: the source of infection, transmission routes, and susceptibility of population. Health care and veterinary supervision systems are responsible for the detection and isolation of diseased animals and leptospira carriers, for vaccination of the animals in the anthropurgic foci. The condition of the water supply system should be supervised. Sources of drinking water should be protected against contamination with animal excrements.

If leptospirosis cases are revealed among people or animals, it is prohibited to use water from open reservoirs for drinking or other domestic needs if these water bodies were the watering place of the diseased animals.

Water from these open bodies can be used again only in 3-4 weeks after elimination of the cause of infection. If water is suspected for being infected with leptospira, it can be used only after boiling. All agricultural workers should be instructed how to prevent abrasion or other minor damage to the skin of the legs and arms (wearing rubber boots, gloves, etc.). Swamps should be irrigated in areas where leptospirosis is revealed.

Deratization should be carried out in cities and towns. Milk of leptospirosis cattle containing the yellow pigment or traces of blood should be decontaminated by boiling and then used for feeding animals. In the absence of visible changes, boiled milk can be used as food. When milking and taking care of leptospirosis cattle, rules of individual protection should be observed. Animals may not be slaughtered during the acute period of the disease. If any changes are found in the organs of slaughtered animals (jaundice, haemorrhage), meat should be used for technical purposes only or after adequate thermal processing.

Hides of the dead or slaughtered animals should be processed with observation of all precautions and then used without any restrictions after drying for 10 days. All persons habitating the areas where there is a danger of leptospirosis infection should be immunized with specific inactivated vaccine; the vaccine is administered in two doses-2 and 2.5 ml (for adults) with a 7-10 day interval between the injections. Children aged over 7 years can be vaccinated too. Revaccination with a single 2 ml dose is necessary in 12 months. Vaccination produces immunity against the commonest pathogenic agents. An attenuated leptospiral vaccine has been recently developed.

Each detected or suspected leptospirosis case should be reported to the higher authority in a given locality. All patients should be registered and hospitalized. Disinfection measures are the same as for intestinal infections.

RICKETTSIAL DISEASES

EPIDEMIC TYPHUS

Aetiology: The causative agent of epidemic typhus is Rickettsia prowazeki. The microorganisms are unstable in the environment but in dry lice faeces they can live from one to several months. The rickettsia can be found in the body of epidemic typhus patient, inside cells of intestinal epithelium of lice and in their faeces. The causative agent of Brill's disease (recrudescent typhus) is the same R. prowazeki which persists in humans as latent infection for long periods of time and causes relapses of the disease at various intervals.

Epidemiology: The only source of infection is a human patient with epidemic typhus who becomes contagious during the last days of the incubation period (2-3 days), during the entire fever period, and till the 7-8th day of the disease after normalization of body temperature. The overall length of the contagious period is 20-21 day. The infection is transmitted by body lice, less frequently by head lice. Body lice deposit their eggs on hair, in pleats and folds of underwear and clothes, while head lice lay them only on hair.

Eggs yield larvae which undergo triple sloughing before they grow to mature insects. This period lasts 7-10 days and should be taken into consideration when observing the focus and prescribing repeated sanitary treatment. When a louse sucks the blood of a typhus patient it becomes contagious in 4-5 days during which rickettsia multiply in the louse intestinal epithelium. After destruction of the epithelial cells the rickettsia gain entrance to the intestinal lumen and are excreted in great amount with faeces. When a louse sucks blood, it excretes a substance that causes itching. As a person scratches the site of a louse bite he rubs the faecal mass with rickettsia into the puncture wound and the scratch site. Contamination can occur when a crushed louse is rubbed into the skin.

An infected louse lives 20-40 days instead of 45-60 days and dies of the ruptured intestine. The incidence of epidemic typhus is characterized by seasonal variations, the highest incidence being during winter and spring. Seasonal variations are absent in Brill's disease; neither can any connection be established between sporadic cases. Head louse and body louse occurs usually in the aged, who often report epidemic typhus in their early history or their stay in the focus of typhus in past life. The quantity of rickettsia is not great in the blood of a Brill's disease patient with the disease in its full swing.

But such patients can become the source of infection if they are affected with pediculosis. Susceptibility to epidemic typhus is high; persons aged from 15 to 40 usually develop the disease. This can be explained by the intensive activity of people at this age. A sufficiently stable immunity develops in those who sustained the disease. The social factor is decisive in epidemiology of this disease. Famine, inadequate housing and sanitary conditions, absence of baths and disinsectants, poor sanitation of population, its intensive migration in connection with war, famine or other disasters promote dissemination of the infection.

Pathogenesis: The pathogenic microorganisms enter the body through scratched or bitten skin. Rickettsia invade the cells of vascular endothelium where they multiply and are carried by the blood stream to cause rickettsaemia. Part of the microorganisms die to release toxin which causes toxaemia. In fine vessels, rickettsia cause thrombi with subsequent proliferation of the vascular wall and around the vessel; thrombophlebitis and specific granuloma thus develop.

Vascular changes become manifest in 4-8 days of the disease in all organs and tissues, especially in the brain, skin, conjunctiva, adrenal glands, myocardium, spleen and the kidneys. These lesions are manifested by specific symptoms on the part of the nervous, psychic, and cardiovascular systems, skin and other organs and tissues. Organic changes develop in 18-20 days and their development terminates by the end of the 4th week and later. Rickettsia are not completely eliminated from some patients, and the process becomes latent with persistence of the microorganisms in the reticuloendothelial cells. Relapses (Brill's disease) can be provoked by overstrain, either physical or psychic, poisoning, variations of temperature, etc.

Clinical picture: The incubation period lasts from 6 to 25 days (usually 12-14 days). The onset of the disease is acute. The body temperature increases; headache, chills, malaise, and thirst develop; the patient loses appetite. Headache intensifies and becomes debilitating; insomnia develops. Irritability and anxiety of the first days are then followed by excitation. Increasing symptoms, especially weakness and fever, force the patient into bed on the 2-3rd day of the disease.

Hyperaemic and swollen face, hyperaemic conjunctiva, injected and dilated scleral vessels (rabbit eyes) are seen during the first days of the disease. The skin of the neck and the upper trunk is also hyperaemic. The tongue is dry and is difficult to protrude (Godelier's sign). The skin is dry and hot to feel. Dyspnoea (central), moderate tachycardia and hypotension are seen. Petechial haemorrhages can develop in 3 days on the conjunctival fold; the haemorrhages also appear on the shoulder or the thigh, below the point where a tourniquet is applied.

Specific rash appears on the 4-5th day of the disease by which the initial period of the disease ends. During the period of the disease in full swing the rash is first represented by roseoles which later change to petechia. Rash develops on the flanks, chest, and the back, covers the whole body. It is intensive and its elements are different in size: from the size of a pin-head to that of a lentil. In moderate cases rash persists till the

12-14th day. As rash develops, fever intensifies and becomes continuous or remitting, and remains so for 6-8 days. The height of the fever period is characterized by moderate neutrophilic leucocytosis (to 9-11 x 109/L), thrombocytopenia and aneosinophilia; ESR is high (18-25 mm/h). The initial symptoms intensify with appearance of skin eruption, and new symptoms supervene. Involvement of the nervous system increases. Consciousness is dimmed, hallucination and delirium develop, the patient is restless, tries to raise in his bed or run. This condition, in the presence of high fever, is known as status typhosus. Symptoms of meningoencephalitis develop: stiff neck,

Kernig and Brudzinski's symptoms, increased tendon reflex, tremor of the extremities, inarticulate speech, throat itching, and difficult swallowing. The heart sounds are dull, heart rate is fast, arterial pressure is low, collapse is possible. The liver and the spleen are enlarged. Constipation develops. Severely ill patients can defaecate and urinate involuntarily, or the urine can be passed in small portions while the bladder is overfilled. In 12-14 days of the disease, body temperature drops and the recovery phase begins. The fever resolves by an accelerated lysis within 2-3 days; less frequently the fall of temperature is critical. Toxaemia decreases and all its symptoms (status typhosus in the first instance) subside gradually.

Rash resolves, consciousness clears, the patient shows interest in the surrounding, sleep and appetite improve, urination normalizes, pulse and arterial pressure normalize as well. But despite the considerable improvement of the patient's general condition, weakness and pain in the legs and by the course of the nerve trunks persist for a long time. The central nervous system remains easily excitable. Mild, moderate and severe forms of epidemic typhus are distinguished. The clinical picture of the disease has considerably changed in recent years (compared with the described classic symptoms). Mild forms of the disease are of greater epidemiologic importance because the specific fever, rash, toxaemia, and nervous and vascular lesions are less pronounced. The body temperature of 38-39°C persists for 7-9 days.

The prevalent elements of the rash are roseoles. Headache and insomnia are pronounced, but other nervous symptoms are either absent or only mild. The status typhosus is usually absent. Brill's disease runs a milder course, the status typhosus is less pronounced and shorter than in epidemic typhus. Other symptoms are not so marked either. The fever period lasts 8-11 days. The onset of the disease is usually acute, the body temperature decreases critically.

Complications: Complications are now rare. They can be divided into 4 groups: (1) lesion of the vessels and the heart-collapse, thromboses, thromboembolism, rupture of the cerebral vessels with hemiparesis or even paralysis, myocarditis, etc.; (2) complications due to involvement of the central and peripheral nervous systems-psychosis, polyradiculitis, neuritis; (3) complications due to secondary infection - pneumonia, otitis, parotitis, furuncles, abscesses; (4) mixed complications - lesion of the vessels and the central nervous system with secondary infection; bedsores, gangrene of the ear lobules, fingers, toes, and nose tip; thrombophlebitis, nephritis, nephrosonephritis, etc.

Diagnosis: The diagnosis is based on clinical, epidemiologic and laboratory findings. Serologic methods of examination are most important diagnostically. Blood specimens (3-5 ml) are tested in the laboratory beginning with the 5-7th day of the disease. Rickettsia agglutination reaction, complement fixation test, indirect haemagglutination and immunofluorescent and allergic tests are among the most sensitive methods. The reaction of rickettsia agglutination with corpuscular rickettsia antigen is considered positive with titres of 1: 160 and higher.

But the use of these reactions is limited because their results are not always trustworthy and cannot be used for retrospective diagnosis. Complement fixation test is conducted with corpuscular or soluble rickettsial antigen. The diagnostic titre is 1: 160 and higher. The maximum quantity of antibodies is found in 12-20 days of the disease (1: 640-1: 1280). Indirect haemagglutination tests are most valuable diagnostically. They are performed on the 3rd-5th day of the disease and the result is considered positive with the titres of 1: 250 and higher. The maximum antibody level is seen in 14-20 days of the disease (1: 1000 and higher).

Treatment: Modern treatment quickly decreases body temperature, eliminates toxaemia, promotes resolution of rash. But antibacterial therapy fails to restore the upset functions of the vascular and nervous systems or eliminate the causative agent from the patient. The following tetracyclines are used during the full swing of the disease, in accordance with the severity of the patient's condition: tetracycline hydrochloride, terramycin, dioxycycline hydrochloride per os, 0.3 g four times a day until normal temperature persists for three days.

Chloramphenicol is inferior to the tetracyclines with respect to its efficacy but whenever necessary it can be given per os in doses of 0.5 g 4 times a day until normal temperature persists for 3 days. In order to decrease toxaemia, a 5 per cent glucose solution or an isotonic sodium chloride solution (800-900 ml each) should be given intravenously. Upset circulation of blood is managed by administration of a 10 per cent glucose solution, Ringer solution, mesaton (1 ml of a 1 per cent solution), strophanthin (0.3-0.5 ml of a 0.5 per cent solution with glucose). The solutions are given intravenously at a low infusion rate. Barbiturates, bromides, aminazine are given to control excitation. In order to prevent thrombosis, anticoagulants (heparin, phenylin) are given.

Patient care is important. Bedsores are likely to develop, and the patient should therefore be helped to change his position in bed; the linen should be stretched to prevent formation of folds. Critical patients should be placed in bed over an inflatable rubber cushion. The sacral region, the buttocks and the shoulder blades should be wiped with camphor alcohol. Rubbing with warm water (37-38°C) and taking warm baths (35-37°C) are sedative. Evacuation of the bowels and urination must be regular.

The patient must rinse his mouth with a 0.5-2 per cent sodium hydrocarbonate solution. If the patient is debilitated by the disease and is unable to do it himself, his mouth should be treated with a cotton tampon wetted with a 2 per cent solution of boric acid and glycerol. The diet must be sparing, sufficiently caloric and rich in vitamins. Meals must be given frequently in small portions. Since the patient is tortured by thirst, drinks should be given without any restriction. The patient is allowed to walk about after 7-8 afebrile days.

Prevention and control: The main measures are aimed at elimination of the source of infection and eradication of pediculosis among population. Patients suspected for epidemic typhus should be hospitalized immediately. Patients with fever in whom the disease is not diagnosed by the 5th day should be hospitalized provisionally. It is very important that patients with epidemic typhus, and also those suspected for this disease be hospitalized during the first 5 days because the infected louse is yet unable to transmit the typhus agent to the surrounding people. Isolation can be discontinued not earlier than in 12 days after normalization of body temperature.

Pediculosis among population shall be controlled by providing all necessary facilities (baths, laundries), by improving sanitary standards, especially among migrating people, such as seasonal workers, builders, etc. Pediculosis can be detected by selective examination of workers at industrial plants, schools, bordering schools, hostels, etc. The screened persons with pediculosis must be given appropriate treatment. Their families and co-workers should be given prophylactic examination and, if necessary, appropriate treatment. Control of pediculosis includes baths at least once in 7-10 days with renewal of the linen and underwear.

Specific prophylaxis should be conducted for special indications. Dry live vaccine should be given. A new vaccine has been developed; it is a chemical vaccine against epidemic typhus consisting of soluble rickettsial antigen. The vaccine is given subcutaneously by a single 0.5 ml dose.

They include immediate hospitalization of the patient, epidemiologic examination, observation of persons who had contacts with the diseased, their laboratory examinations, disinfection of the focus, and examination and, if necessary, appropriate treatment of population in the vicinity of the focus. After hospitalization of the patient, disinsection in the focus should be performed not later than in 3 hours in cities and towns, and 6 hours in rural areas. The patient should not change his underwear before hospitalization. All exposed should be given appropriate treatment in special disinfection units or in common baths transformed into such Units.

All garments, linen and underwear, and also the fomites should be disinsected in steam-formaldehyde or hot air chambers. The rooms and other enclosures should be treated with a 0.5 per cent chlorophos, 0.5 per cent methylacetophos, 5 per cent lysol solution, or 10 per cent dilor (10-15 g per square metre). If special disinsection chambers are not available, soft fomites, linen, underwear should be boiled in a soda-soap solution or soaked in a 0.15 per cent aqueous emulsion of carbophos for 20 minutes, 0.25 per cent aqueous emulsion of dicresyl (20 minutes), 0.5 per cent aqueous emulsion of methylacetophos (30 minutes), the rate of liquid consumption is 4 litres per kg of linen (with subsequent laundry). Garments and clothes can be treated by dusting with a 5 per cent methylacetophos, 1 per cent neopin, or 10 per cent dilor dust, or by spraying with aqueous emulsions used for soaking the linen.

After disinfection, the articles should be wrapped tight in bedcloths for 2-3 hours and then well aired. If head lice are detected (from 1 to 10 species, nits included), they should be eliminated mechanically by combing, or by cutting and shaving the hair on the head. The hair should be collected and burned. If it is necessary to remove nits from hairs, rinsing with a 5-10 per cent acetic acid solution is recommended with subsequent combing (cotton wool or threads must be passed between comb teeth and wetted well with acetic acid solution). If pediculosis is moderate or severe (from 10 lice and more), insecticides should be used. This procedure is however contraindicated to infants under 5 years, pregnant and nursing women, persons with injured skin, etc.

The following insecticides are recommended: a 0.15 per cent aqueous emulsion of carbophos (10-50 ml of the emulsion for a person), a 20 per cent soap suspension of benzyl benzoate. The persons who were exposed to the danger of infection should be observed for 25 days with obligatory daily thermometry.

In order to reveal the source of infection, all persons who had contacts with the diseased, and also persons who sustained a disease with fever within the past three months, should be examined by complement fixation and indirect haemagglutination tests. If the tests are positive, special medical observation must be ensured with repeated serologic testing. If body temperature rises in those who had contacts with the diseased, they should be hospitalized and diagnosis established.

MURINE TYPHUS

Aetiology: The disease is caused by Rickettsia mooseri (the family Rickettsiaceae, the genus Rickettsia).

Epidemiology: The reservoir of infection in nature are rodents (rats, mice) and transmitters of infection among them, fleas and gamasoidea ticks. Infected rodents excrete. R. mooseri with urine. Food contaminated with the urine of infected mice is the main source of infection of humans. Stability of rickettsia to drying provides conditions for air-borne infection. Infection occurs during rubbing of faeces of fleas and ticks into injured skin and mucosa.

Rickettsia are not transmitted by bites of infected fleas, while ticks can thus transmit the infection. Infection is not transmitted from man to man. Murine typhus usually occurs in sea ports and mostly in countries with hot climate. Endemic foci have been reported from the Atlantic, Pacific and Indian coastal areas, and also from the countries around the Mediterranean, Black, Caspian, Baltic and the North seas.

Pathogenesis: The pathogenesis of murine typhus is the same as of epidemic (louse-borne) typhus.

Clinical picture: The incubation period lasts 5-12 days. The body temperature rapidly rises to 38-40°C. Fever persists for about 2 weeks. Characteristic symptoms are pain in the extremities, joints, and in the lumbar region. Headache is another symptom. In 6-7 days of the disease rash develops; roseoles turn into roseole-papular rash in few days. Rash is seen on the face, abdomen, back, and even on the palms and soles. Bradycardia is noted. The clinical picture is similar to that of epidemic (louse-borne) typhus, but the course of the disease is more benign.

Complications: Complications are rare. Diagnosis. The diagnosis is based on clinical and epidemiologic findings. Blood specimens (5 ml) should be tested in the laboratory. The blood is administered to male guinea pigs into the abdominal cavity (3 ml): the testicular tunicae become inflamed. Rickettsial agglutination and complement fixation tests are also conducted. Treatment. Treatment of murine typhus is the same as of louse-borne typhus.

Prevention and control: Planned deratization and disinsection, and also protection of food against contamination with rodents are decisive measures. Vaccination should be performed for epidemiologic indication.

Q FEVER

Aetiology: The disease is caused by Coxiella burnetii. The microorganisms are characterized by high stability to drying and ultraviolet radiation. In tap water they can survive for 160 days, in milk for 125 days, in oil and meat (at low temperature) for 30-40 days.

Epidemiology: The source of infection in natural foci are many animals and birds. The reservoirs and transmitters of the infection are ixodes and other ticks. Infected ticks attack domestic animals; secondary foci of infection thus arise in which the animals are infected due to intimate contacts. The disease in animals is often latent. Domestic animals excreting rickettsia with milk (17-40 days), faeces, urine, placenta, amniotic fluid are the most important source of infection.

Q fever is characterized by a variety of routes by which the infection can be transmitted, e.g. with dust and air, by direct contact with the diseased animal, with food (ingestion of diary products and other infected foods), water (bathing in infected water, drinking it), etc. If pneumonia develops, the patient can excrete the pathogenic agent with sputum, and he can therefore be regarded as a potential source of infection disseminating it by air-borne route and by direct contact. There is no seasonal variations in the incidence of the disease, but in rural areas the morbidity rises in spring when the young animals are delivered. Q fever is reported from all countries.

Pathogenesis: The portal of entry of the infection is the respiratory and eye mucosa, the skin and the alimentary tract. The lymph carries the rickettsia to the blood (primary rickettsaemia) and then to the internal organs (liver, spleen, kidneys), where the rickettsia propagates to cause secondary rickettsaemia and toxaemia.

Clinical picture: The incubation period lasts 12-19 days with extremes of 3 and 32 days. The onset is usually acute: chills and elevation of temperature to 39-40°C. The clinical symptoms are quite varied. The patient complains of weakness, lassitude, hyperhidrosis, severe headache, myalgia, arthralgia, lumbar pain and insomnia. Some patients develop nausea, vomiting, dry cough; the appetite is impaired, nosebleeds are possible. The fever period lasts from 3 to 15 days, most commonly from 7 to 9 days.

Considerable variations in the body temperature are attended by repeated chills and hyperhidrosis. The pulse disagrees with the fever, bradycardia and hypotension develop. The body temperature normalizes by accelerated lysis. Some patients develop the symptoms of involvement of the respiratory organs (tracheitis, bronchitis, pneumonia), which are manifested by dry cough, and chest pain during cough and respiration. X-ray reveals changes in the lungs. When ingested, rickettsia produces dyspepsia and abdominal pain.

Arthralgia, roseoles, petechial rash and other eruptions are associated with allergic manifestations of the disease. Leucopenia, the shift to the left, relative lymphocytosis and monocytosis are seen in the blood; ESR is accelerated. Some patients can develop a severe disease with prolonged fever, inhibition of the nervous and cardiovascular system, and splenic enlargement. The recovery phase lasts 2-4 weeks. Relapses are possible; the disease can also transform into the chronic form.

Diagnosis: The diagnosis is based on clinical, epidemiologic and laboratory findings. Laboratory tests include complement fixation and micro-agglutination tests with specific soluble rickettsial antigen. Blood specimens (5 ml) should be taken beginning with the 7-10th day of the disease. The titres of complement fixation and micro- agglutination tests of 1: 8-1: 16 are positive, but repeated tests are necessary to confirm the diagnosis (by progressively increasing titres).

The immunofluorescent test is a reliable diagnostic method. Intracutaneous tests with purified allergen of the rickettsia are used for direct and retrospective diagnosis. About 5 to 6 ml of blood are taken on the first day of the disease to inoculate two guinea pigs weighing 200-250 g. The temperature of the animals is measured daily; one guinea pig is sacrificed at the height of fever, while the other is left for serologic studies.

Treatment: Treatment is the same as in epidemic (louse-borne) typhus. Since relapses are possible, tetracycline therapy continues for 8-10 days, regardless of the presence or absence of fever, and regardless of the patient's general condition.

Prevention and control: The measures should be directed at eradication of ticks and protection of domestic animals against them. To this end, systematic disinsection should be carried out using carbophos, pyrethrum and other disinsectants during the period of tick activity. The infected animals should be isolated. At farms where Q rickettiosis is reported, quarantine should be established. Animal breeders must observe rules of individual hygiene.

Only persons who sustained Q fever in the past, or vaccinated persons are admitted to take care of infected animals. The personnel should wear special overalls and observe the rules of personal hygiene at animal farms, slaughterhouses, etc. Health education among population is necessary. Milk should be boiled while the diary product prepared only from boiled milk. Wool should be decontaminated. Groups of people or animals should not be admitted to areas endemic for Q fever until these areas are not freed from ticks and rodents (disinsection and deratization measures).

People should be protected from tick bites by wearing protective overalls impregnated with repellants. Patients should be hospitalized for clinical indications. Patient's excrements, garments, dishes and other belongings should be disinfected. The personnel must observe the rules of personal hygiene when taking care of patients. Specific prophylaxis should be carried out among animal breeders, workers of slaughterhouses and meat processing plants in areas dangerous for Q fever. People should be vaccinated with M-44 vaccine. It is diluted with an isotonic sodium chloride solution and rubbed into the skin or given per os. Revaccination is necessary in two years.

PARASITIC ZOONOSES

TAENIASIS

Taeniasis is a tapeworm infection. It is also known as: Pork tapeworm; Beef tapeworm; Tapeworm; Taenia saginata; and Taenia solium.

Aetiology: Tapeworm infection is acquired by eating raw or undercooked meat of infected animals. Beef generally carry Taenia saginata (T. saginata) while pigs carry Taenia solium (T. solium).

Epidemiology: In the human intestine, the larvae from the infected meat develop into the adult tapeworm – which can grow to longer than 12 feet. Tapeworms are segmented, with each segment capable of producing eggs. Eggs are dispersed individually or in groups and can pass out with the stool or through the anus.

Adults and children withT. solium pork tapeworm can, if appropriate hygiene is lacking, become self-infected by ingesting eggs from tapeworm that are picked up on their hands while wiping or scratching the anus. Additionally, these individuals can expose other individuals to T. solium eggs, usually through food handling.

Symptoms: Tapeworm infestation does not usually cause any symptoms. Infection is generally recognized when the infected person passes segments of proglottids in the stool, especially if the segment is moving.

Diagnosis: The stool will be examined for eggs of T. solium or T. saginata.Segments of worm may be seen in stool.

Complications: Rarely, worms may cause obstruction of the intestine. If T. solium larvae migrate to the brain, they can cause seizures and other neurological problems. This condition is called cysticercosis.

Treatment: Tapeworms are treated with medications taken by mouth, usually in a single dose. The drug of choice for tapeworm infections is niclosamide. Praziquantel and albendazole can also be used.

Prevention and control: Feeding practices and inspection of domestic food animals have largely eliminated the problem of tapeworm. Adequate cooking of meat destroys the tapeworm larvae and will prevent infection by tapeworm. Good hygiene and hand washing after using the toilet will prevent self-infection in a person already infected with tapeworms.

VISCERAL LEISHMANIASIS

The following variants are distinguished: Mediterranean (infantile) kala azar, Indian kala azar, East African, Chinese and American leishmaniasis.

Aetiology: Visceral leishmaniasis is caused by various species of Leishmania donovani. For example, Mediterranean littoral leishmaniasis is due to L. donovani infantum, the Indian kala azar is caused by L. donovani donovani. Leishmania readily grow on various media containing animal protein. Various rodents, dogs, cats, monkeys and human beings are susceptible to leishmania.

Epidemiology: The source of infection in the Mediterranean littoral leishmaniasis are dogs, jackals, foxes, possibly rodents; the source of Indian kala azar is a human patient, while the source of East African variant are humans, dogs, jackals, foxes, and rodents. Sandflies of the genus Phlebotomus are the vector of the infection.

After sucking blood from an infected human or animal, female sandflies can transmit the infection in 6-8 days. Mediterranean littoral leishmaniasis afflicts mainly infants aged from 1 to 5 years. Indian and East African visceral leishmaniases affect humans of all ages but young patients dominate. Stable immunity develops after the disease. The disease is reported as sporadic cases and epidemic outbreaks from the Mediterranean littoral, China, Middle East, India, Pakistan, Nepal.

Pathogenesis: The portal of entry of leishmania is the site of sandfly bite. The blood stream carries the microorganisms to the cells of mononuclear phagocytic system of the spleen, liver, bone marrow, and lymph nodes to cause their dysfunction and damage. Some cells die, it is attended by the proliferation of the mononuclear phagocytic system which causes degeneration of the spleen, liver and the lymph nodes.

These organs become enlarged and firm, their function is upset. The gastrointestinal tract and the kidneys are also involved. Destroyed leishmania and their metabolites cause toxaemia and upset metabolism in the macroorganism. Some patients develop a papule at the portal of infection.

Clinical picture: The incubation period of Mediterranean leishmaniasis is from 20 days to 3-5 months and longer, of Indian kala azar 6-8 months on average. Three periods are distinguished in the course of the disease: initial, clinically manifest, and terminal. The onset of the disease is gradual. The patient develops fatigue, malaise, and subfebrile temperature. His appetite is impaired, the skin and visible mucosa are pallid. When the disease is in its full swing, the temperature curve is irregular and undulant. Rises of temperature to 39-40°C are followed by afebrile periods.

Body temperature fluctuates not only within few days but also within 24-hour periods. Temperature variations are attended by chills and sweating. The spleen is firm and enlarged from the first days of the disease. Splenomegaly becomes striking with time. Its lower edges descend to the navel and even lower. The liver and the peripheral lymph nodes are also enlarged. The skin is pallid. Anaemia develops in 2-3 months. It progresses as the bone marrow is involved. Granulocytopenia and agranulocytosis are characteristic.

Haemorrhages into the skin and mucosa are possible, epistaxis and gastrointestinal bleeding occur. Splenohepatomegaly causes portal hypertension, ascites, and oedema. In most patients the red blood cell count is low. Leucopenia (2 x 109/L or lower), neutrophilopenia and eosinophilopenia with relative lymphocytosis, and monocytosis, and also thrombocytopenia are characteristic blood changes. The serum albumin is low while the globulin content is high at the expense of alpha- and beta-globulins; ESR is high (50-90 mm/h). In the absence of timely specific treatment, acute forms of visceral leishmaniasis transform into subacute and protracted forms of the disease.

The skin becomes pale grey. In Indian kala azar the skin is dark, almost black (kala azar in Hindi means black fever); oedema increases, diarrhoea supervenes (often with admixture of mucus and blood). The terminal period is marked by cachexia, marasmus, low muscular tone (frog belly syndrome). In the absence of adequate treatment, the disease lasts from 1 to 2 years. Patients are persistent sources of infection (for years and even decades).

Complications: Untimely treatment can cause death due to secondary infections. Frequent complications of visceral leishmaniasis are pneumonia, otitis, mastoiditis, furunculosis, epistaxis, ulcerative gingivitis and stomatitis, and rupture of the spleen.

Diagnosis: The diagnosis is based on clinical, epidemiologic and laboratory findings. Isolation of leishmania in Romanowsky-Giemsa stained smears of sternal marrow, lymph node bioptate and, less frequently, blood is decisive. The material is also inoculated into NNN medium for growing leishmania cultures.

Serologic tests are also used: fluorescent antibody test, complement fixation test, latex agglutination with leishmania antigents tests. Inoculation of hamsters is also used in biologic studies. Visceral leishmaniasis can be identified by the formol-gel test (2 drops of a 40 per cent formaldehyde solution are added to 1 ml of the patient's blood serum: the serum becomes cloudy and turns into a gel in the presence of leishmania).

Treatment: The specific remedy against visceral leishmaniasis is solusurmin (solustilosan, stibanol, pentostam). It is produced in powder form in sealed vials. Before use, it should be diluted in double-distilled water. The preparation is given once a day intramuscularly or intravenously in the form of 5, 10 or 20 per cent freshly prepared solutions. The course of treatment includes from 7 to 16 such injections. The dose of the preparation (from 0.04 to 0.1 g per kg body weight) should be gradually increased. Treatment can be repeated in a certain lapse of time. Solusurmin is contraindicated in acute nephritis.

Other preparations of pentavalent antimony can also be used: neostibosan, glucantime. If antimony preparations fail, pentamidine should be given daily in a dose of 0.004 g/kg (10-15 injections per course). If secondary infection supervenes, antibiotics should be given. Transfusion of blood and erythrocytes, and also vitamins are indicated for anaemia.

Prevention and control: Leishmaniasis control measures should in the first instance be aimed at elimination of the source of infection. These include extermination of jackals, foxes, stray (especially diseased) dogs; veterinary supervision of dogs in endemic areas is necessary. Timely treatment of visceral leishmaniasis patients with specific preparations is necessary; protection against flying insects is important too. Improvement of populated places helps eradication of insects and sites of their propagation. Enclosures should be treated with insecticides. Population should be protected from insect bites by repellents and other means.

In addition to treatment of patients and elimination of sandflies, the people surrounding the diseased should be given medical supervision. Veterinary supervision of dogs should be conducted. Persons who sustained the disease should be observed for 4-6 months.

CUTANEOUS LEISHMANIASIS

New World and Old World cutaneous leishmaniases are distinguished.

The Old World form: This form is, in turn, divided into two distinct types: an urban (anthroponotic) form (dry leishmaniasis having an incubation period of many months to over a year, and lasting for many months and acute rapidly evolving (zoonotic) form, known also as rural, humid, moist, or wet cutaneous leishmaniasis.

Aetiology: The causative agent of anthroponotic cutaneous leishmaniasis is Leishmania tropica minor, and of the zoonotic form-Leishmania tropica major.

Epidemiology: The source of anthroponotic leishmaniasis is a human being, while in zoonotic forms these are wild rodents. In nature, the causative agent circulates in the system: diseased rodent- sandfly-healthy rodent. The transmitters of leishmania are female sandflies of the genus Phlebotomus: P. papatasii, P. caucasicus, P. sergenti, and others. Anthroponotic leishmaniasis occurs as sporadic cases in towns and cities during the whole year which is due to various incubation periods.

In the zoonotic form, the incidence of the disease increases during the warm season. It occurs only in rural areas. Susceptibility to cutaneous leishmaniasis is universal. The greater portion of population sustains the disease in childhood. Stable immunity is produced only to a specific causative agent. Anthroponotic leishmaniasis occurs in the Middle East, South Europe, India, and Africa, while the zoonotic form in Asia, Africa and South Europe.

Pathogenesis: Leishmania enters a human through a bite of an infected sandfly. After inoculation into the skin, leishmania propagates at the portal of entry to form infiltration. In the anthroponotic form, the papules ulcerate in 3-6 months; in the zoonotic form in 15-16 days.

Clinical picture: The incubation period of the anthroponotic (dry) form is 2-8 months to 11/2-2 years and more. In the zoonotic (moist) form it is from 1 week to 2 months. Cutaneous leishmaniasis affects the face, the neck, the upper and lower extremities, less frequently the trunk. The quantity of ulcers corresponds to the number of bites by infected sandflies. The dry form is characterized by development of a pink papule at the site of a sandfly bite; in 5-6 months the diameter of the papule is 1-2 cm.

The papule is later covered with scale and then crust, and in six months it is affected by necrosis with ulceration (ulcers have a granular bottom). The ulcer diameter increases and can be 4-6 cm. In few months, the ulcer begins healing and a scar is formed in a year. The papule in the wet form is scarlet, looking like a furuncle. In 1 -2 weeks, the centre is necrotized and an ulcer is formed with a diameter of 2-5 cm. It is 1-3 mm deep, and has irregular shape.

New nodules are formed around the ulcer which later are necrotized too. The ulcers fuse into a large ulcer with a diameter of 10-15 cm (Plate VIII). The bottom of the ulcer is granulated. Copious seropurulent exudate dries into a dirty grey crust. In 2-3, sometimes 4-6 months, the ulcer undergoes epithelization and cicatrization (during 3-6 weeks). Scars remain after healing.

Diagnosis: Cutaneous leishmaniasis is diagnosed on the basis of clinical and epidemiologic findings. The laboratory method is also important diagnostically. Smears for laboratory studies are prepared from the exudate which is expressed from a punctured nodule (Romanowsky-Giemsa staining is used). In the presence of ulcers, granulated matter is taken from the bottom of an ulcer after cleaning it with cotton wool. Marginal infiltrate is also used for laboratory examinations.

Treatment: The cutaneous form is treated by local application of solusurmin. The preparation is given under the nodule or in the vicinity of the ulcer. Intracutaneous injection of monomycin and a 4 per cent quinacrine around the ulcer is also helpful. Severe cases should be treated with solusurmin like in visceral leishmaniasis. Ulcerations with lymphangitis and lymphadenitis should be treated with monomycin: 250000 U 3 times a day for 10-12 days. Aminoquinol can be given in a dose of 0.2 g 2-3 times a day for 18-20 days.

Prevention and control: It is necessary to reveal timely patients with cutaneous leishmaniasis. Patients with ulcers on the exposed parts of the body should wear dry bandages. Deratization is obligatory in a given locality and the surrounding areas with a diameter of 1500 m. If a new populated settlement is constructed in a desert, deratization is necessary over an area with a diameter of 3 km.

Population should also be protected from sandfly bites. Whenever necessary, all enclosures should be treated with insecticides. Means of individual protection should be used: repellents, netting and gauzes against flying insects. Specific prophylaxis is performed with a live culture of leishmania which is given intracutaneously in a dose of 0.1-0.2 ml 3 months before activization of sandflies.

The New World form: The disease is known by different names in various countries. Among more common names are American, Brazilian, or mucocutaneous leishmaniasis. The disease is caused by Leishmania braziliensis. The reservoirs of the infection are rodents and domestic animals. The transmitting vector are sandflies of the genus Phlebotomus. Unlike in other forms of cutaneous leishmaniasis, in American leishmaniasis the mucosa is involved in 1-2 years. This causes deformities of the nose, nasopharynx, airways, genitalia and the ears. The disease lasts from 2-3 years to decades. The following complications are possible: infectious sepsis, gangrene, cachexia, and amyloidosis.

SURFACE INFECTIONS

TRACHOMA

Aetiology: Trachoma is the leading infectious cause of ocular morbidity. This disease is a chronic keratoconjunctivitis caused by the obligate intracellular bacterium Chlamydia trachomatis.

Epidemiology: Infection spreads from person to person, and is frequently passed from child to child and from child to mother, especially where there are shortages of water, numerous flies, and crowded living conditions.

Infection often begins during infancy or childhood and can become chronic. If left untreated, the infection eventually causes the eyelid to turn inwards, which in turn causes the eyelashes to rub on the eyeball, resulting in intense pain and scarring of the front of the eye. This ultimately leads to irreversible blindness, typically between 30 and 40 years of age.

Pathogenesis: Trachoma is caused by serovars A, B, Ba, and C of C trachomatis. Different serovars predominate in different families and in different communities.

Chlamydiae are gram-negative, obligate intracellular bacteria. The species C trachomatis causes trachoma and also genital infections (serovars D-K) and lymphogranuloma venereum (serovars L1-L3). Serovars D-K occasionally cause a chronic follicular conjunctivitis that is clinically indistinguishable from trachoma, including follicular conjunctivitis with pannus and, at times, conjunctival scarring. However, these genital serovars do not typically enter stable transmission cycles within communities. Therefore, they are not involved in the genesis of trachoma blindness. Regardless of the serovar (which is determined by polymorphisms in a surface-exposed protein), isolates of C trachomatis obtained from the eye have mutations that inactivate the genes coding for tryptophan synthase, whereas genital isolates have a functional enzyme.

Infection causes inflammation, that is, a predominantly lymphocytic and monocytic infiltrate with plasma cells and macrophages in follicles. The follicles are typical germinal centers with islands of intense B-cell proliferation surrounded by seas of T cells. Recurrent conjunctival reinfection causes the prolonged inflammation that leads to conjunctival scarring. Scarring is associated with atrophy of the conjunctival epithelium, loss of goblet cells, and replacement of the normal, loose, vascular subepithelial stroma with thick compact bands of type IV and type V collagen.

Clinical picture: The bacteria has an incubation period of 5 to 12 days, after which the affected individual experiences symptoms of conjunctivitis, or irritation similar to "pink eye." Blinding endemic trachoma results from multiple episodes of reinfection that maintains the intense inflammation in the conjunctiva. Without reinfection, the inflammation will gradually subside.

The conjunctival inflammation is called "active trachoma" and usually is seen in children, especially pre school children. It is characterized by white lumps in the undersurface of the upper eye lid (conjunctival follicles or lymphoid germinal centres) and by non-specific inflammation and thickening often associated with papillae. Follicles may also appear at the junction of the cornea and the sclera (limbal follicles). Active trachoma will often be irritating and have a watery discharge. Bacterial secondary infection may occur and cause a purulent discharge.

The later structural changes of trachoma are referred to as "cicatricial trachoma". These include scarring in the eye lid (tarsal conjunctiva) that leads to distortion of the eye lid with buckling of the lid (tarsus) so the lashes rub on the eye (trichiasis). These lashes will lead to corneal opacities and scarring and then to blindness. In addition, blood vessels and scar tissue can invade the upper cornea (pannus). Resolved limbal follicles may leave small gaps in pannus (Herbert's Pits).

Diagnosis: The diagnosis of trachoma is made on the basis of the clinical manifestations of the infection. The findings are then used to categorize the severity of disease using the Simplified WHO Trachoma Grading System. Alternative causes of conjunctivitis should also be considered.

In most endemic areas the diagnosis of trachoma is maded clinically. However, laboratory assays are available for the diagnosis of C. trachomatis infection. Tests include immunofluorescent cytology, PCR, Giemsa cytology, and culture. Although these are useful in research studies or for diagnosis in areas with low prevalence, most trachoma control programs rely on the clinical grading scheme. As the positive predictive value of clinical diagnosis for trachoma falls with decreasing prevalence, microbiologic diagnosis may become a more important tool.

Treatment: There is an international commitment led by WHO to eliminate blinding trachoma from the world by 2020, known as the Alliance for the Global Elimination of Trachoma by 2020 (GET 2020).

The SAFE strategy (Surgery, Antibiotics, Facial cleanliness and Environmental improvement) is the core tool of GET 2020 and has been proven effective in reducing the incidence of blindness. Because blindness due to trachoma is irreversible, the strategy focuses on prevention. Surgical correction of trichiasis prevents the development of corneal opacification, while antibiotics, facial cleanliness, and environmental improvements may disrupt the cycle of reinfection.

Mass treatment: Because C. trachomatis is highly infectious and transmitted rapidly in areas of poor hygiene, trachoma is best managed within an entire region rather than on an individual basis.

WHO guidelines recommend that a region should receive mass antibiotic treatment when the prevalence of active trachoma among one to nine year-old children (as assessed clinically) is greater than 10 percent. Subsequent annual treatment should be administered for three years, at which time the prevalence should be reassessed. Annual treatment should continue until the prevalence drops below 5 percent. If the prevalence among one to nine year-old children is less than 10 percent, antibiotic treatment should be administered to households of individuals with active trachoma.

However, it is uncertain whether the WHO strategy described above is always appropriate; one or two treatments may be sufficient, and decline in the prevalence of active trachoma (as assessed clinically) can lag behind the fall in the prevalence of infection detected by PCR testing of conjunctival swabs.

In areas where the prevalence is greater than 50 percent, repeated mass antibiotic distribution may be a viable tool for trachoma elimination. This was illustrated in a study of three Ethiopian villages including 710 patients who received biannual mass oral azithromycin distribution; over a 30-month period, the mean prevalence declined from 43 to <1 percent. In addition, a randomized trial of annual versus biannual mass treatment among over 14,000 individuals demonstrated that biannual distribution leads to a lower trachoma prevalence than annual distribution (6.8 versus 0.9 percent). However, routine biannual antibiotic distribution in endemic areas is not yet part of the WHO guidelines.

Antibiotic selection: WHO recommends azithromycin (single oral dose of 20 mg/kg) or topical tetracycline (1 percent eye ointment twice a day for six weeks) for community-wide distribution. Azithromycin is preferred because it is given as a single oral dose, although it is expensive and generally only available as part of the international donation program organized by Pfizer through the International Trachoma Initiative. Azithromycin is considered safe for use in children from the age of 6 months and during pregnancy.

Topical agents may be a useful alternative in areas where oral azithromycin is not readily available. The WHO recommends topical tetracycline treatment for use in pregnancy. Alternatively, topical azithromycin (1.5 percent) for two or three days may be as effective as oral azithromycin.

Randomized trials have shown that a single dose of oral azithromycin is as effective as a long course of topical tetracycline for the treatment of active trachoma. For initial mass treatment, azithromycin and topical tetracycline are also equally effective.

TETANUS

Aetiology: The disease is due to Clostridium tetani (the family Bacillaceae, the genus Clostridium). This is a motile anaerobic rod which readily forms spores in unfavourable conditions. Vegetative forms of Clostridia are unstable and are killed by boiling for 3 minutes. The spores, on the contrary, are highly resistant to high temperature, drying and disinfectants.

They can be killed only by boiling for 30-50 minutes. The vegetative forms produce specific exotoxin that consists of tetanospasmin having the properties of neurotoxin and tetanohaemolysin that dissolves red blood cells. Tetanus toxin is a strong bacterial poison; by its toxicity it is only inferior to botulinus toxin.

Epidemiology: The tetanus agent and its spores are excreted from animals with their faeces and are accumulated in superficial layers of soil. Humans are infected when dust, soil, and animal faeces get on abraded or otherwise injured skin. Anaerobic conditions are favourable for multiplication of the agent.

Women can be infected during labour or gynaecological manipulations outside hospital. Burns, animal and frost bites also provide beneficial conditions for tetanus infection. Rural residents are mostly affected. The peak of the disease incidence is usually during the warm season. Occurrence increases during war.

Pathogenesis: Clostridia propagate in the human body to produce neurotropic toxin that is carried by the blood stream and the peripheral nerves to the spinal cord and medulla oblongata where it usually causes paralysis of interneurons of the polysynaptic reflex arcs that produce an inhibiting effect on motoneurons. Motoneuron impulses are not coordinated as they pass to the muscles and they cause permanent tonic contraction of the skeletal muscles.

Periodic tetanic muscle spasms are due to intensified efferent and afferent impulses in response to non-specific stimuli (sound, light, tactile, taste, and olfactory). The convulsion syndrome promotes metabolic acidosis and hyperthermia. Heart and respiratory functions are upset. The patient can die of asphyxia, paralysis of the heart and respiratory muscles, and complications (pneumonia, sepsis).

Clinical picture: The incubation period lasts from 2 days to a month. The shorter the incubation period, the severer the course of the disease. During the prodromal period the patient sometimes complains of boring pain in the wound, muscular twitching around the wound, and restlessness. Mild, moderately severe and severe forms of the disease are distinguished.

The disease begins with specific contractions of musticatory muscles, known as trismus (lockjaw): the patient is unable to chew, open his mouth, or talk. Convulsive contractions of the facial muscles produce a characteristic face expression known as risus sardonicus: the mouth is stretched, the eyebrows are high lifted to form deep wrinkles on the forehead. Tonic muscular spasms spread over to the muscles of the neck, back, abdomen and the extremities.

The patient assumes an arching posture resting only against the head and the heels (opisthotonus). The skin is moist with profuse perspiration. Tonic contractions of the respiratory muscles can cause respiratory distress. Dyspnoea and cyanosis develop. The patient can die of apnoea. The abdominal muscles are strained and stiff; they turn as firm as wood. Convulsions last from several seconds to several minutes. Their frequency depends on severity of the disease.

In mild cases they occur 1-2 times a day; in severe cases they are almost continuous. Seizures are debilitating. The patient suffers from insomnia and apprehension. Consciousness is clear. Muscular spasms interfere with deglutition. This, combined with trismus, cause dehydration and wasting. Defaecation and urination are upset. Convulsions intensify due to increased reflex excitation in response to external stimuli (touch, breeze, noise, bright light). Body temperature is either normal or subfebrile. Hyperpyrexia is characteristic of agony (41-42°C).

High leucocyte count and lactic acid of the blood are seen. Tetanus is especially severe in women after extrahospital labour or abortion and in neonates (due to infection during umbilical manipulations). In addition to the described acute tetanus, the following forms are also differentiated:

- Fulminant tetanus that ends in death of the patient in 1-2 days of paralysis of the respiratory muscles;
- Subacute tetanus, characterized by short seizures of convulsion that follow at long intervals;
- Localized tetanus in which muscular spasms first develop around the wound.

The duration of the disease depends on its severity and varies between 2 and 4 weeks. In about 17-18 days, clonic convulsions abate and in 22-25 days tonic strain in the muscles lessens.

Complications: Bronchitis, bronchopneumonia and pneumonia are common complications of tetanus. Muscular rhexis, joint dislocation, and bone fractures are possible.

Diagnosis: The diagnosis is based on clinical findings. Laboratory diagnosis is difficult because the causative agent is hardly detectable in the wound exudate. Biologic tests can be conducted on mice by inoculating them with the material taken from the depth of the wound. The test is considered positive if the animal develops tetanus in 1-2 days.

Treatment: The specific treatment includes intramuscular injection of 100000-200000 U of antitoxic antitetanic serum to adults, 20000-40000 U to neonates, and 80000-100000 U to children. The injections should be given after desensitization. The serum should be warmed before use. The patient is given intramuscularly 1 ml of adsorbed tetanus toxoid 30 minutes before the serum is given. The toxoid should be given repeatedly at 3-5 day intervals (3-5 injections in the course). In addition to horse antitetanic serum, the patient can be given the serum of donors immunized with adsorbed tetanus toxoid, or human antitetanic immunoglobulin in a dose of 900 U (6 ml). The wound must obligatory be treated surgically; the wounds that might heal by the time when the disease develops, should be treated as well. Before treatment of the wound from 3000 to 10000 U of antitetanic serum should be injected in tissues surrounding the wound.

Aminazin (1-2 ml of a 2.5 per cent solution), promedol (1.5 ml of a 2 per cent solution), scopolamine (0.5-1 ml of a 0.05 per cent solution), and dimedrol (3 ml of 1 per cent solution) can be given as neuroplegics. A mixture can be prepared from the mentioned preparations. The following scheme should be followed: chloral hydrate-the lytic mixture-chloral hydrate, etc., at 3-3 1/2 hour intervals. Muscle relaxants (diplacin) are also given to treat severe cases. Doses for children should be decreased according to their age.

Complications should be prevented with antibiotics. Artificial respiration should be used in severe cases. Isotonic sodium chloride solution (to 1500 ml), alkalifying solution (Locke-Ringer solution, to 1000 ml), blood plasma, polyglucin and other solutions should be used to correct liquid loss and acidosis. Mesaton, strophanthin and corglycon should be given to normalize cardiovascular function. Respiratory function can be improved by inhalations of oxygen, or by cytiton (0.5-1 ml), intramuscularly or intravenously. The patient is placed in an intensive care unit. Food must be liquid and caloric. If the mouth would not open and deglutition is difficult, food should be given by a thin gastric tube passed through the nose (during drug-induced sleep).

Prevention and control: Effective prophylaxis of tetanus is attained with anatoxin. Children should be regularly vaccinated with combined vaccine. A complete course of active immunization includes primary vaccination and revaccination. Immunity is maintained by revaccinations at 10-year intervals. Active immunization of susceptible individuals should be done with tetanus toxoid given subcutaneously in a dose of 0.5 ml, two times at a 30-40 day interval.

Revaccinations are necessary at intervals from 6 months to 2 years (one subcutaneous injection of 0.5 ml). Subsequent revaccinations (with the same doses) should be conducted each decade. Depending on previous active immunization, prompt prophylaxis includes thorough debridement of the wound and administration of tetanus toxoid alone or in combination with tetanus serum or antitetanic human immunoglobulin. For example, urgent prophylaxis against tetanus is contraindicated in children and adolescents who received a complete course of vaccination in accordance with their age.

Adults who were not vaccinated, should be given 1 ml of tetanus toxoid and 250 U (3 ml) of antitetanic human immunoglobulin or 3000 U of immune human serum immunoglobulin. Urgent prophylaxis of tetanus is indicated in traumas associated with injuries to the skin and mucosa, in frostbites and burns of the second, third and fourth degree, in extrahospital abortions and labour, in gangrene or necrosis of any type, in abscesses, animal bites, operations on the gastrointestinal tract. Besides, prevention of tetanus includes control of traumatism, surgical treatment of wounds, providing aseptic conditions of labour and abortions, immunization of pregnant against tetanus in areas dangerous for tetanus and health education of population.

LEPROSY

Aetiology: Mycobacterium leprae and Mycobacterium lepromatosis are the causative agents of leprosy. M. lepromatosis is only the causitive agent in diffuse lepromatous leprosy, which can be lethal. An intracellular, acid-fast bacterium, M. leprae is aerobic and rod-shaped, and is surrounded by the waxy cell membrane coating characteristic of Mycobacterium species.

Due to extensive loss of genes necessary for independent growth, M. leprae and M. lepromatosis are unculturable in the laboratory, a factor which leads to difficulty in definitively identifying the organism under a strict interpretation of Koch's postulates. The use of non-culture-based techniques such as molecular genetics has allowed for alternative establishment of causation.

Epidemiology: The exact mechanism of transmission of leprosy is not known: prolonged close contact and transmission by nasal droplet have both been proposed, and, while the latter fits the pattern of disease, both remain unproven. The only other animals besides humans known to contract leprosy are the armadillo, chimpanzee, sooty mangabey, and cynomolgus macaque. The bacterium can also be grown in the laboratory by injection into the footpads of mice. There is evidence that not all people who are infected with M. leprae develop leprosy, and genetic factors have long been thought to play a role, due to the observation of clustering of leprosy around certain families, and the failure to understand why certain individuals develop lepromatous leprosy while others develop other types of leprosy.

It is estimated that due to genetic factors, only 5 percent of the population is susceptible to leprosy. This is mostly because the body is naturally immune to the bacteria, and those persons who do become infected are experiencing a severe allergic reaction to the disease. However, the role of genetic factors is not entirely clear in determining this clinical expression. In addition, malnutrition and prolonged exposure to infected persons may play a role in development of the overt disease. The incubation period for the bacteria can last anywhere from two to ten years.

The most widely held belief is that the disease is transmitted by contact between infected persons and healthy persons. In general, closeness of contact is related to the dose of infection, which in turn is related to the occurrence of disease. Of the various situations that promote close contact, contact within the household is the only one that is easily identified, although the actual incidence among contacts and the relative risk for them appear to vary considerably in different studies. In incidence studies, infection rates for contacts of lepromatous leprosy have varied from 6.2 per 1000 per year in Cebu, Philippines to 55.8 per 1000 per year in a part of Southern India.

Clinical picture: Two exit routes of M. leprae from the human body often described are the skin and the nasal mucosa, although their relative importance is not clear. It is true that lepromatous cases show large numbers of organisms deep down in the dermis. However, whether they reach the skin surface in sufficient numbers is doubtful. Although there are reports of acid-fast bacilli being found in the desquamating epithelium (sloughing of superficial layer of skin) of the skin, Weddell et al. had reported in 1963 that they could not find any acid-fast bacilli in the epidermis, even after examining a very large number of specimens from patients and contacts.

In a recent study, Job et al. found fairly large numbers of M. leprae in the superficial keratin layer of the skin of lepromatous leprosy patients, suggesting that the organism could exit along with the sebaceous secretions.

The importance of the nasal mucosa was recognized as early as 1898 by Schäffer, particularly that of the ulcerated mucosa. The quantity of bacilli from nasal mucosal lesions in lepromatous leprosy was demonstrated by Shepard as large, with counts ranging from 10,000 to 10,000,000. Pedley reported that the majority of lepromatous patients showed leprosy bacilli in their nasal secretions as collected through blowing the nose. Davey and Rees indicated that nasal secretions from lepromatous patients could yield as much as 10 million viable organisms per day.

The entry route of M. leprae into the human body is also not definitely known. The two seriously considered are the skin and the upper respiratory tract. While older research dealt with the skin route, recent research has increasingly favored the respiratory route. Rees and McDougall succeeded in the experimental transmission of leprosy through aerosols containing M. leprae in immune-suppressed mice, suggesting a similar possibility in humans. Successful results have also been reported on experiments with nude mice when M. leprae were introduced into the nasal cavity by topical application. In summary, entry through the respiratory route appears the most probable route, although other routes, particularly broken skin, cannot be ruled out.

In leprosy both the reference points for measuring the incubation period and the times of infection and onset of disease are difficult to define; the former because of the lack of adequate immunological tools and the latter because of the disease's slow onset. Even so, several investigators have attempted to measure the incubation period for leprosy. The minimum incubation period reported is as short as a few weeks and this is based on the very occasional occurrence of leprosy among young infants. The maximum incubation period reported is as long as 30 years, or over, as observed among war veterans known to have been exposed for short periods in endemic areas but otherwise living in non-endemic areas. It is generally agreed that the average incubation period is between 3 and 5 years.

Diagnosis: Diagnosis of leprosy is most commonly based on the clinical signs and symptoms. These are easy to observe and elicit by any health worker after a short period of training. In practice, most often persons with such complaints report on their own to the health centre. Only in rare instances is there a need to use laboratory and other investigations to confirm a diagnosis of leprosy.

In an endemic country or area, an individual should be regarded as having leprosy if he or she shows one of the following cardinal signs:

- Skin lesion consistent with leprosy and with definite sensory loss, with or without thickened nerves.
- Positive skin smears.

The skin lesion can be single or multiple, usually less pigmented than the surrounding normal skin. Sometimes the lesion is reddish or copper-coloured. A variety of skin lesions may be seen but macules (flat), papules (raised), or nodules are common. Sensory loss is a typical feature of leprosy. The skin lesion may show loss of sensation to pin pick and/or light touch. Thickened nerves, mainly peripheral nerve trunks constitute another feature of leprosy. A thickened nerve is often accompanied by other signs as a result of damage to the nerve. These may be loss of sensation in the skin and weakness of muscles supplied by the affected nerve. In the absence of these signs, nerve thickening by itself, without sensory loss and/or muscle weakness is often not a reliable sign of leprosy. The clinical system of classification for the purpose of treatment includes the use of number of skin lesions and nerves involved as the basis for grouping leprosy patients into multibacillary (MB) and paucibacillary (PB) leprosy.

Positive skin smears: In a small proportion of cases, rod-shaped, red-stained leprosy bacilli, which are diagnostic of the disease, may be seen in the smears taken from the affected skin when examined under a microscope after appropriate staining. Leprosy can be classified on the basis of clinical manifestations and skin smear results. In the classification based on skin smears, patients showing negative smears at all sites are grouped as paucibacillary leprosy (PB), while those showing positive smears at any site are grouped as having multibacillary leprosy (MB).

A person presenting with skin lesions or with symptoms suggestive of nerve damage, in whom the cardinal signs are absent or doubtful should be called a "suspect case" in the absence of any immediately obvious alternate diagnosis. Such individuals should be told the basic facts of leprosy and advised to return to the centre if signs persist for more than six months or if at any time worsening is noticed. Suspect cases may be also sent to referral clinics with more facilities for diagnosis.

Treatment: Until the development of dapsone, rifampicin, and clofazimine in the 1940s, there was no effective cure for leprosy. However, dapsone is only weakly bactericidal against M. leprae and it was considered necessary for patients to take the drug indefinitely. Moreover, when dapsone was used alone, the M. leprae population quickly evolved antibiotic resistance; by the 1960s, the world's only known anti-leprosy drug became virtually useless.

The search for more effective anti-leprosy drugs than dapsone led to the use of clofazimine and rifampicin in the 1960s and 1970s. Later, Indian scientist Shantaram Yawalkar and his colleagues formulated a combined therapy using rifampicin and dapsone, intended to mitigate bacterial resistance. Multidrug therapy (MDT) and combining all three drugs was first recommended by a WHO Expert Committee in 1981. These three anti-leprosy drugs are still used in the standard MDT regimens. None of them are used alone because of the risk of developing resistance.

Because this treatment is quite expensive, it was not quickly adopted in most endemic countries. In 1985 leprosy was still considered a public health problem in 122 countries. The 44th World Health Assembly (WHA), held in Geneva in 1991 passed a resolution to eliminate leprosy as a public health problem by the year 2000 - defined as reducing the global prevalence of the disease to less than 1 case per 100,000. At the Assembly, the World Health Organization (WHO) was given the mandate to develop an elimination strategy by its member states, based on increasing the geographical coverage of MDT and patients' accessibility to the treatment.

The WHO Study Group's report on the Chemotherapy of Leprosy in 1993 recommended two types of standard MDT regimen be adopted. The first was a 24-month treatment for multibacillary (MB or lepromatous) cases using rifampicin, clofazimine, and dapsone. The second was a six-month treatment for paucibacillary (PB or tuberculoid) cases, using rifampicin and dapsone. At the First International Conference on the Elimination of Leprosy as a Public Health Problem, held in Hanoi, the global strategy was endorsed and funds provided to WHO for the procurement and supply of MDT to all endemic countries.

Between 1995 and 1999, WHO, with the aid of the Nippon Foundation (Chairman Y?hei Sasakawa, World Health Organization Goodwill Ambassador for Leprosy Elimination), supplied all endemic countries with free MDT in blister packs, channelled through Ministries of Health. This free provision was extended in 2000 with a donation by the MDT manufacturer Novartis, which will run until at least the end of 2010. At the national level, non-government organizations (NGOs) affiliated to the national programme will continue to be provided with an appropriate free supply of this WHO supplied MDT by the government.

MDT remains highly effective and patients are no longer infectious after the first monthly dose. It is safe and easy to use under field conditions due to its presentation in calendar blister packs. Relapse rates remain low, and there is no known resistance to the combined drugs. The Seventh WHO Expert Committee on Leprosy, reporting in 1997, concluded that the MB duration of treatment-then standing at 24 months-could safely be shortened to 12 months "without significantly compromising its efficacy."

Persistent obstacles to the elimination of the disease include improving detection, educating patients and the population about its cause, and fighting social taboos about a disease for which patients have historically been considered "unclean" or "cursed by God" as outcasts. Where taboos are strong, patients may be forced to hide their condition (and avoid seeking treatment) to avoid discrimination. The lack of awareness about Hansen's disease can lead people to falsely believe that the disease is highly contagious and incurable.

Prevention and control: Because leprosy can be cured with medicines, an early diagnosis will often reduce leprosy symptoms and complications. Therefore, while prevention of leprosy is not always possible, especially where leprosy is endemic, control should be possible.

For prevention of leprosy, people who live in the same household as a person with leprosy (household contacts) will need to be examined by a physician. These examinations should be repeated annually for five years. It is important to note that the degree of natural immunity is high, and there is often no need for preventative medicine. However, if you are a household contact and you develop a questionable skin rash, you should have a skin biopsy to determine whether or not leprosy is present.

STD

A sexually transmitted disease (STD) or venereal disease (VD), is an illness that has a significant probability of transmission between humans or animals by means of sexual contact. Increasingly, the term sexually transmitted infection (STI) is used, as it has a broader range of meaning; a person may be infected, and may potentially infect others, without showing signs of disease. Some STIs can also be transmitted via use of an IV drug needle after its use by an infected person, as well as through childbirth or breastfeeding. Sexually transmitted infections have been well known for hundreds of years.

Public health officials originally introduced the term sexually transmitted infection, which clinicians are increasingly using alongside the term sexually transmitted disease in order to distinguish it from the former. Infection simply means that a germ - virus, bacteria, or parasite - that can cause disease or sickness is present inside a person's body. An infected person does not necessarily have any symptoms or signs that the virus or bacteria is actually hurting his or her body; they do not necessarily feel sick. A disease means that the infection is actually causing the infected person to feel sick, or to notice something is wrong. For this reason, the term STI - which refers to infection with any germ that can cause an STD, even if the infected person has no symptoms - is a much broader term than STD." The distinction being made, however, is closer to that between a colonization and an infection, rather than between an infection and a disease.

Specifically, the term STD refers only to infections that are causing symptoms. Because most of the time people do not know that they are infected with an STD until they start showing symptoms of disease, most people use the term STD, even though the term STI is also appropriate in many cases.

Moreover, the term sexually transmissible disease is sometimes used since it is less restrictive in consideration of other factors or means of transmission. For instance, meningitis is transmissible by means of sexual contact but is not labelled as an STI because sexual contact is not the primary vector for the pathogens that cause meningitis. This discrepancy is addressed by the probability of infection by means other than sexual contact. In general, an STI is an infection that has a negligible probability of transmission by means other than sexual contact, but has a realistic means of transmission by sexual contact (more sophisticated means - blood transfusion, sharing of hypodermic needles -are not taken into account). Thus, one may presume that, if a person is infected with an STI, e.g., chlamydia, gonorrhoea, genital herpes, it was transmitted to him/her by means of sexual contact.

Pathology: Many STIs are (more easily) transmitted through the mucous membranes of the penis, vulva, rectum, urinary tract and (less often - depending on type of infection) the mouth, throat, respiratory tract and eyes. The visible membrane covering the head of the penis is a mucous membrane, though it produces no mucus (similar to the lips of the mouth). Mucous membranes differ from skin in that they allow certain pathogens into the body. Pathogens are also able to pass through breaks or abrasions of the skin, even minute ones. The shaft of the penis is particular susceptible due to the friction caused during penetrative sex. The primary sources of infection in ascending order are venereal fluids, saliva, mucosal or skin (particularly the penis), infections may also be transmitted from faeces, urine and sweat (CMV). The amount required to cause infection varies with each pathogen but is always less than you can see with the naked eye.

This is one reason that the probability of transmitting many infections is far higher from sex than by more casual means of transmission, such as non-sexual contact-touching, hugging, shaking hands-but it is not the only reason. Although mucous membranes exist in the mouth as in the genitals, many STIs seem to be easier to transmit through oral sex than through deep kissing. According to this chart, many infections that are easily transmitted from the mouth to the genitals or from the genitals to the mouth, are much harder to transmit from one mouth to another. With HIV, genital fluids happen to contain much more of the pathogen than saliva. Some infections labelled as STIs can be transmitted by direct skin contact. Herpes simplex and HPV are both examples. KSHV, on the other hand, may be transmitted by deep-kissing but also when saliva is used as a sexual lubricant.

Depending on the STD, a person may still be able to spread the infection if no signs of disease are present. For example, a person is much more likely to spread herpes infection when blisters are present (STD) than when they are absent (STI). However, a person can spread HIV infection (STI) at any time, even if he/she has not developed symptoms of AIDS (STD).

All sexual behaviours that involve contact with the bodily fluids of another person should be considered to contain some risk of transmission of sexually transmitted diseases. Most attention has focused on controlling HIV, which causes AIDS, but each STD presents a different situation.

As may be noted from the name, sexually transmitted diseases are transmitted from one person to another by certain sexual activities rather than being actually caused by those sexual activities. Bacteria, fungi, protozoa or viruses are still the causative agents. It is not possible to catch any sexually transmitted disease from a sexual activity with a person who is not carrying a disease; conversely, a person who has an STD got it from contact (sexual or otherwise) with someone who had it, or his/her bodily fluids. Some STDs such as HIV can be transmitted from mother to child either during pregnancy or breastfeeding.

Although the likelihood of transmitting various diseases by various sexual activities varies a great deal, in general, all sexual activities between two (or more) people should be considered as being a two-way route for the transmission of STDs, i.e., "giving" or "receiving" are both risky although receiving carries a higher risk.

Healthcare professionals suggest safer sex, such as the use of condoms, as the most reliable way of decreasing the risk of contracting sexually transmitted diseases during sexual activity, but safer sex should by no means be considered an absolute safeguard. The transfer of and exposure to bodily fluids, such as blood transfusions and other blood products, sharing injection needles, needle-stick injuries (when medical staff are inadvertently jabbed or pricked with needles during medical procedures), sharing tattoo needles, and childbirth are other avenues of transmission. These different means put certain groups, such as medical workers, and haemophiliacs and drug users, particularly at risk.

Recent epidemiological studies have investigated the networks that are defined by sexual relationships between individuals, and discovered that the properties of sexual networks are crucial to the spread of sexually transmitted diseases. In particular, assortative mixing between people with large numbers of sexual partners seems to be an important factor.

It is possible to be an asymptomatic carrier of sexually transmitted diseases. In particular, sexually transmitted diseases in women often cause the serious condition of pelvic inflammatory disease.

Epidemiology: STD incidence rates remain high in most of the world, despite diagnostic and therapeutic advances that can rapidly render patients with many STDs non-infectious and cure most. In many cultures, changing sexual morals and oral contraceptive use have eliminated traditional sexual restraints, especially for women, and both physicians and patients have difficulty dealing openly and candidly with sexual issues. Additionally, development and spread of drug-resistant bacteria (e.g., penicillin-resistant gonococci) makes some STDs harder to cure. The effect of travel is most dramatically illustrated by the rapid spread of the AIDS virus (HIV-1) from Africa to Europe and the Americas in the late 1970s.

Commonly reported prevalence of STIs among sexually active adolescent girls both with and without lower genital tract symptoms include chlamydia trachomatis (10 to 25%), Neisseria gonorrhoeae (3 to 18%), syphilis (0 to 3%), Trichomonas vaginalis (8 to 16%), and herpes simplex virus (2 to 12%). Among adolescent boys with no symptoms of urethritis, isolation rates include C. trachomatis (9 to 11%) and N. gonorrhoeae (2 to 3%).

In 1996, WHO estimated that more than 1 million people were being infected daily. About 60% of these infections occur in young people <25 years of age, and of these 30% are <20 years. Between the ages of 14 and 19, STDs occur more frequently in girls than boys by a ratio of nearly 2: 1; this equalizes by age 20. An estimated 340 million new cases of syphilis, gonorrhea, chlamydia and trichomoniasis occurred throughout the world in 1999.

Prevention: Vaccines are available that protect against some viral STIs, such as Hepatitis B and some types of HPV. Vaccination before initiation of sexual contact is advised to assure maximal protection. The most effective way to prevent sexual transmission of STIs is to avoid contact of body parts or fluids which can lead to transfer, not necessarily any sexual activity with an infected partner. No contact minimizes risk. Not all sexual activities involve contact: cybersex, phonesex or masturbation from a distance are methods of avoiding contact. Proper use of condoms (male or female) reduces contact and risk.

Ideally, both partners should get tested for STIs before initiating sexual contact, or before resuming contact if a partner engaged in contact with someone else. Many infections are not detectable immediately after exposure, so enough time must be allowed between possible exposures and testing for the tests to be accurate. Certain STIs, particularly certain persistent viruses like HPV, may be impossible to detect with current medical procedures.

Many diseases that establish permanent infections can so occupy the immune system that other diseases become more easily transmitted. The innate immune system led by defensins against HIV can prevent transmission of HIV when viral counts are very low, but if busy with other viruses or overwhelmed, HIV can establish itself. Certain viral STI's also greatly increase the risk of death for HIV infected patients.

Condoms: Condoms only provide protection when used properly as a barrier, and only to and from the area that it covers. Uncovered areas are still susceptible to many STDs. In the case of HIV, sexual transmission routes almost always involve the penis, as HIV cannot spread through unbroken skin, thus properly shielding the insertive penis with a properly worn condom from the vagina and anus effectively stops HIV transmission. An infected fluid to broken skin borne direct transmission of HIV would not be considered "sexually transmitted", but can still theoretically occur during sexual contact, this can be avoided simply by not engaging in sexual contact when having open bleeding wounds. Other STDs, even viral infections, can be prevented with the use of latex condoms as a barrier. Some microorganisms and viruses are small enough to pass through the pores in natural skin condoms, but are still too large to pass through latex condoms.

Testing: Prior to the invention of modern medicines, sexually transmitted diseases were generally incurable, and treatment was limited to treating the symptoms of the disease. The first voluntary hospital for venereal diseases was founded in 1746 at London Lock Hospital. The first effective treatment for a sexually transmitted disease was salvarsan, a treatment for syphilis. With the discovery of antibiotics, a large number of sexually transmitted diseases became easily curable, and this, combined with effective public health campaigns against STDs, led to a public perception during the 1960s and 1970s that they have ceased to be a serious medical threat.

During this period, the importance of contact tracing in treating STIs was recognized. By tracing the sexual partners of infected individuals, testing them for infection, treating the infected and tracing their contacts in turn, STI clinics could be very effective at suppressing infections in the general population.

In the 1980s, first genital herpes and then AIDS emerged into the public consciousness as sexually transmitted diseases that could not be cured by modern medicine. AIDS in particular has a long asymptomatic period - during which time HIV (the human immunodeficiency virus, which causes AIDS) can replicate and the disease can be transmitted to others - followed by a symptomatic period, which leads rapidly to death unless treated. Recognition that AIDS threatened a global pandemic led to public information campaigns and the development of treatments that allow AIDS to be managed by suppressing the replication of HIV for as long as possible. Contact tracing continues to be an important measure, even when diseases are incurable, as it helps to contain infection.

Types: Most of the diseases on this list are most commonly transmitted sexually. Some are commonly transmitted in other ways as well; for example, HIV/AIDS is also commonly transmitted through the sharing of infected needles by drug users, while SARS, which can be spread through casual contact such as coughing and sneezing, is very often not associated with sexual activity.

Bacterial

- Bacterial Vaginosis (BV) - not officially an STD but affected by sexual activity.
- Chancroid (Haemophilus ducreyi)
- Donovanosis (Granuloma inguinale or Calymmatobacterium granulomatis)
- Gonorrhea (Neisseria gonorrhoeae)
- Lymphogranuloma venereum (LGV) (Chlamydia trachomatis serotypes L1, L2, L3.)
- Non-gonococcal urethritis (NGU) (Ureaplasma urealyticum or Mycoplasma hominis)
- Staphylococcal infection (Staphylococcus aureus, MRSA) - Sexually transmissible.
- Syphilis (Treponema pallidum)

Fungal

- Tinea cruris "Jock Itch" (Trichophyton rubrum and others). - Sexually transmissible.
- Yeast Infection

Viral

- Adenoviruses thought to contribute to obesity - venereal fluids (also faecal & respiratory fluids)
- Viral hepatitis (Hepatitis B virus) - saliva, venereal fluids.

(Note: Hepatitis A and Hepatitis E are transmitted via the faecal-oral route; Hepatitis C (liver cancer) is rarely sexually transmittable, and the route of transmission of Hepatitis D (only if infected with B) is uncertain, but may include sexual transmission.)

- Herpes Simplex (Herpes simplex virus (1, 2)) skin and mucosal, transmissible with or without visible blisters
  - — Herpes simplex virus 1 may be linked to Alzheimer's disease.
- HIV/AIDS (Human Immunodeficiency Virus) - venereal fluids
- HTLV 1, 2 - venereal fluids

- Genital warts - ("low risk" types of Human papillomavirus HPV) - skin and muscosal, transmissible with or without visible warts
- Cervical cancer, anal cancer - ("high risk" types of Human papillomavirus HPV) - skin and muscosal
- Molluscum contagiosum (molluscum contagiosum virus MCV) - close contact
- mononucleosis
  — (Cytomegalovirus CMV - Herpes 5) - saliva, sweat, urine, feces and venereal fluids.
  — (Epstein-Barr virus EBV - Herpes 4) - saliva
- Kaposi's sarcoma (Kaposi's sarcoma-associated herpes virus KSHV - Herpes 8) - saliva

Parasites

- Pubic lice, colloquially known as "crabs" (Phthirius pubis)
- Scabies (Sarcoptes scabiei)

Protozoal

- Trichomoniasis (Trichomonas vaginalis)

Sexually transmitted enteric infections: Various bacterial (Shigella, Campylobacter, or Salmonella), viral (Hepatitis A, Adenoviruses), or parasitic (Giardia or amoeba) pathogens are transmitted by sexual practices that promote anal-oral contamination (faecal-oral). Sharing sex toys without washing or multiple partnered barebacking can promote anal-anal contamination. Although the bacterial pathogens may coexist with or cause proctitis, they usually produce symptoms (diarrhoea, fever, bloating, nausea, and abdominal pain) suggesting disease more proximal in the GI tract.

Sexually transmissible oral infections: Common colds, influenza, Staphylococcus aureus, E. coli, Adenoviruses, Human Papillomavirus, Oral Herpes (1, 2 & 4, 5, 8), Hepatitis B and the yeast Candida albicans can all be transmitted through the oral route.

YAWS

Aetiology: Yaws also Pétasse tropica, thymosis, polypapilloma tropicum, pian or parangi) is a tropical infection of the skin, bones and joints caused by the spirochete bacterium Treponema pallidum pertenue.

Epidemiology: Yaws is found in humid tropical regions in South America, Africa, Asia and Oceania. Mass treatment campaigns in the

1950s reduced the worldwide prevalence from 50-100 million to fewer than 2 million; however during the 1970s there were outbreaks in south-east Asia and there have been continued sporadic cases in South America. It is unclear how many people worldwide are infected at present. The disease is transmitted by skin-to-skin contact with an infective lesion, the bacterium entering through a pre-existing cut, bite or scratch.

Prior to the mass campaign of the 1950s, Yaws was endemic in Andhra Pradesh, Madhya Pradesh, Maharashtra, Orissa and Tamil Nadu. A recent survey (1985), suggests that Yaws continues to occur in India, although at a lower level, in at least three states, viz. Andhra Pradesh, Madhya Pradesh and Orissa, a total of 1,349 Yaws cases were diagnosed in these three states between 1983 and mid-1985. The affected districts were: West Godavari, Khammam and Vizianagaram in Andhra Pradesh, Bastar in Madhya Pradesh, and Keonjarh, Mayurbhanj, Denkanel, Phulbani, Balasore, and Koraput in Orissa. Whereas, in Andhra Pradesh Yaws occurred exclusively among the tribal population, in Orissa and Madhya Pradesh, both tribal and non-tribal populations were affected. The problem of Yaws now is one of either "Residual yaws" or "Recrudescence" of Yaws due to continued low levels of transmission in some area which has to be controlled and eradicated. Only serological surveys will provide a valid measurement of the problem.

Pathogenesis: Within ninety days (but usually less than a month) of infection a painless but distinctive 'mother yaw' appears, which is a painless nodule which enlarges and becomes warty in appearance. Sometimes nearby 'daughter yaws' also appear simultaneously. This primary stage resolves completely within six months. The secondary stage occurs months to years later, and is characterised by widespread skin lesions of varying appearance, including 'crab yaws' on the palms and soles with desquamation.

These secondary lesions frequently ulcerate (and are then highly infectious), but heal after six months or more. About ten percent of people then go on to develop tertiary disease within five to ten years (during which further secondary lesions may come and go), characterised by widespread bone, joint and soft tissue destruction, which may include extensive destruction of the bone and cartilage of the nose (rhinopharyngitis mutilans or 'gangosa').

Diagnosis: Dark field microscopy of samples taken from early lesions (particularly ulcerative lesions) may show the responsible organism. Blood tests such as RPR and TPHA will also be positive, but there are no current blood tests which distinguish between the four treponematoses.

Treatment: Treatment is normally by a single dose of intramuscular penicillin, or by a course of penicillin, erythromycin or tetracycline tablets. Early lesions may heal completely, but the destructive changes of tertiary yaws are largely irreversible.

Prevention and control: There is no vaccine to prevent Yaws. The principles of prevention are based on the interruption of transmission by early diagnosis and treatment of affected individuals and their contacts.

HIV

Aetiology: The causative agents of the disease are lymphadenopathy associated virus (LAV) isolated in France, and human T-cell lymphotropic virus type III (HTLV III). According to WHO's recommendations, the AIDS virus is called LAV/HTLV-III virus. In 1986, at the International AIDS conference it was suggested that the causative agent of AIDS should be given the name of HIV (human immunodeficiency virus). The virus belongs to the family Retroviridae named so because they contain reverse transcriptase, the enzyme that catalyzes the transcription of RNA to DNA. Oncoviruses also belong to the family of retroviruses. The only oncovirus that has been isolated by the present time is T-cell lymphotropic virus type I (HTLV I) which is the causative agent of lymphosarcoma. The AIDS agent can be found in the blood, semen, urine, saliva and other body fluids of the patient or virus carrier. The infection can thus be transmitted with blood, by sexual intercourse and other contacts. The virus is sensitive to high temperature. At 56°C it is killed in 30 minutes. The virus is sensitive to ether, acetone, and chlorine preparations. It can artificially be grown only in human T-cell cultures.

Epidemiology: The source of infection are human beings. Both patients and virus carriers can be the source. The virus persists in patients for life, while the duration of the carrier state has not yet been established. Virus carriers are especially dangerous because they are not aware of their disease and dissipate the virus among the surrounding people. The virus is transmitted by direct contact during sexual intercourse, through the fomites infected with the patient's or carrier's blood (the virus enters through minor defects on the skin or mucosa), through reuse of carelessly sterilized injection needles or lancets or other tools used in transfusion of blood, blood substitutes, coagulation factors, erythrocytes, leucocytes or, thrombocytes.

The AIDS virus can be transmitted from diseased mothers (or virus carriers) to their foetus. Persons belonging to the so-called risk groups are usually infected. These are homosexual men and bisexuals, drug abusers (intravenous infections by non-sterile syringes), haemophiliacs, persons who receive numerous blood transfusions, and children whose parents belong to the risk groups. Haemophiliacs are often infected by injections of blood coagulating factors VIII and IX (the material is prepared from the blood obtained from at least 2000 donors). AIDS is reported now from many countries of all continents. The endemic areas are believed to be the countries of Central Africa and USA.

Pathogenesis: The AIDS virus enters the blood of a human being and attacks selectively T helpers that include B cells and antibody products which support the function of the immune system. The quantity of T helpers (relative to T suppressors) is reduced in AIDS patients. Besides, the immune control of atypical cell formation decreases and this results in higher occurrence of tumour diseases in AIDS patients. Immune deficiency is the cause of cancer (Kaposi's sarcoma in persons aged under 60, lymphoma of the brain, angioblastic lymphadenopathy). Involvement of the central nervous system causes dementia, multiple sclerosis, etc. Reduced quantity of T helpers decreases bodily resistance to exogenous and endogenous microorganisms, which are otherwise not dangerous.

Clinical picture: It is believed that AIDS can run the following three main forms:

- Asymptomatic
- Systemic lymphadenopathy
- AIDS proper (with secondary infection superimposed upon the specific symptoms of AIDS).

Duration of the asymptomatic infection has not been determined. The signs of the disease are absent, but the specific serologic tests are positive; cases of transmission of the disease by such patients have been reported. The incubation period of AIDS lasts from several months to 5 years. It is followed by the prodromal period (pre-AIDS). This period is usually called generalized (systemic) lymphadenopathy. The specific symptom of this period is enlargement of the lymph nodes on the neck, elbows, and in the armpits. The lymph nodes are moderately tender or painless. They do not fuse with the subcutaneous cellular tissue and are mobile. Their size varies from 1 to 3 cm in diameter.

The body temperature is 37-40°C. Fever can be continuous or intermittent. Profuse sweating, especially during night, and weakness are characteristic. Stool disorders are persistent (at least for 2 months) and resemble those seen in enterocolitis. Unmotivated wasting is characteristic: the patient loses at least 10 per cent of his body weight.

Candidal stomatitis and oesophagitis, suppurative and inflammatory lesions of the genitalia and skin, rash, and frontal alopecia often supervene. Lymphadenopathy can last from 3 months to several years. During the period characterized as AIDS proper, all these symptoms increase. Weakness, fever and diarrhoea intensify; weight loss progresses; hepatomegaly, cough and leucopenia (with possible superimposition of erythroblastopenia) develop.

During the advanced stage of the disease, secondary infection supervenes. Several types of the disease are distinguished in this connection. Pneumocystic pneumonia. The disease is characterized by hypoxaemia, chest pain, and diffuse infiltrations evidenced by x-ray. Pneumonia is often due to Pneumocystis carinii, less frequently due to Legionella Pneumophila. The lungs are involved in more than 50 per cent of AIDS patients.

The central nervous system is involved in about one third of patients. The following forms are differentiated: abscess (due to Toxoplasma gondii), leucoencephalopathy cryptococcal meningitis, subacute encephalitis; tumours (primary and secondary lymphoma of the brain); vascular lesions and lesions of the central nervous system with focal cerebral involvement. Lesions of the central nervous system are associated with the supervening secondary infections.

The gastrointestinal type is characterized by prevalence of diarrhoea, marked wasting, and fever. Secondary infection is usually due to Cryptosporidia and viruses. Other diseases are also possible: ophthalmic lesions (conjunctivitis, keratitis, retinal haemorrhage, etc.), diseases of the kidneys, or skin diseases (usually Kaposi's sarcoma). Secondary infections are usually due to: protozoa and helminths (Pneumocystis carinii) that cause pneumonia; Toxoplasmodia causing pneumonia or lesion of the central nervous system; Cryptosporidia causing intestinal lesions with long-standing diarrhoea; Strongylidiae, causing pneumonia and lesion of the central nervous system; fungi, causing candidiasis, involving the oesophagus and the mouth cavity; cryptococci, causing lesions of the lungs and central nervous system; bacteria (Legionellae), causing pneumonia; mycobacteria, causing disseminated infections; salmonellae, causing enteritis and sepsis; viruses, causing lesions of the lungs, gastrointestinal tract, and the central nervous system; herpesvirus, causing lesions of the lungs, mucosa, and gastrointestinal tract, etc.

Diagnosis: Difficulties in establishing the diagnosis of AIDS are associated with the polymorphous clinical picture of the disease. The diagnosis is based on epidemiologic, clinical, and laboratory findings. The disease usually afflicts homosexual men and bisexuals, prostitutes, drug addicts, and haemophiliacs. Serologic and immunologic tests are used to reveal antibodies to the AIDS virus in the blood of patients and carriers.

Discovery of virus components (antigens, nucleic acid, reverse transcriptase) or virus cultures (blood cultures of human T-cells) are necessary for establishing an accurate diagnosis. A blood specimen (5 ml) of a person suspected for AIDS is taken into 2 sterile test tubes containing 0.7 ml of heparin solution. All precautions should be taken when handling specimens of human material: the laboratory worker must wear gloves and special overalls; syringes, pipettes and laboratory wears must be discarded after a single use. Test tubes containing blood are placed in plastic bags that should be destroyed after use. Serologic tests include reactions with enzyme-labelled antibodies to whole virus, solid-phase radioimmunologic studies, immunofluorescent and immuno-precipitation tests.

The quantity of T helpers decreases relative to the quantity of T supressor cells in AIDS patients. But this index is also low in individuals of the risk groups. Leucopenia and lymphopenia are seen; the quantity of immunoglobulins, especially of IgA and IgG, is low. Skin allergic tests reveal anergia.

Treatment: Specific treatment is not effective. Acyclovir, riboverin and sumarin act on reverse transcriptase. Preparations acting on the virus, such as rifampidine, cyclosporin, and some other preparations are also used. Interferon is given in large doses. Pathogenetic means include hormones of the thymus that act on immunogenesis. These preparations include thymosin, V fractions, T activin, thymostimulin and thymulin. Interleukin-2 is effectively used: it produces effect on maturation, proliferation and differentiation of T-cells. Treatment of secondary infection depends on the nature of the causative agent. The main difficulty of treating AIDS is that one secondary infection may be followed by others.

Prevention and control. Purely medical measures should be combined with measures taken by governmental institutions. The latter include improvement of work at medical and prophylactic institutions where aetiology, epidemiology, pathogenesis, clinic, diagnosis and prevention of AIDS are studied and AIDS patients and carriers are treated. Control of drug abuse, prostitution, homosexualism and other AIDS-promoting phenomena are also important measures. Medical measures include detection, isolation and treatment of AIDS patients and virus carriers. Virus carriers should be detected and observed.

Health education, especially among the young, is very important. Health education must give information on the main symptoms of the disease, measures that may prevent infection, information about the source and ways of infection transmission. Importance of mechanical contraceptive means (condoms) must be emphasized. Donors must undergo thorough serologic and clinical control. AIDS patients and suspected individuals should be placed in separate rooms of infectious hospitals in order to protect them from nosocomial infection and to preclude dissipation of the AIDS virus.

The number of healthy personnel should be minimized. Current disinfection is necessary. Medical personnel should take precautions while examining, treating and attending the patients. Laboratory personnel must be careful as well when handling blood and other materials of AIDS patients. Higher medical authorities should immediately be informed of any new case of AIDS. Carriers must be examined twice a year. If any symptoms are noted, the patient must attend his doctor immediately. Elaboration of the vaccine is a difficult problem because of the high genetic variability of the virus.

Detection of the AIDS virus in the blood, saliva, urine or other body fluids is an indication for current disinfection in the focus of infection and observation of the following rules: it is prohibited to use articles that were used by the patient and through which the blood of AIDS patients or carriers might gain entrance through damaged skin or mucosa of the surrounding people.

REFERENCES

Intersectoral action: Towards population health. Report of the Federal/ Provincial Advisory Committee on Population Health. Ottawa: Health Canada, Communications Directorate, 1999.

Kingdon JW. Agenda, alternatives and public policies. New York: Harper Collins College Publishers. 1995.

Koepsell TD, Wagner EH, Cheadle AC, Patrick DL, Martin DC, Diehr PH, Perrin EB, Kristal AR, Allan-Andrilla CH, Dey LJ. Selected methodological issues in evaluating community-based health promotion and disease prevention programs. Annu Rev Public Health. 1992; 13: 31-57.

Koopman JS, Lynch JW. Individual causal models and population system models in epidemiology. Am J Public Health. 1999; 89(8): 1170-1174.

Kothari A, Birch S. Multilevel health promotion research: Conceptual and analytical considerations. Can J Nurs Res. 2004;36(1): 56-75.

Krauss M, Mueller N, Luke D. Interorganizational relationships within state tobacco control networks: A social network analysis. Prev Chronic Dis. 2004;1(4): 1-25.

Krieger N. Theories for social epidemiology in the 21st century: An ecosocial perspective. Int J Epidemiol. 2001;30(4): 668-677.

Kuhn M, Doucet C, Edwards N. Effectiveness of coalitions in heart health promotion, tobacco use reduction, and injury prevention: A systematic review of the literature 1990-1998. March 1999. Effective Public Health Practice Project.

Kumaranayake L, Watts C. Resource allocation and priority setting of HIV/AIDS interventions: Addressing the generalized epidemic in Sub-Saharan Africa. J Int Dev. 2001;13(4): 451-466.

Labonte R, Schrecker T, Sanders D, Meeus W. Fatal Indifference: The G8, Africa and Global Health. International Development Research Centre. Ottawa. 2004.

Laterveer L, Niessne LW, Yazbeck AS. Pro-poor health policies in poverty reduction strategies. Health Policy Plann. 2003;18(2): 138-145.

Locher AW, Didiion JA. Epidemic to endemic: The impact of HIV on health care policy and nursing practice. Policy, Politics & Nursing Practice. 2003;4(1): 62-70.

Mancini JA, Marek LI. Sustaining community-based programs for families: Conceptualization and measurement. Family Relations. 2004;53: 339-347.

Mathias RG. Death Sentence: Canada's Drug Laws. A public health framework for drug control in Canada. Monograph, Department of Health Care and Epidemiology, University of British Columbia. 2002.

Mayne J. Addressing attribution through contribution analysis: Using performance measures sensibly. Can J Program Eval. 2001;16(1): 1-24.

McCoy D, Sanders D, Baum F, Narayan T, Legge D. Pushing the international health research agenda towards equity and effectiveness. Lancet. 2004;364(9445): 1630-1631.

McDowell I, Spasoff R, Kristjansson B. Evaluation methods and practice: On the classification of population health measurements. Am J Public Health. 2004;94(3): 388-393.

McLaughlin, JA, Jordan, GB. Logic models: A tool for telling your program's performance story. Eval Program Plann. 1999;22(1): 65-72.

McLoughlin E, Fairweather. Influence of free trade on the politics of safety. Inj Prev. 2002; 8(1): 3-5.

Meadows D. Leverage points: Places to Intervene in a System. Sustainability Institute, 1999.

7

Epidemiology and Management of Non-Communicable Diseases

Non-communicable diseases (NCD) include diseases which do not have infectious agents which make them spread from one person to another. WHO (World Health Organisation) cluster of non communicable disease include cardiovascular diseases, Cancer, Diabetes, Chronic obstructive pulmonary disorders (COPD) or chronic respiratory diseases, mental illness and injuries. They are causes of enormous morbidity, premature mortality and a threat to the economic resources of many countries.

Understanding the differences is crucial in terms of finding appropriate cost effective strategies for prevention and control. The communicable diseases usually have a single causative agent, sudden onset of symptoms, respond to short course treatments and are curable whereas non-communicable diseases are multi factorial, have a long course with gradual onset of symptoms, require prolonged care & treatment and affect the quality of life.

It is estimated that by 2020, over 70% of the global burden of disease will be caused by non-communicable diseases, mental health disorders and injuries.' Alcohol related problems were the leading cause of male disability and the tenth leading cause of female disability in developed nations. Tobacco use was predicted to cause more disease and disability than any other single cause and to a greater extent in underdeveloped nations by the year 2020.

Chronic diseases are already the major cause of morbidity and mortality in the developed countries. The rapid rise of non-communicable diseases represents one of the major public health challenge that all the countries in the, would face. The world health report 1999 shows that in 1998 non communicable diseases accounted for 77% of global mortality and 85% of the global burden of disease was, from the low and middle income countries.

Most of the non-communicable diseases are linked to common risk factors, namely, tobacco use, alcohol abuse, unhealthy diet, physical inactivity and environmental carcinogens.

NUTRITION

The importance of diet and nutrition on the development of chronic non-communicable diseases are well proven. It leads to increased incidence of CVDS, various forms of cancers, diabetes, osteoporosis and also has adverse impact on oral health. The consumption of starch as staple food has declined and that of meat, eggs and diary foods have increased considerably. Frequent eating outside home and snacking often facilitate this increase in the consumption of high fat, animal products. Foods that are processed with high saturated fats, have become common and accessible to a wider section of the population.

Man kind eats to satisfy the feeling of hunger. Nutrition plays an important role in the promotion and maintenance of health and in the prevention of disease in order to keep well our bodies, need nourishment. Just as a plant will not grow without water sun shine and proper manure, human beings also need food stuffs of different kinds of nourish to the body. Malnutrition and under nutrition are the greatest international health problems of the present day. A sound knowledge of nutrition is therefore essential for all community health workers. Nutrition deals with the way in which the human body receives and uses all the substances or materials necessary for its growth and development and for keeping it is good condition.

A person who does not eats the right foods or does not eat enough is malnourished and we call this s malnutrition also means that a child is less clever than he should be. The trouble may start even before birth if his mother does not have the right foods when she is pregnant. The malnourished child does not play but sits doing nothing.

MALNUTRITION

This condition is wide spread in India among children 6 months to 3 years. Malnutrition is a condition which occurs when the body does not get the proper kind of food in the amounts needed for maintaining health or child is getting too little of energy foods (calories) as well as the little of body building (proteins) foods. in fact there is starvation or under nutrition.

India is home to the greatest population of severely malnourished children in the world. Four hundred million children suffer daily, which is a greater problem than in Sub-Saharan Africa. Childhood malnutrition is a massive crisis caused by a combination of factors including inadequate or inappropriate food intake, childhood diseases, harmful childcare practices, and improper care during illness: all contributing to poor health and millions of deaths annually. It affects growth potential and the risk of mortality and morbidity in later years of life.

Substantial improvements have been made in health and well being since India's independence in 1947 but still more than half of all children under the age of four are malnourished, 30 percent of newborns are significantly underweight, and 60 percent of women are anaemic. The early years of life are the most crucial because it is when the body develops the most mentally and physically and is most vulnerable to disease and illness.

The children of India are malnourished because of factors attributed to overpopulation, poverty, destruction of the environment, lack of education, gender inequality, and inaccessible medical care. Poverty is a major cause of malnourishment because it limits the amount of food available to children causing wasting and a lack of vitamins, minerals and nutritional value leading to stunting and low weight. Overpopulation is a serious problem linked to competition for food, shelter and medical care and leads to malnutrition amongst children, especially in rural areas where access to medical care and food is limited.

Protein-energy malnutrition (PEM) is a potentially fatal body-depletion disorder. It is the leading cause of death in children in developing countries. PEM is also referred to as protein-calorie malnutrition. It develops in children and adults whose consumption of protein and energy (measured by calories) is insufficient to satisfy the body's nutritional needs. While pure protein deficiency can occur when a person's diet provides enough energy but lacks the protein minimum, in most cases the deficiency will be dual. PEM may also occur in persons who are unable to absorb vital nutrients or convert them to energy essential for healthy tissue formation and organ function.

Types of PEM: Primary PEM results from a diet that lacks sufficient sources of protein and/or energy. Secondary PEM is more common in the United States, where it usually occurs as a complication of AIDS, cancer, chronic kidney failure, inflammatory bowel disease, and other illnesses that impair the body's ability to absorb or use nutrients or to compensate for nutrient losses. PEM can develop gradually in a patient who has a chronic illness or experiences chronic semi-starvation. It may appear suddenly in a patient who has an acute illness.

The main factors causing PEM are:

- Poverty and poor environmental sanitation.
- Ignorance, illiteracy, food fads and habits.
- Repeated infections such as diarrhoea and respiratory infections.
- Large families with not enough foods.
- Low birth weight and an anaemic mother.
- Infections, worm infections.

Signs and symptoms: The signs and symptoms of malnutrition in children are:

- Growth failure or the child loses weight.
- Skin changes - skin dry, scaly or rough, loss of sub coetaneous fat (elasticity).
- Eye changes - dryness, night blindness.
- Hair changes - light colour, brittle.
- Oedema.
- Anaemia.
- Others: Apathy, listlessness, soreness of mouth, bowing of legs, frequent episodes of illness etc.

Methods to identify malnutrition: There are several methods to identify malnutrition in children:

- Height and weight: The best way to identify children who are malnourished is to take their height and weight regularly. The growth chart shows the child's health and nutritional status.
- Mid arm circumference: Another simple and useful methods is to measure the mid arm circumference. Any child between 1-5 years considered to be malnourished, if the measurement is less than 12.8 cms.
- Clinical and laboratory examination: The examination of child from head to foot for signs of malnutrition (i.e. protein, vitamin and mineral deficiencies) is another approach for detecting malnutrition. Such examinations may be supplemented by laboratory tests such as estimation of haemoglobin.

Problems of Malnutrition

The important problems of malnutrition in India are:

Kwashiorkor and Marasmus: These are serious diseases of PEM. which develop in young children between 1-3 years of age. They are due to (a). An inadequate diet, that is a diet lacking in proteins and calories and (b) Infections such as diarrhoea, measles, bronchitis which lead the child into malnutrition.

The signs of Kwashiorkor are:

- Oedema.
- Growth failure
- Diarrhoea
- Hair and skin changes

The signs of Marasmus are:

- Marked wasting of muscles and
- Loss of subcutaneous fat.
- The child is reduced to "skin and bones". Kwashiorkor and Marasmus affect not only the physical growth but also mental development of the child. They can also cause death.

PEM need to be prevented by means of:

- Proper antenatal care of mothers, because a healthy mother give birth to a healthy baby.
- Promotion of breast feeding.
- Proper weaning of the child. The child should be given nutrition supplement starting around the age 4-6 months as breast milk alone is not sufficient to sustain the growth of the child. Nutritional supplements can be easily prepared at home using low cost locally available foods such as cereals, millets, pulses groundnuts, sugar and jaggery. Proper use of these supplements help in preventing malnutrition during the weaning period.
- Nutrition education of the mother.
- Immunization of the child against child hood diseases.
- Food hygiene practices to prevent infections.
- Economic development to decrease poverty.
- Improved environmental sanitation.

- Nutrition and health education.
- Family planning.

OVER NUTRITION

Over nutrition is a form of malnutrition in which nutrients are oversupplied relative to the amounts required for normal growth, development, and metabolism. The term can refer to obesity brought on by general overeating of foods high in caloric content, as well as the oversupply of a specific nutrient or categories of nutrients, such as mineral or vitamin poisoning due to excessive intake of dietary supplements, or nutritional imbalances caused by various fad diets.

Over nutrition results from eating too much, eating too many of the wrong things, not exercising enough, or taking too many vitamins or other dietary replacements. Risk of over nutrition is also increased by being more than 20% overweight, consuming a diet high in fat and salt, and taking high doses of:

- Nicotinic acid (niacin) to lower elevated cholesterol levels
- Vitamin B6 to relieve premenstrual syndrome
- Vitamin A to clear up skin problems
- Iron or other trace minerals not prescribed by a doctor

Nutritional disorders can affect any system in the body and the senses of sight, taste, and smell. Malnutrition begins with changes in nutrient levels in blood and tissues. Alterations in enzyme levels, tissue abnormalities, and organ malfunction may be followed by illness and death.

NUTRITIONAL DEFICIENCIES

Nutritional deficiencies occur when a person's nutrient intake consistently falls below the recommended requirement. Nutritional deficiencies can lead to a variety of health problems, the most prevalent of which are anaemia, beriberi, osteoporosis, pellagra, and rickets. Anaemia occurs when the body does not have enough red blood cells to transport oxygen from the lungs to the body's cells. The most common symptom of anaemia is a constant feeling of fatigue. Making sure that one's diet contains the proper amounts of iron, foliate, and vitamin B12 can prevent anaemia.

Prolonged thiamine deficiency can result in one of the more serious nutritional deficiencies, beriberi. Thiamine plays a major role in nerve processes, and a prolonged deficiency can result in nerve damage as well as heart and other muscle damage. Beriberi can be prevented by eating a diet containing foods rich in thiamine, such as meats, legumes, and whole-wheat breads.

Osteoporosis is an asymptomatic condition in which the loss of minerals can cause the body's bones to become porous and fragile. Making sure that one's diet contains the recommended amount of calcium and vitamin D can reduce the risk of developing osteoporosis. The niacin-deficiency disease, pellagra, can produce symptoms such as dermatitis, dementia, diarrhoea, and even death. Pellagra can be prevented through eating almost any protein-rich foods.

Nutritional Deficiency and Its Symptoms:

Nutrient	Typical Symptoms and Diseases
Biotin	Dermatitis, eye inflammation, hair loss, loss of muscle control, insomnia, muscle weakness
Calcium	Brittle nails, cramps, delusions, depression, insomnia, irritability, osteoporosis, palpitations, peridontal disease, rickets, tooth decay
Chromium	Anxiety, fatigue, glucose intolerance, adult-onset diabetes
Copper	Anaemia, arterial damage, depression, diarrhoea, fatigue, fragile bones, hair loss, hyperthyroidism, weakness
Essential fatty acids	Diarrhoea, dry skin and hair, hair loss, immune impairment, infertility, poor wound healing, premenstrual syndrome, acne, eczema, gall stones, liver degeneration
Folic acid	Anaemia, apathy, diarrhoea, fatigue, headaches, insomnia, loss of appetite, neural tube defects in foetus, paranoia, shortness of breath, weakness
Iodine	Cretinism, fatigue, hypothyroidism, weight gain
Magnesium	Anxiety, confusion, heart attack, hyperactivity, insomnia, nervousness, muscular irritability, restlessness, weakness
Manganese	Atherosclerosis, dizziness, elevated cholesterol, glucose intolerance, hearing loss, loss of muscle control, ringing in ears

Niacin	Bad breath, canker sores, confusion, depression, dermatitis, diarrhoea, emotional instability, fatigue, irritability, loss of appetite, memory impairment, muscle weakness, nausea, skin eruptions and inflammation
Pantothenic acid (B5)	Abdominal pains, burning feet, depression, eczema, fatigue, hair loss, immune impairment, insomnia, irritability, low blood pressure, muscle spasms, nausea, poor coordination
Potassium	Acne, constipation, depression, oedema, excessive water consumption, fatigue, glucose intolerance, high cholesterol levels, insomnia, mental impairment, muscle weakness, nervousness, poor reflexes
Pyridoxine (B6)	Acne, anaemia, arthritis, eye inflammation, depression, dizziness, facial oiliness, fatigue, impaired wound healing, irritability, loss of appetite, loss of hair, mouth lesions, nausea
Riboflavin	Blurred vision, cataracts, depression, dermatitis, dizziness, hair loss, inflamed eyes, mouth lesions, nervousness, neurological symptoms (numbness, loss of sensation, "electric shock" sensations), seizures. sensitivity to light, sleepiness, weakness
Selenium	Growth impairment, high cholesterol levels, increased incidence of cancer, pancreatic insufficiency (inability to secrete adequate amounts of digestive enzymes), immune impairment, liver impairment, male sterility
Thiamin	Confusion, constipation, digestive problems, irritability, loss of appetite, memory loss, nervousness, numbness of hands and feet, pain sensitivity, poor coordination, weakness
Vitamin A	Acne, dry hair, fatigue, growth impairment, insomnia, hyperkeratosis (thickening and roughness of skin), immune impairment, night blindness, weight loss

Vitamin B-12	Anaemia, constipation, depression, dizziness, fatigue, intestinal disturbances, headaches, irritability, loss of vibration sensation, low stomach acid, mental disturbances, moodiness, mouth lesions, numbness, spinal cord degeneration
Vitamin C	Bleeding gums, depression, easy bruising, impaired wound healing, irritability, joint pains, loose teeth, malaise, and tiredness.
Vitamin D	Burning sensation in mouth, diarrhoea, insomnia, myopia, nervousness, osteomalacia, osteoporosis, rickets, scalp sweating
Vitamin E	Gait disturbances, poor reflexes, loss of position sense, loss of vibration sense, shortened red blood cell life
Vitamin K	Bleeding disorders
Zinc	Acne, amnesia, apathy, brittle nails, delayed sexual maturity, depression, diarrhoea, eczema, fatigue, growth impairment, hair loss, high cholesterol levels, immune impairment, impotence, irritability, lethargy, loss of appetite, loss of sense of taste, low stomach acid, male infertility, memory impairment, night blindness, paranoia, white spots on nails, wound healing impairment

ANAEMIA

Among the many blood related syndromes people suffer from, Anaemia is a significant one. In this disorder, the blood haemoglobin count falls below the regular level. This haemoglobin molecule performs the task of carrying oxygen in the body. It stays in the red blood cells. When a person turns anaemic, his body tissues get lesser amount of oxygen. The consequence is fatigue, listlessness and a host of other medical complications in due course of time.

Insufficient iron in the diet is a common cause of anaemia. Those who lack iron look pale easily get out breath and feel tired. Children who are anaemic are often sick.

Normally the iron in our bodies is used over and over again and we need little extra from our diet, but in the following circumstances iron is lost and anaemia is caused unless more iron is taken into the body:

- Bleeding of any kind, including menstruation, piles trouble and dysentery.
- Disease such as malaria and hook worm, when blood is destroyed.
- In pregnancy because the foetus takes iron from the mother.

Growing children need extra iron to make blood, and anaemia is common especially after the age of 3or 4 months when the iron stored in the liver is used up. There is very little iron in milk and other foods must be given to these young children.

People suffering from anaemia often do not show any prominent symptoms for a long time. However the people suffering from this blood disorder often complain of weakness, lethargy, dizziness etc. When the disease reaches an acute stage, some other perceptible signs appear. These include palpitations, short breath, sourness of gums and mouth and headaches. In some cases, the skin colour appears to be pale.

As a matter of fact, almost anybody can fall prey to this menace. Usually pregnant women are susceptible to this disorder. However anaemia can also affect elderly men and women, teenagers and even children. In most of the cases, it is seen that the affected people followed a diet that did not have adequate nutrients like vitamin B12, iron as well as folic acid.

The treatments for anaemia are largely dependent on the causes. If the disease has stemmed from a deficiency of iron intake then eating food imbued with iron will be a good idea. There are some food and vegetables that are rich in iron. Examples include eggs, red meat, dried apricots, spinach, sardines and wholemeal bread. One should also consume foods rich in Vitamin B12 like poultry, eggs, fish, meat, cheese and milk etc. Apart from these, broccoli, pulses, wheat germ etc needs to be taken since they have folic acid that helps in iron absorption. Often, taking iron supplements can prove to be beneficial. Vitamin C rich foods can also help the iron absorption by the body. In severe cases of the disease, blood transfusion becomes mandatory

HYPERTENSION

Hypertension is synonymous with high blood pressure. Blood pressure is a measure of the force of blood against the walls of the arteries, which are the conduits that carry blood from the heart to other parts of the body.

In some people, the blood cannot flow easily through these arteries. For example, if the arteries are narrowed for some reason, the pressure will go up to keep the blood flowing. This is high blood pressure.

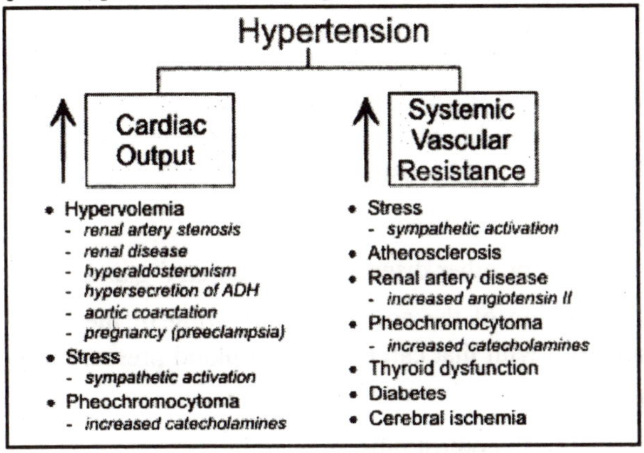

Fig. Hypertension Causes

When the heart pumps blood into the arteries, the blood flows with a force pushing against the walls of the arteries. Blood pressure is the product of the flow of blood times the resistance in the blood vessels. High blood pressure is also called hypertension.

What makes high blood pressure important is that initially it may cause no symptoms but can still cause serious long-term complications. The key complications of high blood pressure include heart disease, heart attack, congestive heart failure, stroke, kidney failure, peripheral artery disease, and aortic aneurysms (outpouchings of the aorta). Public awareness of these dangers has increased. High blood pressure has become the second most common reason for medical office visits in the United States.

Blood pressure is measured with a blood pressure cuff and recorded as two numbers, such as 120/80 mm Hg (millimeters of mercury). The top, larger number is called the systolic pressure. This is the pressure generated when the heart contracts (pumps). It reflects the pressure of the blood against arterial walls. The bottom, smaller number is called the diastolic pressure. This reflects the pressure in the arteries while the heart is filling and resting between heartbeats.

Scientists have determined a normal range for both systolic and diastolic blood pressure after examining the blood pressure of many people.

Those whose blood pressure is consistently higher than this norm are said to have high blood pressure or hypertension. High blood pressure in adults is defined as a consistently elevated blood pressure of 140 mm Hg systolic and 90 mm Hg diastolic or higher.

Causes

In about 10% of people, high blood pressure is caused by another disease (this is called secondary hypertension). In such cases, when the root cause is treated, blood pressure usually returns to normal. These causes of secondary hypertension include the following conditions:

- Chronic kidney disease
- Tumours or other diseases of the adrenal gland
- Coarctation of the aorta - A narrowing of the aorta that you are born with that can cause high blood pressure in your arms
- Pregnancy
- Use of birth control pills
- Alcohol addiction
- Thyroid dysfunction

In the other 90% of cases, the cause of high blood pressure is not known (referred to as primary hypertension). Although the specific cause is unknown, certain factors are recognized as contributing to high blood pressure.

- Age: The older you get, the greater the likelihood that you will develop high blood pressure, especially systolic, as your arteries get stiffer. This is largely due to arteriosclerosis, or "hardening of the arteries."
- Race: Blacks have high blood pressure more often than whites. They develop high blood pressure at a younger age and develop more severe complications sooner.
- Socioeconomic status: High blood pressure is also more common among the less educated and lower socioeconomic groups.
- Family history (heredity): The tendency to have high blood pressure appears to run in families.
- Gender: Generally men have a greater likelihood of developing high blood pressure than women. This likelihood varies according to age and among various ethnic groups.

- Overweight (obesity): Obesity is defined as having a body mass index (BMI) greater than 30 kg/m2. It is very closely related to high blood pressure. Medical professionals strongly recommend that all obese people with high blood pressure lose weight until they are within 15% of their healthy body weight. Your health care provider can help you calculate your BMI and healthy range of body weight.
- Sodium (salt) sensitivity: Some people have high sensitivity to sodium (salt), and their blood pressure goes up if they use salt. Reducing sodium intake tends to lower their blood pressure. Indians consume 10-15 times more sodium than they need. Fast foods and processed foods contain particularly high amounts of sodium. Many over-the-counter medicines, such as painkillers, also contain large amounts of sodium. Read labels to find out how much sodium is contained in food items. Avoid those with high sodium levels.
- Alcohol use: Drinking more than one to two drinks of alcohol per day tends to raise blood pressure in those who are sensitive to alcohol.
- Birth control pills (oral contraceptive use): Some women who take birth control pills develop high blood pressure.
- Lack of exercise (physical inactivity): A sedentary lifestyle contributes to the development of obesity and high blood pressure.
- Drugs: Certain drugs, such as amphetamines (stimulants), diet pills, and some pills used for cold and allergy symptoms, tend to raise blood pressure.

Symptoms

High blood pressure usually causes no symptoms. Even if high blood pressure does cause symptoms, the symptoms are usually mild and nonspecific (vague, or suggesting many different disorders). Thus, high blood pressure often is labeled "the silent killer." People who have high blood pressure typically don't know it until their blood pressure is measured.

Sometimes people with high blood pressure have the following symptoms:

- Headache
- Dizziness
- Blurred vision
- Nausea

People often do not seek medical care until they have symptoms arising from the organ damage caused by chronic (ongoing, long-term) high blood pressure. The following types of organ damage are commonly seen in chronic high blood pressure:

- Heart attack
- Heart failure
- Stroke or "mini stroke" (transient ischemic attack, TIA)
- Kidney failure
- Eye damage with loss of vision
- Peripheral arterial disease
- Outpouchings of the aorta, called aneurysms

About 1% of people with high blood pressure do not seek medical care until the high blood pressure is very severe, a condition known as malignant hypertension.

- In malignant hypertension, the diastolic blood pressure (the lower number) often exceeds 140 mm Hg.
- Malignant hypertension may be associated with headache, light-headedness, or nausea.
- This degree of high blood pressure requires emergency hospitalization and lowering of blood pressure to prevent brain haemorrhage or stroke.

It is of utmost importance to realize that high blood pressure can be unrecognized for years, causing no symptoms but causing progressive damage to the heart, other organs, and blood vessels.

Diagnosis

The only way to tell whether you have high blood pressure is to have it measured with a blood pressure cuff (sphygmomanometer). This device consists of a gauge and a rubber cuff that is placed around your arm and inflated. Having your blood pressure measured is painless and takes just a few minutes.

Blood pressure (BP) is classified as follows:

- Normal BP - Systolic less than 120 mm Hg; diastolic less than 80 mm Hg
- Prehypertension - Systolic 120-139 or diastolic 80-89 mm Hg
- High BP

- Stage 1 - Systolic 140-159; diastolic 90-99 mm Hg
- Stage 2 - Systolic more than 160; diastolic more than 100 mm Hg

Tests will be ordered to check for causes of high blood pressure and to assess any organ damage from high blood pressure or its treatment. These tests may include the following:

- Blood tests including measurement of electrolytes, blood urea, and creatinine levels (to assess potential kidney damage)
- Lipid profile for levels of various kinds of cholesterol
- Special tests for hormones of the adrenal gland or thyroid gland
- Urine tests for electrolytes and hormones

A noninvasive, painless eye examination with an ophthalmoscope will look for ocular damage. Ultrasound of the kidneys, CT scan of the abdomen, or both may be done to assess damage or enlargement of the kidneys and adrenal glands. Any of the following may be performed to detect damage to the heart or blood vessels:

- Electrocardiogram(ECG) is a noninvasive test that detects the electrical activity of the heart and records it on paper. ECG is helpful for quantitating any damage of the heart muscle, such as heart attack, and/or thickening/hypertrophy of the heart wall/ muscle, common complications of high blood pressure.
- Echocardiogram is an ultrasound examination of the heart taken through the chest. Sound waves take a picture of the heart as it beats and relaxes and then transmits these images to a video monitor. The echo can detect problems with the heart such as enlargement, abnormalities in motion of the heart wall, blood clots, and heart valve abnormalities. It also gives a good measurement of the strength of the heart muscle (ejection fraction). The echocardiogram is more accurate than an ECG, but also more expensive.
- A plain chest x-ray primarily provides an estimate of the size of the heart, but it is much less specific than echocardiography, which looks inside the heart.
- Doppler ultrasound is used to check blood flow through arteries at pulse points in your arms, legs, hands, and feet. This is an accurate way to detect peripheral vascular disease, which can be associated with high blood pressure. It also can depict the arteries to both kidneys and sometimes depicts narrowings that can lead to high BP in a minority of patients.

Treatment

The goal of hypertension treatment is to get to a blood pressure reading of 135-140/85-90 mm Hg. Before determining the right medication to treat hypertension, lab tests must be done as well as an electrocardiogram to review heart function. Typical drugs used to treat hypertension include:

- Diuretics - diuretics have been prescribed for more than 30 years, and are widely used today to treat hypertension in conjunction with lifestyle modifications. Diuretics promote fluid passing out of the body.
- Vasodilators - Vasodilators are commonly used with diuretics and beta blockers to reduce peripheral vascular resistance.
- Beta Blockers - The next most widely used type of drug used to treat hypertension after diuretics. Beta Blockers decrease the stress on the heart, and basically smooth out the stresses in the blood pumping system by reducing peripheral vascular resistance.
- ACE inhibitors - ACE inhibitors are used to lower peripheral vascular resistance by affecting complex enzymes.
- Calcium Channel Blockers - Calcium Channel Blockers are used to block calcium from entering the smooth muscle, causing vasodilation and decreased peripheral vascular resistance.

Over treatment of hypertension can be dangerous, leading to Hypotension. Hypotension (low blood pressure) may result in falls. It is important to obtain a blood pressure test while the person is standing. Orthostatic Hypotension occurs when someone stands up and their blood pressure drops 10 points (10 mm Hg). This may cause one to fall.

It is important to take a blood pressure test about one hour after eating. After a meal, a hormone is released that dilates the blood vessels and causes one's blood pressure to decrease. Any headaches, dizziness, or double vision/blurred vision should be immediately reported, as these are late danger signs of high blood pressure that may result in a stroke if not treated immediately.

Blood pressure drugs should not be withdrawn, and no doses should be skipped without doctor's orders. The body adjusts to and depends on the drugs. If you monitor your blood pressure at home, periodically validate the readings at your doctor's office. A cuff that is too small for your arm will result in a blood pressure reading that is higher than the real pressure.

Prevention and Control

Once hypertension is diagnosed, it can usually be controlled. Thus, the many potential negative outcomes of unmanaged high blood pressure such as strokes and heart attacks can be prevented or at least reduced in severity. Lifestyle modifications reduce the amount of medication that must be used to control hypertension.

Examples of lifestyle modifications for hypertension prevention are:

- Weight reduction
- Sodium restriction
- Decrease intake of saturated fats
- Regular exercise (aerobic-type)
- Restrict alcohol
- Restrict caffeine
- Relaxation
- Quieting of smoking.

STROKE

A stroke is the rapidly developing loss of brain functions due to a disturbance in the blood vessels supplying blood to the brain. This can be due to ischemia (lack of blood supply) caused by thrombosis or embolism or due to a haemorrhage. As a result, the affected area of the brain is unable to function, leading to inability to move one or more limbs on one side of the body, inability to understand or formulate speech or inability to see one side of the visual field. In the past, stroke was referred to as cerebrovascular accident or CVA, but the term "stroke" is now preferred.

A stroke is a medical emergency and can cause permanent neurological damage, complications and death. It is the leading cause of adult disability in the United States and Europe. In the UK, it is the second most common cause of death, the first being heart attacks and third being cancer. It is the number two cause of death worldwide and may soon become the leading cause of death worldwide. Risk factors for stroke include advanced age, hypertension (high blood pressure), previous stroke or transient ischemic attack (TIA), diabetes, high cholesterol, cigarette smoking and atrial fibrillation. High blood pressure is the most important modifiable risk factor of stroke.

The traditional definition of stroke, devised by the World Health Organization in the 1970s is a "neurological deficit of cerebrovascular cause that persists beyond 24 hours or is interrupted by death within 24 hours". This definition was supposed to reflect the reversibility of tissue damage and was devised for the purpose, with the time frame of 24 hours being chosen arbitrarily. The 24-hour limit divides stroke from transient ischemic attack, which is a related syndrome of stroke symptoms that resolve completely within 24 hours. With the availability of treatments that, when given early, can reduce stroke severity, many now prefer alternative concepts, such as brain attack and acute ischemic cerebrovascular syndrome (modelled after heart attack and acute coronary syndrome respectively), that reflect the urgency of stroke symptoms and the need to act swiftly.

Classification

Strokes can be classified into two major categories: ischemic and hemorrhagic. Ischemia is due to interruption of the blood supply, while haemorrhage is due to rupture of a blood vessel or an abnormal vascular structure. 80% of strokes are due to ischemia; the remainder are due to haemorrhage. Some haemorrhages develop inside areas of ischemia ("hemorrhagic transformation"). It is unknown how many haemorrhages actually start off as ischemic stroke.

Ischemic stroke: In an ischemic stroke, blood supply to part of the brain is decreased, leading to dysfunction of the brain tissue in that area. There are four reasons why this might happen: thrombosis (obstruction of a blood vessel by a blood clot forming locally), embolism, systemic hypoperfusion (general decrease in blood supply, e.g. in shock) and venous thrombosis. Stroke without an obvious explanation is termed "cryptogenic" (of unknown origin); this constitutes 30-40% of all ischemic strokes.

There are various classification systems for acute ischemic stroke. The Oxford Community Stroke Project classification (OCSP, also known as the Bamford or Oxford classification) relies primarily on the initial symptoms; based on the extent of the symptoms, the stroke episode is classified as total anterior circulation infarct (TACI), partial anterior circulation infarct (PACI), lacunar infarct (LACI) or posterior circulation infarct (POCI). These four entities predict the extent of the stroke, the area of the brain affected, the underlying cause, and the prognosis. The TOAST (Trial of Org 10172 in Acute Stroke Treatment) classification is based on clinical symptoms as well as results of further investigations; on this basis, a stroke is classified as being due to (1) thrombosis or embolism due to atherosclerosis of a large artery, (2) embolism of cardiac origin, (3) occlusion of a small blood vessel, (4) other determined cause,

(5) undetermined cause (two possible causes, no cause identified, or incomplete investigation).

Hemorrhagic stroke: Intracranial haemorrhage is the accumulation of blood anywhere within the skull vault. A distinction is made between intra-axial haemorrhage (blood inside the brain) and extra-axial haemorrhage (blood inside the skull but outside the brain). Intra-axial haemorrhage is due to intraparenchymal haemorrhage or intraventricular hemorrhage (blood in the ventricular system). The main types of extra-axial haemorrhage are epidural hematoma (bleeding between the dura mater and the skull), subdural hematoma (in the subdural space) and subarachnoid hemorrhage (between the arachnoid mater and pia mater). Most of the hemorrhagic stroke syndromes have specific symptoms (e.g. headache, previous head injury). Intracerebral hemorrhage (ICH) is bleeding directly into the brain tissue, forming a gradually enlarging hematoma (pooling of blood).

Symptoms

Stroke symptoms typically start suddenly, over seconds to minutes, and in most cases don't progress further. The symptoms depend on the area of the brain affected. The more extensive the area of brain affected, the more functions that are likely to be lost. Some forms of stroke can cause additional symptoms: in intracranial hemorrhage, the affected area may compress other structures. Most forms of stroke are not associated with headache, apart from subarachnoid hemorrhage and cerebral venous thrombosis and occasionally intracerebral hemorrhage.

Various systems have been proposed to increase recognition of stroke by patients, relatives and emergency first responders. Sudden-onset face weakness, arm drift, and abnormal speech are the findings most likely to lead to the correct identification of a case of stroke. Proposed systems include FAST (face, arm and speech test), the Los Angeles Prehospital Stroke Screen (LAPSS) and the Cincinnati Prehospital Stroke Scale (CPSS). Use of these scales is recommended by professional guidelines.

For people referred to the emergency room, early recognition of stroke is deemed important as this can expedite diagnostic tests and treatments. A scoring system called ROSIER (recognition of stroke in the emergency room) is recommended for this purpose; it is based on features from the medical history and physical examination.

Loss of consciousness, headache, and vomiting usually occurs more often in hemorrhagic stroke than in thrombosis because of the increased intracranial pressure from the leaking blood compressing on the brain. If symptoms are maximal at onset, the cause is more likely to be a subarachnoid hemorrhage or an embolic stroke.

Pathophysiology

Ischemic: Ischemic stroke occurs due to a loss of blood supply to part of the brain, initiating the ischemic cascade. Brain tissue ceases to function if deprived of oxygen for more than 60 to 90 seconds and after a few hours will suffer irreversible injury possibly leading to death of the tissue, i.e., infarction.

Atherosclerosis may disrupt the blood supply by narrowing the lumen of blood vessels leading to a reduction of blood flow, by causing the formation of blood clots within the vessel, or by releasing showers of small emboli through the disintegration of atherosclerotic plaques. Embolic infarction occurs when emboli formed elsewhere in the circulatory system, typically in the heart as a consequence of atrial fibrillation, or in the carotid arteries. These break off, enter the cerebral circulation, then lodge in and occlude brain blood vessels.

Due to collateral circulation, within the region of brain tissue affected by ischemia there is a spectrum of severity. Thus, part of the tissue may immediately die while other parts may only be injured and could potentially recover. The ischemia area where tissue might recover is referred to as the ischemic penumbra.

As oxygen or glucose becomes depleted in ischemic brain tissue, the production of high energy phosphate compounds such as adenosine triphosphate (ATP) fails leading to failure of energy dependent processes (such as ion pumping) necessary for tissue cell survival. This sets off a series of interrelated events that result in cellular injury and death. A major cause of neuronal injury is release of the excitatory neurotransmitter glutamate.

The concentration of glutamate outside the cells of the nervous system is normally kept low by so-called uptake carriers, which are powered by the concentration gradients of ions (mainly Na) across the cell membrane. However, stroke cuts off the supply of oxygen and glucose which powers the ion pumps maintaining these gradients. As a result the transmembrane ion gradients run down, and glutamate transporters reverse their direction, releasing glutamate into the extracellular space. Glutamate acts on receptors in nerve cells (especially NMDA receptors), producing an influx of calcium which activates enzymes that digest the cells' proteins, lipids and nuclear material. Calcium influx can also lead to the failure of mitochondria, which can lead further toward energy depletion and may trigger cell death due to apoptosis.

Ischemia also induces production of oxygen free radicals and other reactive oxygen species. These react with and damage a number of cellular and extracellular elements. Damage to the blood vessel lining or endothelium is particularly important. In fact, many antioxidant neuroprotectants such as uric acid and NXY-059 work at the level of the endothelium and not in the brain per se. Free radicals also directly initiate elements of the apoptosis cascade by means of redox signaling.

These processes are the same for any type of ischemic tissue and are referred to collectively as the ischemic cascade. However, brain tissue is especially vulnerable to ischemia since it has little respiratory reserve and is completely dependent on aerobic metabolism, unlike most other organs.

Brain tissue survival can be improved to some extent if one or more of these processes is inhibited. Drugs that scavenge Reactive oxygen species, inhibit apoptosis, or inhibit excitotoxic neurotransmitters, for example, have been shown experimentally to reduce tissue injury due to ischemia. Agents that work in this way are referred to as being neuroprotective. Until recently, human clinical trials with neuroprotective agents have failed, with the probable exception of deep barbiturate coma. However, more recently NXY-059, the disulfonyl derivative of the radical-scavenging spintrap phenylbutylnitrone, is reported be neuroprotective in stroke. This agent appears to work at the level of the blood vessel lining or endothelium. Unfortunately, after producing favorable results in one large-scale clinical trial, a second trial failed to show favorable results.

In addition to injurious effects on brain cells, ischemia and infarction can result in loss of structural integrity of brain tissue and blood vessels, partly through the release of matrix metalloproteases, which are zinc- and calcium-dependent enzymes that break down collagen, hyaluronic acid, and other elements of connective tissue. Other proteases also contribute to this process. The loss of vascular structural integrity results in a breakdown of the protective blood brain barrier that contributes to cerebral edema, which can cause secondary progression of the brain injury.

As is the case with any type of brain injury, the immune system is activated by cerebral infarction and may under some circumstances exacerbate the injury caused by the infarction. Inhibition of the inflammatory response has been shown experimentally to reduce tissue injury due to cerebral infarction, but this has not proved out in clinical studies.

Hemorrhagic: Hemorrhagic strokes result in tissue injury by causing compression of tissue from an expanding hematoma or hematomas. This can distort and injure tissue. In addition, the pressure may lead to a loss of blood supply to affected tissue with resulting infarction, and the blood released by brain hemorrhage appears to have direct toxic effects on brain tissue and vasculature.

Diagnosis

Stroke is diagnosed through several techniques: a neurological examination, CT scans (most often without contrast enhancements) or MRI scans, Doppler ultrasound, and arteriography. The diagnosis of stroke itself is clinical, with assistance from the imaging techniques. Imaging techniques also assist in determining the subtypes and cause of stroke. There is yet no commonly used blood test for the stroke diagnosis itself, though blood tests may be of help in finding out the likely cause of stroke.

For detecting chronic hemorrhages, MRI scan is more sensitive. For the assessment of stable stroke, nuclear medicine scans SPECT and PET/CT may be helpful. SPECT documents cerebral blood flow and PET with FDG isotope the metabolic activity of the neurons.

When a stroke has been diagnosed, various other studies may be performed to determine the underlying etiology. With the current treatment and diagnosis options available, it is of particular importance to determine whether there is a peripheral source of emboli. Test selection may vary, since the cause of stroke varies with age, comorbidity and the clinical presentation. Commonly used techniques include:

- An ultrasound/doppler study of the carotid arteries (to detect carotid stenosis) or dissection of the precerebral arteries
- An electrocardiogram (ECG) and echocardiogram (to identify arrhythmias and resultant clots in the heart which may spread to the brain vessels through the bloodstream)
- A Holter monitor study to identify intermittent arrhythmias
- An angiogram of the cerebral vasculature (if a bleed is thought to have originated from an aneurysm or arteriovenous malformation)
- Blood tests to determine hypercholesterolemia, bleeding diathesis and some rarer causes such as homocysteinuria

Treatment

Prompt treatment of stroke and medical problems related to stroke, such as high blood sugar and pressure on the brain, may minimize brain damage and improve the chances of survival. Starting a rehabilitation program as soon as possible after a stroke increases your chances of recovering some of the abilities you lost.

Initial treatment for a stroke varies depending on whether it's caused by a blood clot (ischemic) or bleeding in the brain (hemorrhagic). Initial treatment focuses on restoring blood flow for an ischemic stroke or controlling bleeding for a hemorrhagic stroke. As with a heart attack, permanent damage from a stroke often occurs within the first few hours. The quicker you receive treatment, the less damage will occur.

RHEUMATIC HEART DISEASE

Rheumatic heart disease is a condition in which permanent damage to heart valves is caused by rheumatic fever. The heart valve is damaged by a disease process that generally begins with a strep throat caused by streptococcus A bacteria, that may eventually cause rheumatic fever.

Rheumatic heart disease is the most serious complication of rheumatic fever. As many as 39% of patients with acute rheumatic fever may develop varying degrees of pancarditis with associated valve insufficiency, heart failure, pericarditis, and even death. With chronic rheumatic heart disease, patients develop valve stenosis with varying degrees of regurgitation, atrial dilation, arrhythmias, and ventricular dysfunction.

Rheumatic heart disease is a complication of rheumatic fever in which the heart valves are damaged. Rheumatic fever is an inflammatory disease that begins with a strep throat. It can affect connective tissue throughout the body, especially in the heart, joints, brain and skin. Although rheumatic fever can strike people of all ages, it is most common in children between 5 and 15 years old. The best way to prevent rheumatic fever is to treat strep throat with antibiotics.

The symptoms of rheumatic heart disease vary and damage to the heart often is not readily noticeable. When symptoms do appear, they may depend on the extent and location of the heart damage.

Typically, symptoms of rheumatic fever appear about two weeks after the onset of an untreated strep throat infection. Apart from the sore throat caused by the strep infection, children have a fever and feel ill. Commonly, the child will have a very painful, swollen and red joint – usually a large joint like a knee, ankle, elbow or shoulder – that goes away after a day or two only to be replaced by the same findings in another joint. Short-lived skin rashes may occur, but are not common. Even if the heart is affected, it is usually not sever enough to cause symptoms, and occasionally the child may be short of breath.

Most cases of strep throat, including untreated infections, do not cause rheumatic fever. However, if rheumatic fever affects the heart valves, it can disrupt normal blood flow through the heart and cause damage to the heart.

Pathophysiology

Rheumatic fever is a systemic disease affecting the peri-arteriolar connective tissue and can occur after an untreated Group A Beta hemolytic streptococcal pharyngeal infection. It is believed to be caused by antibody cross-reactivity. This cross-reactivity is a Type II hypersensitivity reaction and is termed molecular mimicry. Usually, self reactive B cells remain anergic in the periphery without T cell co-stimulation. During a Strep. infection activated antigen presenting cells such as macrophages present the bacterial antigen to helper T cells. Helper T cells subsequently activate B cells and induce the production of antibodies against the cell wall of Streptococcus. However the antibodies may also react against the myocardium and joints, producing the symptoms of rheumatic fever.

Group A streptococcus pyogenes has a cell wall composed of branched polymers which sometimes contain "M proteins" that are highly antigenic. The antibodies which the immune system generates against the "M proteins" may cross react with cardiac myofiber protein myosin and smooth muscle cells of arteries, inducing cytokine release and tissue destruction. This inflammation occurs through direct attachment of complement and Fc receptor-mediated recruitment of neutrophils and macrophages. Characteristic Aschoff bodies, composed of swollen eosinophilic collagen surrounded by lymphocytes and macrophages can be seen on light microscopy. The larger macrophages may become Aschoff giant cells. Acute rheumatic valvular lesions may also involve a cell-mediated immunity reaction as these lesions predominantly contain T-helper cells and macrophages.

In acute RF, these lesions can be found in any layer of the heart and is hence called pancarditis. The inflammation may cause a serofibrinous pericardial exudates described as "bread-and-butter" pericarditis, which usually resolves without sequelae. Involvement of the endocardium typically results in fibrinoid necrosis and verrucae formation along the lines of closure of the left-sided heart valves. Warty projections arise from the deposition, while subendothelial lesions may induce irregular thickenings called MacCallum plaques.

Chronic rheumatic heart disease is characterized by repeated inflammation with fibrinous resolution. The cardinal anatomic changes of the valve include leaflet thickening, commissural fusion and shortening and thickening of the tendinous cords.

Symptoms

The symptoms of rheumatic fever usually start about one to five weeks after patient has been infected with Streptococcus bacteria. The following are the most common symptoms of rheumatic fever. However, each person may experience symptoms differently. Symptoms may include:

- Joint inflammation - including swelling, tenderness, and redness over multiple joints. The joints affected are usually the larger joints in the knees or ankles. The inflammation "moves" from one joint to another over several days.
- Small nodules or hard, round bumps under the skin
- A change in neuromuscular movements (this is usually noted by a change in your child's handwriting and may also include jerky movements)
- Rash (a pink rash with odd edges that is usually seen on the trunk of the body or arms and legs)
- Fever
- Weight loss
- Fatigue
- Stomach pains

Diagnosis

The first step in diagnosing rheumatic heart disease is establishing that patient recently had a strep infection. The doctor may order a throat culture and/or a blood test to check for the presence of strep antibodies. However, it is likely that signs of the strep infection may be gone by the time patient goes to the doctor. In that case, the doctor will need you to try to remember if your child recently had a sore throat or other symptoms of a strep infection.

The doctor will do a physical examination and check your child for signs of rheumatic fever, including joint pain and inflammation. The doctor also will listen to your child's heart to check for abnormal rhythms or murmurs that may signify that the heart has been strained.

In addition, there are a couple of tests that may be used to check the heart and assess damage, including:

- Chest X-ray – This allows your child's doctor to check the size of the heart and to see if there is excess fluid in the heart or lungs.
- Echocardiogram – This test uses sound waves to measure the heart's size and shape and creates an image of the heart.

Treatment

The management of acute rheumatic fever is geared toward the reduction of inflammation with anti-inflammatory medications such as aspirin or corticosteroids. Individuals with positive cultures for strep throat should also be treated with antibiotics. Aspirin is the drug of choice and should be given at high doses of 100mg/kg/day. One should watch for side effects like gastritis, salicylate poisoning etc. Steroids are reserved for cases where there is evidence of involvement of heart. The use of steroids may prevent further scarring of tissue and may prevent development of sequelae such as Mitral stenosis. Monthly injections of Longacting Penicillin must be given for a period of 5 years in patients having one attack of Rheumatic fever. If there is evidence of carditis, the length of Penidure therapy may be up to 40 years. Another important cornerstone in treating rheumatic fever includes the continual use of low dose antibiotics (such as penicillin, sulfadiazine, or erythromycin) to prevent recurrence.

Patients with positive cultures for Streptococcus pyogenes should be treated with penicillin as long as allergy is not present. This treatment will not alter the course of the acute disease.

Patients with significant symptoms may require corticosteroids. Salicylates are useful for pain.

Some patients develop significant carditis which manifests as congestive heart failure. This requires the usual treatment for heart failure: diuretics and digoxin. Unlike normal heart failure, rheumatic heart failure responds well to corticosteroids.

Prevention and Control

Prevention of recurrence is achieved by eradicating the acute infection and prophylaxis with antibiotics.

Nurses also have a role in prevention, primarily in screening school-aged children for sore throats that may be caused by Group A streptococci (especially Group A ? Hemolytic Streptococcus pyogenes).

A more cost-effective and attainable goal is the prevention of recurrent attacks of rheumatic fever (secondary prevention), and this should be the first priority of prevention. Although oral antibiotic regimens can be effective, it has been known for almost 50 years that monthly injections of benzathine penicillin G are the most effective method for preventing recurrences. The change in the morbidity and mortality rates for patients with rheumatic heart disease in economically developed countries has been due largely to the decrease of rheumatic fever recurrences.

The World Health Organization has instituted trial rheumatic fever prevention in 16 Third World countries. These programs involve early detection of rheumatic fever and rheumatic heart disease, secondary prophylaxis, and health education of the population and health care providers. Preliminary results from this cooperative study have shown a decrease in rheumatic fever recurrences among patients maintained on secondary prophylaxis of monthly injections of benzathine penicillin G. The fear of serious allergic reactions has been a barrier to the use of this agent in many Third World countries, but a recent international study showed that anaphylaxis is rare in patients with rheumatic fever receiving long-term benzathine penicillin G.

CORONARY HEART DISEASE

Coronary heart disease (CHD) (or atherosclerotic heart disease) is the end result of the accumulation of atheromatous plaques within the walls of the coronary arteries that supply the myocardium (the muscle of the heart) with oxygen and nutrients.

CHD is the leading cause of death worldwide. While the symptoms and signs of coronary artery disease are noted in the advanced state of disease, most individuals with coronary artery disease show no evidence of disease for decades as the disease progresses before the first onset of symptoms, often a "sudden" heart attack, finally arises. After decades of progression, some of these atheromatous plaques may rupture and (along with the activation of the blood clotting system) start limiting blood flow to the heart muscle. The disease is the most common cause of sudden death, and is also the most common reason for death of men and women over 20 years of age. According to the Guinness Book of Records, Northern Ireland is the country with the most occurrences of CAD. By contrast, the Maasai of Africa have almost no heart disease.

As the degree of coronary artery disease progresses, there may be near-complete obstruction of the lumen of the coronary artery, severely restricting the flow of oxygen-carrying blood to the myocardium. Individuals with this degree of coronary artery disease typically have suffered from one or more myocardial infarctions (heart attacks), and may have signs and symptoms of chronic coronary ischemia, including symptoms of angina at rest and flash pulmonary oedema.

A distinction should be made between myocardial ischemia and myocardial infarction. Ischemia means that the amount of oxygen supplied to the tissue is inadequate to supply the needs of the tissue. When the myocardium becomes ischemic, it does not function optimally. When large areas of the myocardium becomes ischemic, there can be impairment in the relaxation and contraction of the myocardium. If the blood flow to the tissue is improved, myocardial ischemia can be reversed. Infarction means that the tissue has undergone irreversible death due to lack of sufficient oxygen-rich blood.

An individual may develop a rupture of an atheromatous plaque at any stage of the spectrum of coronary artery disease. The acute rupture of a plaque may lead to an acute myocardial infarction (heart attack).

Pathophysiology

Limitation of blood flow to the heart causes ischemia (cell starvation secondary to a lack of oxygen) of the myocardial cells. When myocardial cells die from lack of oxygen, this is called a myocardial infarction (commonly called a heart attack). It leads to heart muscle damage, heart muscle death and later scarring without heart muscle regrowth.

Myocardial infarction usually results from the sudden occlusion of a coronary artery when a plaque ruptures, activating the clotting system and atheroma-clot interaction fills the lumen of the artery to the point of sudden closure. The narrowing of the lumen of the heart artery before sudden closure is often not severe, according to clinical research completed in the late 1990s and using IVUS examinations within 6 months prior to a heart attack. High grade stenoses as such exceeding 75% blockage, such as detected by stress testing while carrying much higher individual risk for sudden closure, were found to be responsible for only 14% of acute heart attacks because they are rarer compared to less severe narrowings. The events leading up to plaque rupture are not understood despite many theories. Myocardial infarction is almost never caused by temporary spasm of the artery wall occluding the lumen, a condition also associated with atheromatous plaque and CHD.

CHD is associated with smoking, diabetes, and hypertension. A family history of early CAD is one of the less important predictors of CHD. Most of the familial association of coronary artery disease are related to common dietary habits. Screening for CHD includes evaluating high-density and low-density lipoprotein (cholesterol) levels and triglyceride levels. Despite much press, most of the alternative risk factors including homocysteine, C-reactive protein (CRP), Lipoprotein (a), coronary calcium and more sophisticated lipid analysis have added little if any additional value to the conventional risk factors of smoking, diabetes and hypertension.

Symptoms

The most common symptom is angina. Angina can be described as a discomfort, heaviness, pressure, aching, burning, fullness, squeezing or painful feeling in your chest. It can be mistaken for indigestion or heartburn. Angina is usually felt in the chest, but may also be felt in the shoulders, arms, neck, throat, jaw or back.

Other symptoms that can occur with coronary artery disease include:

- Shortness of breath
- Palpitations (irregular heart beats, skipped beats or a "flip-flop" feeling in your chest)
- A faster heartbeat
- Weakness or dizziness
- Nausea
- Sweating

Myocardial Infarction

Symptoms can include:

- Discomfort, pressure, heaviness, or pain in the chest, arm or below the breastbone
- Discomfort radiating to the back, jaw, throat or arm
- Fullness, indigestion or choking feeling (may feel like heartburn)
- Sweating, nausea, vomiting or dizziness
- Extreme weakness, anxiety or shortness of breath
- Rapid or irregular heartbeats

During a heart attack, symptoms typically last 30 minutes or longer and are not relieved by rest or oral medications (medications taken by mouth). Initial symptoms can start as a mild discomfort that progresses to significant pain.

Some people have a heart attack without having any symptoms (a "silent" MI). A silent MI can occur among all people, though it occurs more often among diabetics.

If you think you are having a heart attack, DO NOT DELAY. Call for emergency help (dial 911 in most areas). Immediate treatment of a heart attack is very important to lessen the amount of damage to your heart.

Arrhythmias

When symptoms of arrhythmias are present, they may include:

- Palpitations (a feeling of skipped heart beats, fluttering or "flip-flops," or feeling that your heart is "running away").
- Pounding in your chest.
- Dizziness or feeling light-headed.
- Fainting.
- Shortness of breath.
- Chest discomfort.
- Weakness or fatigue (feeling very tired).

Atrial Fibrillation

Atrial fibrillation (AF) is a type of arrhythmia. Most people with AF experience one or more of the following symptoms:

- Heart palpitations (a sudden pounding, fluttering, or racing feeling in the heart).
- Lack of energy; tired.
- Dizziness (feeling faint or light-headed).
- Chest discomfort (pain, pressure, or discomfort in the chest).
- Shortness of breath (difficulty breathing during activities of daily living).

Some patients with atrial fibrillation have no symptoms. Sometimes these episodes are briefer.

Heart Valve Disease

Symptoms of Heart valve disease can include:

- Shortness of breath and/or difficulty catching your breath. You may notice this most when you are active (doing your normal daily activities) or when you lie down flat in bed.
- Weakness or dizziness.
- Discomfort in your chest. You may feel a pressure or weight in your chest with activity or when going out in cold air.
- Palpitations (this may feel like a rapid heart rhythm, irregular heartbeat, skipped beats or a flip-flop feeling in your chest).
- If valve disease causes heart failure, symptoms may include:
- Swelling of your ankles, feet or abdomen. Swelling may also occur in your belly, which may cause you to feel bloated.
- Quick weight gain (a weight gain of two or three pounds in one day is possible).

Symptoms do not always relate to the seriousness of your valve disease. You may have no symptoms at all and have severe valve disease, requiring prompt treatment. Or, as with mitral valve prolapse, you may have severe symptoms, yet tests may show minor valve disease.

Diagnosis

The diagnosis of coronary artery disease requires a careful history, physical examination, and an electrocardiogram (ECG). Once the initial evaluation is performed, imaging and laboratory studies, stress testing, and cardiac catheterization may be necessary to obtain further information.

To determine if coronary artery disease is present, physician may obtain medical history, listen to heart, take pulse and check blood pressure. An electrocardiogram, or ECG, may be run. With this test, electrodes connected to a recording machine are attached to the chest, wrist and ankles to measure changes in electrical activity of the heart with every beat. If the ECG reading is abnormal, other tests may be ordered such as stress testing, cardiac ultrasound, cardiac catheterization, or nuclear imaging.

In addition to evaluating risk factors, there are also noninvasive imaging techniques available to detect coronary artery disease at its earliest stage. Young or old, it is extremely important to be aware of coronary artery disease. It is a progressive disease that can lead to death or heart failure. There are many treatment options which can slow the progression or in some cases reverse the effects of the disease. The non-invasive and catheterization technique available to detect coronary artery disease are listed below:

- An EKG - An EKG is a record of the heart's electrical impulses. It can identify abnormalities in heart rate and rhythm, and it can provide clues that part of your heart muscle isn't getting enough blood.
- Blood test for heart enzymes - When heart muscle is damaged, even a little, enzymes leak out of the damaged muscle cells into the bloodstream. Elevated heart enzymes suggest a heart problem.
- An exercise stress test on a treadmill - An exercise stress test monitors the effects of treadmill exercise on blood pressure and EKG and can identify heart problems.
- An echocardiogram - This test uses ultrasound to produce images of the heart's movement with each beat.
- Imaging test with radioactive tracers - In this test, a radioactive material is injected and is taken up by the heart muscle, which helps certain features show up on images taken with special cameras.
- A coronary angiogram (a series of X-rays of the coronary arteries) - The coronary angiogram is considered the most accurate way to measure the severity of coronary disease. During an angiogram, a thin, long, flexible tube called a catheter is inserted into an artery in the forearm or groin, and then threaded through the circulatory system into the coronary arteries. Dye is injected to show the blood flow within the coronary arteriés and to identify any areas of narrowing or blockage.

Treatment

Medications must be taken as directed. Drugs can have side effects. If side effects occur, they should be reported to the doctor. Often, a change in the dose or type of a medication, or the use of a combination of drugs, can stop the side effect.

Drugs used to treat Coronary Heart Disease and its risk factors include:

- Aspirin: helps to lower the risk of a heart attack for those who have already had one. It also helps to keep arteries open in those who have had a previous heart bypass or other artery-opening procedure such as coronary angioplasty.

Because of its risks, aspirin is not approved by the Food and Drug Administration for the prevention of heart attacks in healthy persons. It may be harmful for some persons, especially those with no risk of heart disease. Patients must be assessed carefully to make sure the benefits of taking aspirin outweigh the risks. Each person should talk to his or her doctor about whether or not to take aspirin.

Aspirin also is given to patients who arrive at a hospital emergency department with a suspected heart attack.

- Digitalis: helps the heart contract better and is used when the heart's pumping function has been weakened; it also slows some fast heart rhythms.
- ACE (angiotensin converting enzyme) inhibitor: stops production of a chemical produced by the body that makes blood vessels narrow. It is used for high blood pressure and damaged heart muscle. It also can prevent kidney damage in some patients with diabetes.
- Beta blocker: slows the heart and makes it beat with less force, lowering blood pressure and making the heart work less hard. It is used for high blood pressure, chest pain, and to prevent a repeat heart attack.
- Nitrate (including nitroglycerine): relaxes blood vessels and stops chest pain/angina.
- Calcium-channel blocker: relaxes blood vessels, and is used for high blood pressure and chest pain/angina.
- Diuretic: decreases fluid in the body and is used for high blood pressure. Diuretics are sometimes referred to as "water pills."
- Blood cholesterol-lowering agents: decrease LDL levels in the blood. Some can increase HDL.
- Thrombolytic agents: also called "clot-busting drugs," they are given during a heart attack to dissolve a blood clot in a coronary artery in order to restore blood flow. They must be given immediately after heart attack symptoms begin. To be most effective, they need to be given within 1 hour of the start of heart attack symptoms.

Special Procedures: Advanced atherosclerosis may require a special procedure to open an artery and improve blood flow. This is usually done to ease severe chest pain, or to clear major or multiple blockages in blood vessels.

Two commonly used procedures are coronary angioplasty and coronary artery bypass graft operation:

- Coronary angioplasty, or balloon angioplasty: In this procedure, a fine tube, or catheter, is threaded through an artery into the narrowed heart vessel. The catheter has a tiny balloon at its tip. The balloon is repeatedly inflated and deflated to open and stretch the artery, improving blood flow. The balloon is then deflated, and the catheter is removed.

  Doctors often insert a stent during the angioplasty. A wire mesh tube, the stent is used to keep an artery open after an angioplasty. The stent stays in the artery permanently.

  Angioplasty is not surgery. It is done while the patient is awake and may last 1 to 2 hours.

  In about a third of those who have an angioplasty, the blood vessel becomes narrowed or blocked again within 6 months. Vessels that reclose may be opened again with another angioplasty or a coronary artery bypass graft. An artery with a stent also can reclose.

- Coronary artery bypass graft operation: Also known as "bypass surgery," the procedure uses a piece of vein taken from the leg, or of an artery taken from the chest or wrist. This piece is attached to the heart artery above and below the narrowed area, thus making a bypass around the blockage. Sometimes, more than one bypass is needed.

  Bypass surgery may be needed due to various reasons, such as an angioplasty that did not sufficiently widen the blood vessel, or blockages that cannot be reached by, or are too long or hard for, angioplasty. In certain cases, bypass surgery may be preferred to angioplasty. For instance, it may be used for persons who have both Coronary Heart Disease and diabetes.

  A bypass also can close again. This happens in about 10 percent of bypass surgeries, usually after 10 or more years.

Other procedures also may be used to open coronary arteries:

- Atherectomy: A specially equipped catheter is threaded through an artery to a blockage, where thin strips of plaque are shaved off and removed. Balloon angioplasty or insertion of a stent may be done as well.

- Laser angioplasty: A catheter with a laser tip is inserted into an artery to burn, vaporize, or break down plaque. The procedure may be used alone or along with balloon angioplasty.

It is important to understand that these procedures relieve the symptoms of Coronary Heart Disease but do not cure the disease. Lifestyle changes must still be followed and any necessary medications must continue to be taken

Prevention and Control

Lifestyle: Six key steps can help prevent or control Coronary. Heart Disease: stop smoking cigarettes, lower high blood pressure, reduce high blood cholesterol, lose extra weight, become physically active, and manage diabetes.

Here's more on each step:

- Cigarette smoking: There is no safe way to smoke. Although low-tar and low-nicotine cigarettes may somewhat reduce the risk for lung cancer, they do not lessen the risk for Coronary Heart Disease. In fact, smoking accelerates atherosclerosis. It also increases the risk for stroke.

  The risk for Coronary Heart Disease increases along with the number of cigarettes smoked daily. Quitting sharply lowers the risk, even in the first year and no matter what a person's age. Quitting also reduces the risk for a second heart attack in those who have already had one.

- High blood pressure: Also known as hypertension, high blood pressure usually has no symptoms. Once developed, it typically lasts a lifetime. If uncontrolled, it can lead to heart and kidney diseases, and stroke.

  Blood pressure is given as two numbers-the systolic pressure over the diastolic pressure-and both are important. A measurement of 140/90 mmHg (millimeters of mercury) or above is called high blood pressure-but if either number is high, that too is hypertension. A healthy blood pressure is around 120/80.

  Lifestyle steps often can prevent or control high blood pressure: lose excess weight, become physically active, follow a healthy eating plan, including foods lower in salt and sodium, and limit alcohol intake. Some of these steps are the same as those needed to reduce the risk for Coronary Heart Disease and are discussed later.

A key ingredient of healthy eating is choosing foods lower in salt (sodium chloride) and other forms of sodium. Most Indians should consume no more than 2,400 milligrams of sodium (which equals about 6 grams of salt, or about 1 teaspoon) in a day. This is the amount listed as a Daily Value on the Nutrition Facts label on food items. Recent research shows that it's even better to consume no more than 1,500 milligrams of sodium (which equals about 4 grams of salt, or about 2/3 teaspoon) in a day. This includes ALL salt-that in processed foods or added in cooking or at the table.

An overall eating plan also should be low in saturated fat and cholesterol, and moderate in total fat. It also should include plenty of fruits and vegetables-most are naturally low in salt and calories.

Those who consume alcoholic beverages should do so in moderation. Alcoholic beverages supply calories but few nutrients. They are harmful when consumed in excess, and some persons should not drink at all. Furthermore, drinking alcoholic beverages increases the risk of some serious health problems. For example, even one drink a day can slightly raise the risk of breast cancer. While drinking alcoholic beverages in moderation may lower the risk of Coronary Heart Disease-mainly among men over age 45 and women over age 55-there are other factors that reduce the risk of heart disease. These include a healthy diet, physical activity, avoidance of smoking, and maintenance of a healthy weight.

Moderate drinking is defined as no more than two drinks a day for men and no more than one drink a day for women. One drink equals 1.5 ounces of 80-proof whiskey, or 5 ounces of wine, or 12 ounces of beer (regular or light).

Those who drink alcoholic beverages should be aware that they may affect medications taken. They should check about this with their doctor or pharmacist.

- High blood cholesterol: Cholesterol is a soft, waxy substance involved in normal cell function. Normally, the body makes all the cholesterol it needs. Excess saturated fat and cholesterol in the diet cause the fatty buildup in blood vessels, which contributes to atherosclerosis.

  Cholesterol travels through the blood in packages called lipoproteins. There are two main types of lipoprotein that affect the risk for Coronary Heart Disease: low-density lipoprotein (LDL), also called the "bad" cholesterol, which causes deposits in blood vessels; and high-density lipoprotein (HDL), also called the "good" cholesterol, which helps remove cholesterol from the blood. It's important to have a low level of LDL and a high level of HDL.

Healthy adults age 20 and older should have a lipoprotein analysis once every 5 years to measure their levels of total cholesterol, LDL, HDL, and triglycerides, another fatty substance in the blood.

To help prevent or control high blood cholesterol, follow a healthy eating plan such as that mentioned previously, become physically active, and lose excess weight. Those who already have Coronary Heart Disease should be especially careful to control their cholesterol and may need to follow an eating plan more restricted in saturated fat and cholesterol.

- Overweight/obesity: About 65 percent of adults are overweight or obese. Being overweight or obese increases the risk not only for heart disease, but also for other conditions, including stroke, gallbladder disease, arthritis, and breast, colon, and other cancers.

  Overweight and obesity are determined by two key measures-body mass index, or BMI, and waist circumference. BMI relates height to weight. A normal BMI is 18.5-24.9; an overweight BMI is 25-29.9; and an obese BMI is 30 and over. For waist circumference, heart disease risk increases if it is greater than 35 inches for women or greater than 40 inches for men.

- Physical activity: Physical activity is one of the best ways to help prevent and control Coronary Heart Disease. It can lower LDL and raise HDL. It also lowers blood pressure for those who are overweight.

  To become physically active, do 30 minutes of a moderate activity on most and, preferably, all days. Examples of moderate activities are brisk walking and dancing. If 30 minutes is too much time, break it up into periods of at least 10 minutes each. Those who have been inactive should start slowly. Begin at a lower level of physical activity and slowly increase the time and intensity of the effort.

Those with Coronary Heart Disease or who have a high risk for it should check with their doctor before starting a physical activity program. Others who should consult a doctor first include those with chronic health problems, men over age 40, and women over age 50. The doctor can give advice on how rigorous the exercise should be.

Those who have had a heart attack benefit greatly from physical activity. Many hospitals have a cardiac rehabilitation program. The doctor can offer advice about a suitable program.

- Diabetes: It damages blood vessels, including the coronary arteries of the heart. Up to 75 percent of those with diabetes develop heart and blood vessel diseases. Diabetes also can lead to stroke, kidney failure, and other problems.

Diabetes occurs when the body is not able to use sugar as it should for growth and energy. The body gets sugar when it changes food into glucose (a form of sugar). A hormone made in the pancreas and called insulin is needed for the glucose to be taken up and used by the body. In diabetes, the body cannot make use of the glucose in the blood because either the pancreas cannot make enough insulin or the insulin that is available is not effective.

Symptoms of diabetes include: increased thirst and urination (including at night), weight loss, and blurred vision, hunger, fatigue, frequent infections, and slow healing of wounds or sores.

There are two main types of diabetes-type 1 and type 2. Type 1 usually appears suddenly and most commonly in those under age 30. Type 2 diabetes occurs gradually and most often in those over age 40. Up to 95 percent of those with diabetes have type 2.

You're more likely to develop type 2 if you are overweight or obese, especially with extra weight around the middle, over age 40, or have high blood pressure or a family history of diabetes.

Because of the link with heart disease, it's important for those with diabetes to prevent or control heart disease and its risk factors. Fortunately, new research shows that the same steps that reduce the risk of Coronary Heart Disease also lower the chance of developing type 2 diabetes. And, for those who already have diabetes, those steps, along with taking any prescribed medication, also can delay or prevent the development of complications of diabetes, such as eye or kidney disease and nerve damage.

According to the research, a 7 percent loss of body weight and 150 minutes of moderate physical activity a week can reduce the chance of developing diabetes by 58 percent in those who are at high risk. The lifestyle changes cut the risk of developing type 2 diabetes regardless of age, ethnicity, gender, or weight.

CANCER

Cancer is a class of diseases in which a group of cells display uncontrolled growth (division beyond the normal limits), invasion (intrusion on and destruction of adjacent tissues), and sometimes metastasis (spread to other locations in the body via lymph or blood). These three malignant properties of cancers differentiate them from benign tumours, which are self-limited, do not invade or metastasize. Most cancers form a tumour but some, like leukaemia, do not. The branch of medicine concerned with the study, diagnosis, treatment, and prevention of cancer is oncology.

Cancer may affect people at all ages, even foetuses, but the risk for most varieties increases with age. Cancer causes about 13% of all deaths.

Nearly all cancers are caused by abnormalities in the genetic material of the transformed cells. These abnormalities may be due to the effects of carcinogens, such as tobacco smoke, radiation, chemicals, or infectious agents. Other cancer-promoting genetic abnormalities may be randomly acquired through errors in DNA replication, or are inherited, and thus present in all cells from birth. The heritability of cancers are usually affected by complex interactions between carcinogens and the host's genome. New aspects of the genetics of cancer pathogenesis, such as DNA methylation, and microRNAs are increasingly recognized as important.

Genetic abnormalities found in cancer typically affect two general classes of genes. Cancer-promoting oncogenes are typically activated in cancer cells, giving those cells new properties, such as hyperactive growth and division, protection against programmed cell death, loss of respect for normal tissue boundaries, and the ability to become established in diverse tissue environments. Tumour suppressor genes are then inactivated in cancer cells, resulting in the loss of normal functions in those cells, such as accurate DNA replication, control over the cell cycle, orientation and adhesion within tissues, and interaction with protective cells of the immune system.

Nomenclature

The following closely related terms may be used to designate abnormal growths:

- Tumour: originally, it meant any abnormal swelling, lump or mass. In current English, however, the word tumour has become synonymous with neoplasm, specifically solid neoplasm. Note that some neoplasms, such as leukaemia, do not form tumours.
- Neoplasm: the scientific term to describe an abnormal proliferation of genetically altered cells. Neoplasms can be benign or malignant:
- Malignant neoplasm or malignant tumour: synonymous with cancer.
- Benign neoplasm or benign tumour: a tumour (solid neoplasm) that stops growing by itself, does not invade other tissues and does not form metastases.
- Invasive tumour: The name refers to invasion of surrounding tissues.
- Pre-malignancy, pre-cancer or non-invasive tumour: A neoplasm that is not invasive but has the potential to progress to cancer (become invasive) if left untreated. These lesions are, in order of increasing potential for cancer, atypia, dysplasia and carcinoma in situ.

Classification

Cancers are classified by the type of cell that resembles the tumour and, therefore, the tissue presumed to be the origin of the tumour. Examples of general categories include:

- Carcinoma: Malignant tumours derived from epithelial cells. This group represents the most common cancers, including the common forms of breast, prostate, lung and colon cancer.
- Sarcoma: Malignant tumours derived from connective tissue, or mesenchymal cells.
- Lymphoma and leukaemia: Malignancies derived from hematopoietic (blood-forming) cells

- Germ cell tumour: Tumours derived from totipotent cells. In adults most often found in the testicle and ovary; in foetuses, babies, and young children most often found on the body midline, particularly at the tip of the tailbone; in horses most often found at the poll (base of the skull).
- Blastic tumour or blastoma: A tumour (usually malignant) which resembles an immature or embryonic tissue. Many of these tumours are most common in children.
- Malignant tumours: are usually named using -carcinoma, -sarcoma or -blastoma as a suffix, with the Latin or Greek word for the organ of origin as the root. For instance, a cancer of the liver is called hepatocarcinoma; a cancer of the fat cells is called liposarcoma. For common cancers, the English organ name is used. For instance, the most common type of breast cancer is called ductal carcinoma of the breast or mammary ductal carcinoma. Here, the adjective ductal refers to the appearance of the cancer under the microscope, resembling normal breast ducts.
- Benign tumours (which are not cancers) are named using -oma as a suffix with the organ name as the root. For instance, a benign tumour of the smooth muscle of the uterus is called leiomyoma (the common name of this frequent tumour is fibroid). Unfortunately, some cancers also use the -oma suffix, examples being melanoma and seminoma.

Causes

Cancer is a diverse class of diseases which differ widely in their causes and biology. The common thread in all known cancers is the acquisition of abnormalities in the genetic material of the cancer cell and its progeny. Research into the pathogenesis of cancer can be divided into three broad areas of focus. The first area of research focuses on the agents and events which cause or facilitate genetic changes in cells destined to become cancer. Second, it is important to uncover the precise nature of the genetic damage, and the genes which are affected by it. The third focus is on the consequences of those genetic changes on the biology of the cell, both in generating the defining properties of a cancer cell, and in facilitating additional genetic events, leading to further progression of the cancer.

Mutation: Cancer pathogenesis is traceable back to DNA mutations that impact cell growth and metastasis. Substances that cause DNA mutations are known as mutagens, and mutagens that cause cancers are known as carcinogens. Particular substances have been linked to specific types of cancer. Tobacco smoking is associated with many forms of cancer, and causes 90% of lung cancer. Prolonged exposure to asbestos fibers is associated with mesothelioma.

Many mutagens are also carcinogens, but some carcinogens are not mutagens. Alcohol is an example of a chemical carcinogen that is not a mutagen. Such chemicals may promote cancers through stimulating the rate of cell division. Faster rates of replication leaves less time for repair enzymes to repair damaged DNA during DNA replication, increasing the likelihood of a mutation.

Decades of research has demonstrated the link between tobacco use and cancer in the lung, larynx, head, neck, stomach, bladder, kidney, oesophagus and pancreas. Tobacco smoke contains over fifty known carcinogens, including nitrosamines and polycyclic aromatic hydrocarbons. Tobacco is responsible for about one in three of all cancer deaths in the developed world, and about one in five worldwide. Indeed, lung cancer death rates in the United States have mirrored smoking patterns, with increases in smoking followed by dramatic increases in lung cancer death rates and, more recently, decreases in smoking followed by decreases in lung cancer death rates in men. However, the numbers of smokers worldwide is still rising, leading to what some organizations have described as the tobacco epidemic.

Sources of ionizing radiation, such as radon gas, can cause cancer. Prolonged exposure to ultraviolet radiation from the sun can lead to melanoma and other skin malignancies.

Radio-frequency radiation from mobile phones has been proposed as a cause of cancer, but there is little evidence of such a link. Nevertheless, some experts caution against prolonged exposure.

Viral or bacterial infection: Some cancers can be caused by infection with pathogens. Many cancers originate from a viral infection; this is especially true in animals such as birds, but also in humans, as viruses are responsible for 15% of human cancers worldwide. The main viruses associated with human cancers are human papillomavirus, hepatitis B and hepatitis C virus, Epstein-Barr virus, and human T-lymphotropic virus. Experimental and epidemiological data imply a causative role for viruses and they appear to be the second most important risk factor for cancer development in humans, exceeded only by tobacco usage. The mode of virally-induced tumours can be divided into two, acutely-transforming or slowly-transforming. In acutely transforming viruses, the virus carries an overactive oncogene called viral-oncogene (v-onc), and the infected cell is transformed as soon as v-onc is expressed. In contrast, in slowly-transforming viruses, the virus genome is inserts near a proto-oncogene in the host genome. The viral promoter or other transcription regulation elements then cause overexpression of that proto-oncogene. This induces uncontrolled cell division. Because the site of insertion is not specific to proto-oncogenes and the chance of insertion near any proto-oncogene is low, slowly-transforming viruses will cause tumours much longer after infection than the acutely-transforming viruses.

Hepatitis viruses, including hepatitis B and hepatitis C, can induce a chronic viral infection that leads to liver cancer in 0.47% of hepatitis B patients per year (especially in Asia), and in 1.4% of hepatitis C carriers per year. Liver cirrhosis, whether from chronic viral hepatitis infection or alcoholism, is associated with the development of liver cancer, and the combination of cirrhosis and viral hepatitis presents the highest risk of liver cancer development. Worldwide, liver cancer is one of the most common, and most deadly, cancers due to a huge burden of viral hepatitis transmission and disease.

In addition to viruses, researchers have noted a connection between bacteria and certain cancers. The most prominent example is the link between chronic infection of the wall of the stomach with Helicobacter pylori and gastric cancer. Although only a minority of those infected with Helicobacter go on to develop cancer, since this pathogen is quite common it is probably responsible for the majority of these cancers.

Hormonal imbalances: Some hormones can act in a similar manner to non-mutagenic carcinogens in that they may stimulate excessive cell growth. A well-established example is the role of hyperestrogenic states in promoting endometrial cancer.

Immune system dysfunction: HIV is associated with a number of malignancies, including Kaposi's sarcoma, non-Hodgkin's lymphoma, and HPV-associated malignancies such as anal cancer and cervical cancer. AIDS-defining illnesses have long included these diagnoses. The increased incidence of malignancies in HIV patients points to the breakdown of immune surveillance as a possible etiology of cancer. Certain other immune deficiency states (e.g. common variable immunodeficiency and IgA deficiency) are also associated with increased risk of malignancy.

Heredity: Most forms of cancer are "sporadic", and have no basis in heredity. There are, however, a number of recognised syndromes of cancer with a hereditary component, often a defective tumour suppressor allele.

Other causes: Excepting the rare transmissions that occur with pregnancies and only a marginal few organ donors, cancer is generally not a transmissible disease. The main reason for this is tissue graft rejection caused by MHC incompatibility. In humans and other vertebrates, the immune system uses MHC antigens to differentiate between "self" and "non-self" cells because these antigens are different from person to person. When non-self antigens are encountered, the immune system reacts against the appropriate cell. Such reactions may protect against tumour cell engraftment by eliminating implanted cells. The development of donor-derived tumours from organ transplants is exceedingly rare. The main cause of organ transplant associated tumours seems to be malignant melanoma, that was undetected at the time of organ harvest.

A few types of cancer in non-humans have been found to be caused by transmission of the tumour cells themselves. This phenomenon is seen in dogs with Sticker's sarcoma, also known as canine transmissible venereal tumour, as well as Devil facial tumour disease in Tasmanian devils.

Pathophysiology

Cancer is fundamentally a disease of regulation of tissue growth. In order for a normal cell to transform into a cancer cell, genes which regulate cell growth and differentiation must be altered. Genetic changes can occur at many levels, from gain or loss of entire chromosomes to a mutation affecting a single DNA nucleotide. There are two broad categories of genes which are affected by these changes. Oncogenes may be normal genes which are expressed at inappropriately high levels, or altered genes which have novel properties. In either case, expression of these genes promotes the malignant phenotype of cancer cells.

Tumour suppressor genes are genes which inhibit cell division, survival, or other properties of cancer cells. Tumour suppressor genes are often disabled by cancer-promoting genetic changes. Typically, changes in many genes are required to transform a normal cell into a cancer cell.

There is a diverse classification scheme for the various genomic changes which may contribute to the generation of cancer cells. Most of these changes are mutations, or changes in the nucleotide sequence of genomic DNA. Aneuploidy, the presence of an abnormal number of chromosomes, is one genomic change which is not a mutation, and may involve either gain or loss of one or more chromosomes through errors in mitosis.

Large-scale mutations involve the deletion or gain of a portion of a chromosome. Genomic amplification occurs when a cell gains many copies (often 20 or more) of a small chromosomal locus, usually containing one or more oncogenes and adjacent genetic material. Translocation occurs when two separate chromosomal regions become abnormally fused, often at a characteristic location. A well-known example of this is the Philadelphia chromosome, or translocation of chromosomes 9 and 22, which occurs in chronic myelogenous leukaemia, and results in production of the BCR-abl fusion protein, an oncogenic tyrosine kinase.

Small-scale mutations include point mutations, deletions, and insertions, which may occur in the promoter of a gene and affect its expression, or may occur in the gene's coding sequence and alter the function or stability of its protein product. Disruption of a single gene may also result from integration of genomic material from a DNA virus or retrovirus, and such an event may also result in the expression of viral oncogenes in the affected cell and its descendants.

Diagnosis

Most cancers are initially recognized either because signs or symptoms appear or through screening. Neither of these lead to a definitive diagnosis, which usually requires the opinion of a pathologist, a type of physician (medical doctor) who specializes in the diagnosis of cancer and other diseases.

Investigation: People with suspected cancer are investigated with medical tests. These commonly include blood tests, X-rays, CT scans and endoscopy.

Biopsy: A cancer may be suspected for a variety of reasons, but the definitive diagnosis of most malignancies must be confirmed by histological examination of the cancerous cells by a pathologist. Tissue can be obtained from a biopsy or surgery. Many biopsies (such as those of the skin, breast or liver) can be done in a doctor's office. Biopsies of other organs are performed under anesthesia and require surgery in an operating room.

The tissue diagnosis given by the pathologist indicates the type of cell that is proliferating, its histological grade and other features of the tumour. Together, this information is useful to evaluate the prognosis of this patient and to choose the best treatment. Cytogenetics and immunohistochemistry are other types of testing that the pathologist may perform on the tissue specimen. These tests may provide information about future behavior of the cancer (prognosis) and best treatment.

Treatment

Cancer can be treated by surgery, chemotherapy, radiation therapy, immunotherapy, monoclonal antibody therapy or other methods. The choice of therapy depends upon the location and grade of the tumour and the stage of the disease, as well as the general state of the patient (performance status). A number of experimental cancer treatments are also under development.

Complete removal of the cancer without damage to the rest of the body is the goal of treatment. Sometimes this can be accomplished by surgery, but the propensity of cancers to invade adjacent tissue or to spread to distant sites by microscopic metastasis often limits its effectiveness. The effectiveness of chemotherapy is often limited by toxicity to other tissues in the body. Radiation can also cause damage to normal tissue.

Because "cancer" refers to a class of diseases, it is unlikely that there will ever be a single "cure for cancer" any more than there will be a single treatment for all infectious diseases.

Surgery: In theory, non-hematological cancers can be cured if entirely removed by surgery, but this is not always possible. When the cancer has metastasized to other sites in the body prior to surgery, complete surgical excision is usually impossible. In the Halstedian model of cancer progression, tumours grow locally, then spread to the lymph nodes, then to the rest of the body. This has given rise to the popularity of local-only treatments such as surgery for small cancers. Even small localized tumours are increasingly recognized as possessing metastatic potential.

Examples of surgical procedures for cancer include mastectomy for breast cancer and prostatectomy for prostate cancer. The goal of the surgery can be either the removal of only the tumour, or the entire organ. A single cancer cell is invisible to the naked eye but can regrow into a new tumour, a process called recurrence. For this reason, the pathologist will examine the surgical specimen to determine if a margin of healthy tissue is present, thus decreasing the chance that microscopic cancer cells are left in the patient.

In addition to removal of the primary tumour, surgery is often necessary for staging, e.g. determining the extent of the disease and whether it has metastasized to regional lymph nodes. Staging is a major determinant of prognosis and of the need for adjuvant therapy.

Occasionally, surgery is necessary to control symptoms, such as spinal cord compression or bowel obstruction. This is referred to as palliative treatment.

Radiation therapy: Radiation therapy (also called radiotherapy, X-ray therapy, or irradiation) is the use of ionizing radiation to kill cancer cells and shrink tumours. Radiation therapy can be administered externally via external beam radiotherapy (EBRT) or internally via brachytherapy. The effects of radiation therapy are localised and confined to the region being treated. Radiation therapy injures or destroys cells in the area being treated (the "target tissue") by damaging their genetic material, making it impossible for these cells to continue to grow and divide. Although radiation damages both cancer cells and normal cells, most normal cells can recover from the effects of radiation and function properly. The goal of radiation therapy is to damage as many cancer cells as possible, while limiting harm to nearby healthy tissue. Hence, it is given in many fractions, allowing healthy tissue to recover between fractions.

Radiation therapy may be used to treat almost every type of solid tumour, including cancers of the brain, breast, cervix, larynx, lung, pancreas, prostate, skin, stomach, uterus, or soft tissue sarcomas. Radiation is also used to treat leukaemia and lymphoma. Radiation dose to each site depends on a number of factors, including the radiosensitivity of each cancer type and whether there are tissues and organs nearby that may be damaged by radiation. Thus, as with every form of treatment, radiation therapy is not without its side effects.

Chemotherapy: Chemotherapy is the treatment of cancer with drugs ("anticancer drugs") that can destroy cancer cells. In current usage, the term "chemotherapy" usually refers to cytotoxic drugs which affect rapidly dividing cells in general, in contrast with targeted therapy. Chemotherapy drugs interfere with cell division in various possible ways, e.g. with the duplication of DNA or the separation of newly formed chromosomes.

Most forms of chemotherapy target all rapidly dividing cells and are not specific for cancer cells, although some degree of specificity may come from the inability of many cancer cells to repair DNA damage, while normal cells generally can. Hence, chemotherapy has the potential to harm healthy tissue, especially those tissues that have a high replacement rate (e.g. intestinal lining). These cells usually repair themselves after chemotherapy.

Because some drugs work better together than alone, two or more drugs are often given at the same time. This is called "combination chemotherapy"; most chemotherapy regimens are given in a combination.

The treatment of some leukaemias and lymphomas requires the use of high-dose chemotherapy, and total body irradiation (TBI). This treatment ablates the bone marrow, and hence the body's ability to recover and repopulate the blood. For this reason, bone marrow, or peripheral blood stem cell harvesting is carried out before the ablative part of the therapy, to enable "rescue" after the treatment has been given. This is known as autologous stem cell transplantation. Alternatively, hematopoietic stem cells may be transplanted from a matched unrelated donor (MUD).

Targeted therapies: Targeted therapy, which first became available in the late 1990s, has had a significant impact in the treatment of some types of cancer, and is currently a very active research area. This constitutes the use of agents specific for the deregulated proteins of cancer cells. Small molecule targeted therapy drugs are generally inhibitors of enzymatic domains on mutated, overexpressed, or otherwise critical proteins within the cancer cell. Prominent examples are the tyrosine kinase inhibitors imatinib (Gleevec/Glivec) and gefitinib (Iressa).

Monoclonal antibody therapy is another strategy in which the therapeutic agent is an antibody which specifically binds to a protein on the surface of the cancer cells. Examples include the anti-HER2/neu antibody trastuzumab (Herceptin) used in breast cancer, and the anti-CD20 antibody rituximab, used in a variety of B-cell malignancies.

Targeted therapy can also involve small peptides as "homing devices" which can bind to cell surface receptors or affected extracellular matrix surrounding the tumour. Radionuclides which are attached to this peptides (e.g. RGDs) eventually kill the cancer cell if the nuclide decays in the vicinity of the cell. Especially oligo- or multimers of these binding motifs are of great interest, since this can lead to enhanced tumour specificity and avidity.

Prevention and Control

Cancer prevention is defined as active measures to decrease the incidence of cancer. This can be accomplished by avoiding carcinogens or altering their metabolism, pursuing a lifestyle or diet that modifies cancer-causing factors and/or medical intervention (chemoprevention, treatment of pre-malignant lesions). The epidemiological concept of "prevention" is usually defined as either primary prevention, for people who have not been diagnosed with a particular disease, or secondary prevention, aimed at reducing recurrence or complications of a previously diagnosed illness.

Observational epidemiological studies that show associations between risk factors and specific cancers mostly serve to generate hypotheses about potential interventions that could reduce cancer incidence or morbidity. Randomized controlled trials then test whether hypotheses generated by epidemiological trials and laboratory research actually result in reduced cancer incidence and mortality. In many cases, findings from observational epidemiological studies are not confirmed by randomized controlled trials.

About a third of the twelve most common cancers worldwide are due to nine potentially modifiable risk factors. Men with cancer are twice as likely as women to have a modifiable risk factor for their disease. The nine risk factors are tobacco smoking, excessive alcohol use, diet low in fruit and vegetables, limited physical exercise, human papillomavirus infection (unsafe sex), urban air pollution, domestic use of solid fuels, and contaminated injections (hepatitis B and C).

Lifestyle risk factors: The vast majority of cancer risk factors are environmental or lifestyle-related in nature, leading to the claim that cancer is a largely preventable disease. Examples of modifiable cancer risk factors include alcohol consumption (associated with increased risk of oral, esophageal, breast, and other cancers), smoking (although 20% of women with lung cancer have never smoked, versus 10% of men), physical inactivity (associated with increased risk of colon, breast, and possibly other cancers), and being overweight (associated with colon, breast, endometrial, and possibly other cancers). Based on epidemiologic evidence, it is now thought that avoiding excessive alcohol consumption may contribute to reductions in risk of certain cancers; however, compared with tobacco exposure, the magnitude of effect is modest or small and the strength of evidence is often weaker. Other lifestyle and environmental factors known to affect cancer risk (either beneficially or detrimentally) include certain sexually transmitted diseases (such as those conveyed by the human papillomavirus), the use of exogenous hormones, exposure to ionizing radiation and ultraviolet radiation, and certain occupational and chemical exposures.

Chemoprevention: The concept that medications could be used to prevent cancer is an attractive one, and many high-quality clinical trials support the use of such chemoprevention in defined circumstances.

Daily use of tamoxifen, a selective estrogen receptor modulator (SERM), typically for 5 years, has been demonstrated to reduce the risk of developing breast cancer in high-risk women by about 50%. A recent study reported that the selective estrogen receptor modulator raloxifene has similar benefits to tamoxifen in preventing breast cancer in high-risk women, with a more favorable side effect profile.

Raloxifene is a SERM like tamoxifen; it has been shown (in the STAR trial) to reduce the risk of breast cancer in high-risk women equally as well as tamoxifen. In this trial, which studied almost 20,000 women, raloxifene had fewer side effects than tamoxifen, though it did permit more DCIS to form.

Finasteride, a 5-alpha-reductase inhibitor, has been shown to lower the risk of prostate cancer, though it seems to mostly prevent low-grade tumours. The effect of COX-2 inhibitors such as rofecoxib and celecoxib upon the risk of colon polyps have been studied in familial adenomatous polyposis patients and in the general population. In both groups, there were significant reductions in colon polyp incidence, but this came at the price of increased cardiovascular toxicity.

Genetic testing: Genetic testing for high-risk individuals is already available for certain cancer-related genetic mutations. Carriers of genetic mutations that increase risk for cancer incidence can undergo enhanced surveillance, chemoprevention, or risk-reducing surgery. Early identification of inherited genetic risk for cancer, along with cancer-preventing interventions such as surgery or enhanced surveillance, can be lifesaving for high-risk individuals.

DIABETES MELLITUS

Diabetes mellitus is a syndrome of disordered metabolism, usually due to a combination of hereditary and environmental causes, resulting in abnormally high blood sugar levels (hyperglycemia). Blood glucose levels are controlled by a complex interaction of multiple chemicals and hormones in the body, including the hormone insulin made in the beta cells of the pancreas. Diabetes mellitus refers to the group of diseases that lead to high blood glucose levels due to defects in either insulin secretion or insulin action.

Diabetes develops due to a diminished production of insulin (in type 1) or resistance to its effects (in type 2 and gestational). Both lead to hyperglycaemia, which largely causes the acute signs of diabetes: excessive urine production, resulting compensatory thirst and increased fluid intake, blurred vision, unexplained weight loss, lethargy, and changes in energy metabolism. Monogenic forms, e.g. MODY, constitute 1-5 % of all cases.

All forms of diabetes have been treatable since insulin became medically available in 1921, but there is no cure. The injections by a syringe, insulin pump, or insulin pen deliver insulin, which is a basic treatment of type 1 diabetes. Type 2 is managed with a combination of dietary treatment, exercise, medications and insulin supplementation.

Pathophysiology

Insulin production is more or less constant within the beta cells, irrespective of blood glucose levels. It is stored within vacuoles pending release, via exocytosis, which is primarily triggered by food, chiefly food containing absorbable glucose. The chief trigger is a rise in blood glucose levels after eating.

Insulin is the principal hormone that regulates uptake of glucose from the blood into most cells (primarily muscle and fat cells, but not central nervous system cells). Therefore deficiency of insulin or the insensitivity of its receptors plays a central role in all forms of diabetes mellitus.

Most of the carbohydrates in food are converted within a few hours to the monosaccharide glucose, the principal carbohydrate found in blood and used by the body as fuel. The most significant exceptions are fructose, most disaccharides (except sucrose and in some people lactose), and all more complex polysaccharides, with the outstanding exception of starch. Insulin is released into the blood by beta cells (?-cells), found in the Islets of Langerhans in the pancreas, in response to rising levels of blood glucose, typically after eating. Insulin is used by about two-thirds of the body's cells to absorb glucose from the blood for use as fuel, for conversion to other needed molecules, or for storage.

Insulin is also the principal control signal for conversion of glucose to glycogen for internal storage in liver and muscle cells. Lowered glucose levels result both in the reduced release of insulin from the beta cells and in the reverse conversion of glycogen to glucose when glucose levels fall. This is mainly controlled by the hormone glucagon which acts in an opposite manner to insulin. Glucose thus recovered by the liver re-enters the bloodstream; muscle cells lack the necessary export mechanism.

Higher insulin levels increase some anabolic ("building up") processes such as cell growth and duplication, protein synthesis, and fat storage.

Insulin (or its lack) is the principal signal in converting many of the bidirectional processes of metabolism from a catabolic to an anabolic direction, and vice versa. In particular, a low insulin level is the trigger for entering or leaving ketosis (the fat burning metabolic phase).

If the amount of insulin available is insufficient, if cells respond poorly to the effects of insulin (insulin insensitivity or resistance), or if the insulin itself is defective, then glucose will not be absorbed properly by those body cells that require it nor will it be stored appropriately in the liver and muscles. The net effect is persistent high levels of blood glucose, poor protein synthesis, and other metabolic derangements, such as acidosis.

Symptoms

The classical triad of diabetes symptoms is polyuria, polydipsia and polyphagia, which are, respectively, frequent urination, increased thirst and consequent increased fluid intake, and increased appetite. Symptoms may develop quite rapidly (weeks or months) in type 1 diabetes, particularly in children. However, in type 2 diabetes symptoms usually develop much more slowly and may be subtle or completely absent. Type 1 diabetes may also cause a rapid yet significant weight loss (despite normal or even increased eating) and irreducible fatigue. All of these symptoms except weight loss can also manifest in type 2 diabetes in patients whose diabetes is poorly controlled.

When the glucose concentration in the blood is raised beyond its renal threshold, reabsorption of glucose in the proximal renal tubuli is incomplete, and part of the glucose remains in the urine (glycosuria). This increases the osmotic pressure of the urine and inhibits reabsorption of water by the kidney, resulting in increased urine production (polyuria) and increased fluid loss. Lost blood volume will be replaced osmotically from water held in body cells and other body compartments, causing dehydration and increased thirst.

Prolonged high blood glucose causes glucose absorption, which leads to changes in the shape of the lenses of the eyes, resulting in vision changes; sustained sensible glucose control usually returns the lens to its original shape. Blurred vision is a common complaint leading to a diabetes diagnosis; type 1 should always be suspected in cases of rapid vision change, whereas with type 2 change is generally more gradual, but should still be suspected.

Patients (usually with type 1 diabetes) may also initially present with diabetic ketoacidosis (DKA), an extreme state of metabolic dysregulation characterized by the smell of acetone on the patient's breath; a rapid, deep breathing known as Kussmaul breathing; polyuria; nausea; vomiting and abdominal pain; and any of many altered states of consciousness or arousal (such as hostility and mania or, equally, confusion and lethargy). In severe DKA, coma may follow, progressing to death. Diabetic ketoacidosis is a medical emergency and requires immediate hospitalization.

A rarer but equally severe possibility is hyperosmolar nonketotic state, which is more common in type 2 diabetes and is mainly the result of dehydration due to loss of body water. Often, the patient has been drinking extreme amounts of sugar-containing drinks, leading to a vicious circle in regard to the water loss.

Diagnosis

The diagnosis of type 1 diabetes, and many cases of type 2, is usually prompted by recent-onset symptoms of excessive urination (polyuria) and excessive thirst (polydipsia), often accompanied by weight loss. These symptoms typically worsen over days to weeks; about a quarter of people with new type 1 diabetes have developed some degree of diabetic ketoacidosis by the time the diabetes is recognized. The diagnosis of other types of diabetes is usually made in other ways. These include ordinary health screening; detection of hyperglycemia during other medical investigations; and secondary symptoms such as vision changes or unexplainable fatigue. Diabetes is often detected when a person suffers a problem that is frequently caused by diabetes, such as a heart attack, stroke, neuropathy, poor wound healing or a foot ulcer, certain eye problems, certain fungal infections, or delivering a baby with macrosomia or hypoglycemia.

Diabetes mellitus is characterized by recurrent or persistent hyperglycemia, and is diagnosed by demonstrating any one of the following:

- Fasting plasma glucose level at or above 126 mg/dL (7.0 mmol/l).
- Plasma glucose at or above 200 mg/dL (11.1 mmol/l) two hours after a 75 g oral glucose load as in a glucose tolerance test.
- Symptoms of hyperglycemia and casual plasma glucose at or above 200 mg/dL (11.1 mmol/l).

A positive result, in the absence of unequivocal hyperglycemia, should be confirmed by a repeat of any of the above-listed methods on a different day. Most physicians prefer to measure a fasting glucose level because of the ease of measurement and the considerable time commitment of formal glucose tolerance testing, which takes two hours to complete. According to the current definition, two fasting glucose measurements above 126 mg/dL (7.0 mmol/l) is considered diagnostic for diabetes mellitus.

Patients with fasting glucose levels from 100 to 125 mg/dL (6.1 and 7.0 mmol/l) are considered to have impaired fasting glucose. Patients with plasma glucose at or above 140 mg/dL or 7.8 mmol/l, but not over 200, two hours after a 75 g oral glucose load are considered to have impaired glucose tolerance. Of these two pre-diabetic states, the latter in particular is a major risk factor for progression to full-blown diabetes mellitus as well as cardiovascular disease.

While not used for diagnosis, an elevated level of glucose irreversibly bound to hemoglobin (termed glycosylated hemoglobin or HbA1c) of 6.0% or is considered abnormal by most labs; HbA1c is primarily used as a treatment-tracking test reflecting average blood glucose levels over the preceding 90 days (approximately). However, some physicians may order this test at the time of diagnosis to track changes over time. The current recommended goal for HbA1c in patients with diabetes is <7.0%, which is considered good glycemic control, although some guidelines are stricter (<6.5%). People with diabetes who have HbA1c levels within this range have a significantly lower incidence of complications from diabetes, including retinopathy and diabetic nephropathy.

Treatment

Diabetes mellitus is currently a chronic disease, without a cure, and medical emphasis must necessarily be on managing/avoiding possible short-term as well as long-term diabetes-related problems. There is an exceptionally important role for patient education, dietetic support, sensible exercise, self monitoring of blood glucose, with the goal of keeping both short-term blood glucose levels, and long term levels as well, within acceptable bounds. Careful control is needed to reduce the risk of long term complications.

Prevention

Type 1 diabetes risk is known to depend upon a genetic predisposition based on HLA types (particularly types DR3 and DR4), an unknown environmental trigger (suspected to be an infection, although none has proven definitive in all cases), and an uncontrolled autoimmune response that attacks the insulin producing beta cells. Some research has suggested that breastfeeding decreased the risk in later life; various other nutritional risk factors are being studied, but no firm evidence has been found. Giving children 2000 IU of Vitamin D during their first year of life is associated with reduced risk of type 1 diabetes, though the causal relationship is obscure.

Children with antibodies to beta cell proteins (i.e., at early stages of an immune reaction to them) but no overt diabetes, and treated with vitamin B-3 (niacin), had less than half the diabetes onset incidence in a 7-year time span as did the general population, and an even lower incidence relative to those with antibodies as above, but who received no vitamin B3.

Type 2 diabetes risk can be reduced in many cases by making changes in diet and increasing physical activity. The ADA does not recommend alcohol consumption as a preventive, but it is interesting to note that moderate alcohol intake may reduce the risk (though heavy consumption absolutely and clearly increases damage to bodily systems significantly); a similarly confused connection between low dose alcohol consumption and heart disease is termed the French Paradox.

There is inadequate evidence that eating foods of low glycemic index is clinically helpful despite recommendations and suggested diets emphasizing this approach.

There are numerous studies which suggest connections between some aspects of Type II diabetes with ingestion of certain foods or with some drugs. Some studies have shown delayed progression to diabetes in predisposed patients through prophylactic use of metformin, rosiglitazone, or valsartan. In patients on hydroxychloroquine for rheumatoid arthritis, incidence of diabetes was reduced by 77% though causal mechanisms are unclear. Breastfeeding may also be associated with the prevention of type 2 of the disease in mothers. Clear evidence for these and any of many other connections between foods and supplements and diabetes is sparse to date; none, despite secondary claims for (or against), is sufficiently well established to justify as a standard clinical approach.

BLINDNESS

Blindness is the condition of lacking visual perception due to physiological or neurological factors. Various scales have been developed to describe the extent of vision loss and define "blindness." Total blindness is the complete lack of form and visual light perception and is clinically recorded as "NLP," an abbreviation for "no light perception." Blindness is frequently used to describe severe visual impairment with residual vision.

Those described as having only "light perception" have no more sight than the ability to tell light from dark. A person with only "light projection" can tell the general direction of a light source.

In order to determine which people may need special assistance because of their visual disabilities, various governmental jurisdictions have formulated more complex definitions referred to as legal blindness. Legal blindness is defined as visual acuity (vision) of 20/200 (6/60) or less in the better eye with best correction possible. This means that a legally blind individual would have to stand 20 feet (6.1 m) from an object to see it-with vision correction-with the same degree of clarity as a normally sighted person could from 200 feet (61 m).

In many areas, people with average acuity who nonetheless have a visual field of less than 20 degrees (the norm being 180 degrees) are also classified as being legally blind. Approximately ten percent of those deemed legally blind, by any measure, have no vision. The rest have some vision, from light perception alone to relatively good acuity. Low vision is sometimes used to describe visual acuities from 20/70 to 20/200.

By the 10th Revision of the WHO International Statistical Classification of Diseases, Injuries and Causes of Death, low vision is defined as visual acuity of less than 6/18, but equal to or better than 3/60, or corresponding visual field loss to less than 20 degrees, in the better eye with best possible correction. Blindness is defined as visual acuity of less than 3/60, or corresponding visual field loss to less than 10 degrees, in the better eye with best possible correction.

It should be noted that blind people with undamaged eyes may still register light non-visually for the purpose of circadian entrainment to the 24-hour light/dark cycle. Light signals for this purpose travel through the retinohypothalamic tract (RHT), so a damaged optic nerve beyond where the RHT exits it is no hindrance.

Causes

Serious visual impairment has a variety of causes:

Diseases: Most visual impairment is caused by disease and malnutrition. According to WHO estimates in 2002, the most common causes of blindness around the world are:

- Cataracts (47.8%),
- Glaucoma (12.3%),
- Uveitis (10.2%),

- Age-related macular degeneration (AMD) (8.7%),
- Trachoma (3.6%),
- Corneal opacity (5.1%), and
- Diabetic retinopathy (4.8%), among other causes.

People in developing countries are significantly more likely to experience visual impairment as a consequence of treatable or preventable conditions than are their counterparts in the developed world. While vision impairment is most common in people over age 60 across all regions, children in poorer communities are more likely to be affected by blinding diseases than are their more affluent peers.

The link between poverty and treatable visual impairment is most obvious when conducting regional comparisons of cause. Most adult visual impairment is related to age-related macular degeneration and diabetic retinopathy. While both of these conditions are subject to treatment, neither can be cured. Another common cause is retinopathy of prematurity.

In developing countries, wherein people have shorter life expectancies, cataracts and water-borne parasites-both of which can be treated effectively-are most often the culprits. Of the estimated 40 million blind people located around the world, 70-80% can have some or all of their sight restored through treatment. In developed countries where parasitic diseases are less common and cataract surgery is more available, age-related macular degeneration, glaucoma, and diabetic retinopathy are usually the leading causes of blindness.

Abnormalities and injuries: Eye injuries, most often occurring in people under 30, are the leading cause of monocular blindness (vision loss in one eye) throughout the United States. Injuries and cataracts affect the eye itself, while abnormalities such as optic nerve hypoplasia affect the nerve bundle that sends signals from the eye to the back of the brain, which can lead to decreased visual acuity. People with injuries to the occipital lobe of the brain can, despite having undamaged eyes and optic nerves, still be legally or totally blind.

Genetic defects: People with albinism often suffer from visual impairment to the extent that many are legally blind, though few of them actually cannot see. Leber's congenital amaurosis can cause total blindness or severe sight loss from birth or early childhood.

Recent advances in mapping of the human genome have identified other genetic causes of low vision or blindness. One such example is Bardet-Biedl syndrome.

Poisoning: Rarely, blindness is caused by the intake of certain chemicals. A well-known example is methanol, which ironically is only mildly toxic and minimally intoxicating, but when not competing with ethanol for metabolism, methanol breaks down into the substances formaldehyde and formic acid which in turn can cause blindness, an array of other health complications, and death. Methanol is commonly found in methylated spirits, denatured ethyl alcohol, to avoid paying taxes on selling ethanol intended for human consumption. Methylated spirits are sometimes used by alcoholics as a desperate and cheap substitute for regular ethanol alcoholic beverages.

Treatment

A 2008 study tested the effect of using gene therapy to help restore the sight of patients with a rare form of inherited blindness, known as Leber Congenital Amaurosis or LCA. Leber Congenital Amaurosis damages the light receptors in the retina and usually begins affecting sight in early childhood, with worsening vision until complete blindness around the age of 30.

The study used a common cold virus to deliver a normal version of the gene called RPE65 directly into the eyes of affected patients. Remarkably all 3 patients aged 19, 26 and 26 responded well to the treatment and reported improved vision following the procedure. Due to the age of the patients and the degenerative nature of LCA the improvement of vision in gene therapy patients is encouraging for researchers. It is hoped that gene therapy may be even more effective in younger LCA patients who have experienced limited vision loss as well as in other blind or partially blind individuals.

REFERENCES

Essential of community health Nursing 3rd edition, K. Park

Community health Nursing – Kasturi Sunder Rao

Social and preventive medicine – K. Park

M/S Banarsidas Bhanot publishers, Jabalpur

A new text book for Nurses in India vol – I

The foundation of Nursing – Veerak pitman, Zwemer Annamme by Rajah and Co – printers, Madras.

A textbook for health worker (ANM)by A.M. Chalkley vol – I and vol – II, new age international publishes, New Delhi

The text book of community health for Nurses by J.E. Park and K.Park, Asrani publishers, Jabalpur.

General psychology by Hans Raj bhattia Oxford and BH publishing CO. PVT. LTD – Calcutta

General psychology, published by SV University

Social psychology, published by SV University

Psycho pathology, published by SV University

Developmental psychology, published by SV University

An introduction to sociology by Sachdeva, Vidya Bhushan, Kitab Mahal, Allahabad

The pocket medical Dictionary by L.M. Harrison CBBS publishers-New Delhi.

8

Population and its Control

For most of human history, up to around 10 thousand years ago (generally accepted by science, although some place the time a few thousand years earlier), Earth's human population remained stabilized at around 8 to 10 million. Since then it has grown, at varying rates, to reach its present level of over 6,200 million (6.2 billion). This growth started when people began to grow crops and domesticate animals, which initiated the change from a hunter/gatherer subsistence (natural food supply) to a technology-driven food supply (agriculture).

We note that about 620 (or more) humans are alive today (most supported by agricultural technology) for every one human who was supported by the natural food supply of early non-technological Earth. The more recent "explosive" growth, which causes serious human population problems and environmental problems, is due to much more than just advances in agricultural technology. Among other factors is the decrease in the death rate due to advances in medicine and sanitation.

POPULATION EXPLOSION

Population explosion or overpopulation denotes a situation in which the number of people living in a country rapidly exceeds its carrying or sustaining capabilities. It is not just the quantity of people but the ratio of it in connection with the natural or artificial resources at hand. Population explosion can occur due to a number of reasons such as a step-up of birth rates, down slope of mortality rates with the advent of modern medical sciences, a simultaneous increase in immigration and decrease in emigration and so on.

Although India occupies only 2.4% of the world's total land area, Indian demography comprises of nearly 1.12 billion people, which is roughly one-sixth of the world's population and second largest in the world next to China.

Distribution of World Population in 2005

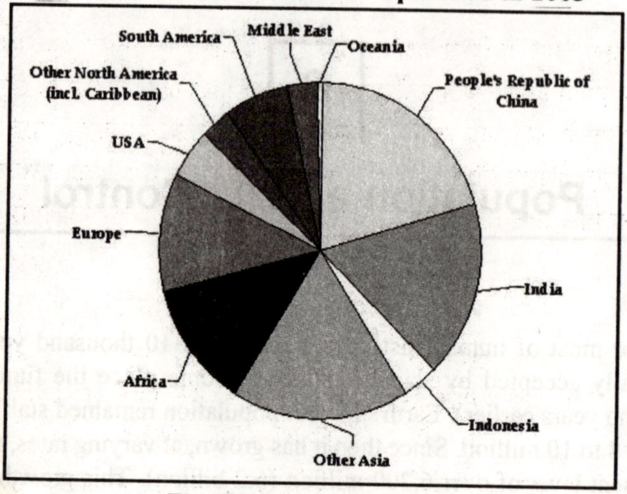

Fig. Population Explosion

India is facing intense problem of population outburst. People are experiencing the crisis such as climate change, shortage of food and also severe energy crisis that are all related to the ever-increasing population. Our civilization is being squeezed between rising population densities. It can be said that if such trends continue, there will be a severe shortage of food supply.

The government should impose a population control system upon every person living in the country by limiting them to have one child. The eruption of population has affected the standard of living of the people. The time has come when future citizens while in educational institutions should understand various issues related to the population problem. It has been observed that in some places, there is a shortage of drinking water. Village people started migrating to cities where they can get some water and employment. Today, in some places, people have start fighting for food, water and place to live.

The heavy centralization of India's family planning programs often prevents due consideration from being given to regional differences. Centralization is encouraged to a large extent by reliance on central government funding. As a result, many of the goals and assumptions of national population control programs do not correspond exactly with local attitudes toward birth control. In large part of India, people have strong preference for sons which leads to population growth. They have a feeling that sons will assist with farm labour as they are growing up. Son will also serve as their parent's only security in old age.

The government should implement program to reduce unplanned pregnancies, lowering fertility rates to the sun replacement levels and also they should try to provide assistance to people. An important family planning program in India is the Project for Community Action in Family Planning. Located in Karnataka, the project operates in 154 project villages and 255 control villages. All project villages are of sufficient size to have a health sub centre, although this advantage is offset by the fact that those villages are the most distant from the area's primary health centres. The project is much assisted by local voluntary groups, such as the women's clubs. The local voluntary groups either provide or secure sites suitable as distribution depots for condoms and birth control pills and also make arrangements for the operation of sterilization camps. Data provided by the Project for Community Action in Family Planning show that important achievements have been realized in the field of population control.

Population control program is essential because of the energy crisis. If this issue is ignored, it will have dangerous consequences.. Many factors are also directly or indirectly associated with over population. People often experience a shortage of employment opportunities, but they should understand that job opportunity is not related to population. Many young men and women do not get employment according to their education therefore they involve in criminal activities and become drug peddler. Most people are not aware of the fact that the environmental problem is associated with population. Many people believe that there is a strong link between the growing global population and climate change. Resources are limited in the environment and if people keep using them all then there will be crisis for future generation. Others believe that unmanaged population growth could lead to catastrophe because of the Earth's finite resources. Therefore, it can be said that majority of population is concerned about the impact of overpopulation on their lives, the Earth and the future.

Global warming is also related to overpopulation. To control global warming, population must be controlled. As the population grows, the demand for the consumption of energy such as electricity, cars and other energy resources increases which in turn affects the nature. If population growth is controlled, people can control the ever increasing of burning energy that might hamper their future. Many countries in the world are global warming polluter, contributing greenhouse gas emissions primarily from transportation, industry and power plant sources. The other thing that people should be concerned about is the infrastructure. All of us should understand that places are getting smaller and smaller as the population grows. Places, which once held beautiful landscape, have been turned into mega complexes to house the increasing number of people.

Population also affects on the education system. Today, education is very expensive and few people can afford to attend colleges or even high school. The shortage of seats in the colleges and universities are limited and many parents afford to bear the cost of education of more than two children. Hence this is another reason that people should keep smaller families so that they can afford the better facilities for all of them. Over population can cause many problems that people are not aware. Some issues are relating to nature, other relates to crime growth and also less of employment opportunities. Today, many younger generations understand that having few children can help protect the environment. The disparity that lies here is that many younger people feel that they have the right to have as many children they want. Therefore, the only best thing to do in such a case is to better educate them with the merits of smaller family.

People live a world that has given us an ample of resources to sustain them and it is up to human beings on how they use the same. As the number of people grows, the amount of earth space is reduced. It should be remembered that people live in a world that has three parts water and one part land and if that falls short than they have no other option but to build man made islands to accommodate the ever increasing rise of population. The need to address the family planning scenario has become a very important concern and many countries have joined hand in taking up the matter to educate the general public about the consequences of having a large family.

Younger generations today are more concerned about the environment because the way people are continuing, they have no idea what the world will be if the population keeps growing. Therefore, government should impose the law that a family shall not have more than one or two kids so that they can curb the population growth and also save the environment from the misuse of the energy by millions of people. Resources are dying out because human needs are increasing day-by-day. Sea levels are rising due to global warming. People survive on food and water. If stern action is not taken from the government to regulate population control then the country will become unrecognizable slums filled with broken-down housing, bad transportation, and hungry and thirsty people living on the filthy edge of human survival. Population contributes to a vast number of problems however, many countries have adopted family planning which is both successful and unsuccessful but they have managed to put the word across to many about the issues and concerns that they should be aware of and that prevention is better than cure.

Population growth is an important issue for any country. If better facilitates are not provided then many young people take up the path of crime just to sustain themselves and this also becomes a major concern of the government as the inmate population also increase and they have to build various other infrastructure to hold them. However, the major concern regarding over population is that of nature and shortage of food and water. Developing countries like India, Pakistan should take better precaution to curb the increasing number of people as many would thing that they might find opportunities in these areas because they are still yet to be developed. The government should therefore be strict with laws to limit over population without hurting the feeling of the general public.

The literal meaning of population is "the whole number of people or inhabitants in a country or region" (Webster's dictionary), and the literal meaning of population explosion is "a pyramiding of numbers of a biological population" (Webster's dictionary).As the number of people in a pyramid increases, so do the problems related to the increased population. The main factors affecting the population change are the birth rate, death rate and migration. The birth rate is the ratio between births and individuals in a specified population and time (Miller, 253). The death rate is the ratio between the number of deaths and individuals in a specified population and time (Miller, 253). Migration is the number of people moving in (immigration) or out (emigration) of a country, place or locality.

The population change is calculated by the formula:

Population change = (Births + Immigration) – (Deaths + Emigration)

The recent increase in the world population has been caused due to the following major reasons:

- The increase in birth rates due to medical improvements
- The decrease in death rates due to better medical facilities and advancements in the field of medicine.
- Immigration to better developed countries due to several reasons like better job opportunities, war, and natural causes like hurricanes, earthquakes, and so forth.

India, being a developing country, has had to face several economic and political challenges. One of the most important problems is the population explosion. India's population hit 1 billion in May 2000, increasing the urgency for the country to moderate its population growth. Some of the reasons for this population explosion are poverty, better medical facilities, and immigration from the neighboring countries of Bangladesh and Nepal.

The population density of India in 1996 was about 287 persons per square kilometer (Encyclopedia Britannica). Several solutions to decrease the rate of population increase have been tried by the government, some successful, some unsuccessful. Although the rate of increase has decreased, the rate has not reached the satisfactory level yet. The population in India continues to increase at an alarming rate. The effects of this population increase are evident in the increasing poverty, unemployment, air and water pollution, and shortage of food, health resources and educational resources.

REASONS FOR POPULATION EXPLOSION

Birth Rate

Poverty: According to ABC News, India currently faces approximately "... 33 births a minute, 2,000 an hour, 48,000 a day, which calculates to nearly 12 million a year". Unfortunately, the resources do not increase as the population increases. Instead the resources keep decreasing, leading to making survival for a human being more and more competitive even for the basic necessities of life like food, clothing and shelter.

India currently faces a vicious cycle of population explosion and poverty. One of the most important reasons for this population increase in India is poverty. More than 300 million Indians earn less than US $1 everyday and about 130 million people are jobless. The people, who have to struggle to make two ends meet produce more children because more children mean more earning hands. Also, due to poverty, the infant mortality rate among such families is higher due to the lack of facilities like food and medical resources. Thus, they produce more children assuming that not all of them would be able to survive. The end result is a mounting increase in the population size of India. Due to the increase in population, the problems of scarce resources, jobs, and poverty increases. Thus the cycle continues leading to an ever-increasing population that we see today. This cycle in fact might be considered as a positive feedback, in that the increase in one results in the increase of the other factor. As the poverty and the population both increase, the development of the country and the society seems even more far-fetched.

Traditions: India's culture runs very deep and far back in history. Due to the increased population, the educational facilities are very scarce. As a result, most people still strictly follow ancient beliefs. According to ABC News, the famous Indian author, Shobha De said, "God said 'Go forth and produce' and we just went ahead and did exactly that." In addition, a lot of families prefer having a son rather than a daughter. As a result, a lot of families have more children than they actually want or can afford, resulting in increased poverty, lack of resources, and most importantly, an increased population.

Another one of India's cultural norms is for a girl to get married at an early age. In most of the rural areas and in some urban areas as well, families prefer to get their girls married at the age of 14 or 15. Although child marriage is illegal in India, the culture and the society surrounding the girls in India does not allow them to oppose such decisions taken by their family. For many, giving a girl child in marriage is done not by choice, but rather out of compulsion. The poor economic status of tribal villagers is attributed as one of the primary factors responsible for the prevalence of child marriages in India.

Death Rate

Although poverty has increased and the development of the country continues to be hampered, the improvements in medical facilities have been tremendous. This improvement might be considered positive, but as far as population increase is considered, it has only been positive in terms of increasing the population further. The crude death rate in India in 1981 was approximately 12.5, and that decreased to approximately 8.7 in 1999. Also, the infant mortality rate in India decreased from 129 in 1981 to approximately 72 in 1999. These numbers are clear indications of the improvements in the medical field. This development is good for the economy and society of India, but strictly in terms of population, this advancement has further enhanced the increase in population.

The average life expectancy of people in India has increased from 52.9 in 1975-80 to 62.4 in 1995-00. Although our near and dear ones would live longer, due to the increase in the population, the resources available per person would be much less, leading to a decrease in the curvature of the slope of development instead of a higher gradient. In addition, abortion is not allowed by several religions that are followed in India. In fact, in Islam, one of the leading religions of India, children are considered to be gifts of God, and so the more children a woman has, the more she is respected in her family and society. As a result, although the

As we can observe, the increased population size is leading to increased pollution, which in turn is leading to a more hostile environment for human beings themselves.

Unemployment and Illiteracy

Suppose we forget about the environment, and only worry about ourselves. Nonetheless, with the increasing population, even that is not possible because with the increasing number of people, we have to share our resources with even more people. Resources of all types are limited, even employment, especially in India. India, being a developing country, has a limited number of jobs available. Due to the increasing number of people, the competition for the most menial jobs is also tremendous. In 1972-73, unemployment rates in rural areas were 1.2 for males and 0.5 for females, and in urban areas, it was 4.8 for males and 6.0 for females. This unemployment rate rose to 2.3 for males and 1.5 for females in rural areas and 4.9 for males and 8.2 for females in urban areas in 1998-99. With the increasing population, unemployment rates are bound to rise even further. Several highly educated people with Bachelors and Master's degrees in India sit at home, because they cannot find jobs. This, we believe, is the major reason for Indians to migrate to developed countries.

Such unemployment and underemployment leads to corruption and exploitation of people by the richer classes of the society. This lack of resources further leads to lack of educational resources. Due to the unavailability of resources, parents cannot afford to educate their children to higher levels. Some parents simply cannot afford to teach their children further, and in some families, children need to work along with their parents in order to bring food to the table. According to the World Bank Group, "about 32 million primary school-age children, mostly girls or those from the poorest households and disadvantaged groups, are not in school; more than half of rural students drop out before completing the primary cycle, and only one-third of females make it to the secondary level." In addition, "nearly half the population over 15 years old and about 60 percent of all women over 15 years old is illiterate."

Also, basic education has become a commodity that acts on the basis of supply and demand. Basic education has become too expensive in India for a commoner to afford for his/her children. Lack of education further leads to even more unemployment. Due to these reasons, a major part of the population is either illiterate or has the most minimum education leading them to accept minimal work in which they cannot even support themselves.

Unemployment, or underemployment, further leads to poverty. This again starts the vicious cycle of poverty and population explosion discussed above. Poverty leads to an increase in the population, because poverty leads people to produce more children to increase the earning members of the family. This increases the population size of India, which further increases the unemployment rate and lack of educational facilities leading to poverty that started this whole cycle.

Food Resources

Resources are always limited. And in a developing and highly populous country like India, resources are even scarcer. Population explosion results in the shortage of even the most basic resources like food. According to an article by World Bank Group, "...more than half of all children under the age of four are malnourished, 30 percent of newborns are significantly underweight, and 60 percent of women are anemic." Resources are limited everywhere. Thus, unless we can develop a technology that would enable us to live on just one grain of wheat, the population increase remains a serious problem in India. India spends approximately $10 billion each year on malnutrition (World Bank Group), and even then the government of India cannot provide the everyday nutritional requirements to everybody in India.

MEASURES TO CONTROL POPULATION

Population control is the practice of limiting population increase, usually by reducing the birth rate. The practice has sometimes been voluntary, as a response to poverty, environmental concerns, or out of religious ideology, but in some times and places it has been socially mandated. This is generally conducted to improve quality of life for a society or as a solution to overpopulation. While population control can involve measures that improve people's lives, giving them greater control of their reproduction some programs have exposed them to exploitation.

The population control movement was active throughout the 1960s and 1970s driving many reproductive health and family planning programs. In the 1980s tension grew between population control advocates and feminist women's health activists who advance women's reproductive rights as part of a human rights-based approach. Growing opposition to the narrow population control focus led to a significant change in population policies in the early 1990s.

Population control may use one or more of the following practices:

- Contraception
- Abstinence

- Abortion
- Emigration to other areas
- Decreasing immigration
- Increasing death rate

The methods chosen can be strongly influenced by the religious and cultural beliefs of the community's members. Failures of the other methods can lead to the use of abortion or infanticide, in which case it is regarded as a necessary drastic last resort.

REFERENCES

St Leger L. Health and nature – new challenges for health promotion. Health Promot Int. 2003;18(3): 173-175.

Setting priorities in injury prevention: The application of an incidence based cost model. Inj Prev. 2002;8(1): 74-78.

Spasoff R A. (1999), Epidemiologic methods for Health Policy, Oxford University Press, new York, especially chapter 1 "Policy, Public Policy and Health Policy", and chapter 7 "Policy Implementation" p. 169-173.

Spasoff RA. (1999), "Allocating health resources" (p. 172-179. World Health Organization (2000)

Stahl T, Rutten A, Nutbeam D, Kannas L. The importance of policy orientation and environment on physical activity participation – a comparative analysis between Eastern Germany, Western Germany and Finland. Health Promot Int. 2002;17(3): 235-246.

Stokols D. Translating social ecological theory into guidelines for community health promotion. Am J Health Promot. 1996;10(4): 282-298.

Stone D. Policy Paradox: The art of political decision-making. WW. Norton & Company. New York. 2002. p. 17-85.

Thompson D, Litthejohns LB, Smith N. Caught in the web: Piloting a methodology to assess community capacity in a rural heart health project. Can J Program Eval. 2000;15(2): 35-55.

Towner E, Dowswell T. Community-based childhood injury prevention interventions: what works? Health Promot Int. 2002;17(3): 273-284.

Treasury Board Secretariat. The development of results-based management and accountability frameworks for horizontal initiatives. Ottawa: Author, June 2002.

Treasury Board Secretariat (TBS) (2001), Guide for the development of results-based management and accountability frameworks, TBS, Ottawa, and TBS (2002).

Vernon IS, Jumper-Thurman P. Prevention of HIV/AIDS in Native American Communities: Promising interventions. Public Health Rep. 2002;117(1): S96-S103.

Wandersman, A. Community mobilization for prevention and health promotion can work. In N. Schneiderman, MA Speers, JM Silva, H Tomes, & JH Gentry (Eds.), Integrating behavioral and social sciences with public health. Washington, D.C.: American Psychological Association; 2001. p. 231-247.

Warner KE. The need for, and value of, a multi-level approach to disease prevention: The case of tobacco control. In Promoting Health: Intervention strategies from social and behavioural research. BD Smedley & SL Syme (Eds.), National Academy Press, Washington, D.C., 2000. p. 417-449.

Weed DL. Beyond black box epidemiology. Am J Public Health. 1998;88(1): 12-14.

Wisotzky M, Albuquerque M, Pechacek RF, Park BZ. The national tobacco control program: Focusing on policy to broaden impact. Public Health Rep. 2004;119(3): 303-310.

Bibliography

Alexander H, MacDonald E. Evaluating policy-driven multi-agency partnership working: A cancer prevention strategy group and a multi-agency domestic abuse group. Presentation to the United Kingdom Evaluation Society Annual Conference, December 2001.

Anderson L, Shinn C, Fullilove M et al. The effectiveness of early childhood development programs: A systemic review. Am J Prev Med. 2003;24(S3): 32-46.

Angus et al, (1995), Sustainable Health Care for Canada, Queen's-University of Ottawa Economic Projects, Ottawa (available at www.cprn.org), and Auer et al. (1995).

Billings J. Community development: A critical review of approaches to evaluation. J Adv Nurs. 2000;31(2): 472-480.

Birch S, Stoddart G, Beland F. Modeling the community as a determinant of health. Can J Public Health. 1998;89(6): 402-405.

Bryant T. Role of knowledge in public health and health promotion policy change. Health Promot Int. 2002;17(1): 89-98.

Coday M, Klesges LM, Garrison RJ, Johnson KC, O'Toole M, Morris GS. Health opportunities with physical exercise (HOPE): Social contextual interventions to reduce sedentary behaviour in urban settings. Health Educ Res. 2002;17(5): 637-647.

Cook A, Jardine A, Weinstein P. Using human disease outbreaks as a guide to multilevel ecosystem interventions. Environ Health Perspect. 2004; 112(11): 1143-1146.

Cummins SK, Jackson RJ. The Built Environment and Children's Health. Pediatr Clin North Am. 2001;48(5): 1241-1252.

Deschesnes M, Martin C, Jomphe-Hill A. Comprehensive approaches to school health promotion: how to achieve broader implementation? Health Promot Int. 2003;18(4): 387-396.

Dianne Watkins; Judy Edwards; Pam Gastrell; "Community Health Nursing" Frameworks for Practice"; Elsevier Health Sciences- 2003

Donaldson C C, Halma L, Gall N, (2002) "Setting Priorities and Allocating Resources in Regional Health Authorities: A Report from Two Pilot Exercises Using Program Budgeting and Marginal Analysis".

Ebrahim S, Smith GD. Exporting failure? Coronary heart disease and stroke in developing countries. Int J Epidemiol. 2001;30(2): 201-205.

Edwards N, Mill J, Kothari A. Multiple Intervention Research Programs in Community Health. Can J Nurs Res. 2004;36(1): 40-55.

Edwards N. Population health: Determinants and interventions. Can J Public Health. 1999; 90(1): 10-11.

Ensor T, Cooper S. Resource allocation and purchasing: influencing the demand side. The University of York, Centre for Health Economics. Heslington, University of York.

Farquharson K. Influencing policy transnationally: Pro- and anti-tobacco global advocacy networks. Aust J Pub Admin. 2003;62(4): 80-92.

Frankish J, Kwan B, Flores J. Assessing the health of communities: Indicator projects and their impacts. Institute of Health Promotion Research, UBC, Sept 2002.

Frankish J. Study on the implementation of health goals in Canada. Institute of Health Promotion Research, UBC, 2000.

Glasgow RE, Vogt TM, Boles SM. Evaluating the public health impact of Health Promotion Interventions: The RE-AIM Framework. Am J Public Health. 1999;89(8): 1322-1327.

Goodman RM. Bridging the gap in effective program implementation: From concept to application. J Community Psychol. 2000;28(3): 309-321.

Goyer KC, Gow J. Alternatives to current HIV/AIDS policies and practices in South African prinsons. J Public Health Policy. 2002;23(3): 303-323.

Green LW, Richard L, Potvin L. Ecological foundations of health promotion. Am J Health Promot. 1996;10(4): 270-281.

Hancock T, Labonte R, Edwards R. Indicators that count: Measuring population health at the community level. Can J Public Health. 1999;90(1): S22-S26.

Hawe P, Noort M, King L, Jordens C. Multiplying health gains: The critical role of capacity-building within health promotion programs. Health Policy. 1997;39(1): 29-42.

Hawe P, Shiell A. Social capital and health promotion. Soc Sci Med. 2000;51(6): 871-885.

Hawe P. Needs assessment must become more change-focused. Aust NZ J of Public Health 1996;20(5): 473-478.

Jenny little wood; "Current issues in Community Nursing" Primary Health Care in practice"; Elsevier Health Sciences ; 1999.

Kamalam S; "Essentials in Community Health Nursing Practice"; Jaypee Brothers, Medical Publishers (P) Ltd, New Delhi.

Karon Saucier Lundy; Sharyn James; "Caring for the Public Health" Jones & Barlett Publishers -2001

Kingdon JW. Agenda, alternatives and public policies. New York: Harper Collins College Publishers. 1995.

Koepsell TD, Wagner EH, Cheadle AC, Patrick DL, Martin DC, Diehr PH, Perrin EB, Kristal AR, Allan-Andrilla CH, Dey LJ. Selected methodological issues in evaluating community-based health promotion and disease prevention programs. Annu Rev Public Health. 1992; 13: 31-57.

Koopman JS, Lynch JW. Individual causal models and population system models in epidemiology. Am J Public Health. 1999; 89(8): 1170-1174.

Kothari A, Birch S. Multilevel health promotion research: Conceptual and analytical considerations. Can J Nurs Res. 2004;36(1): 56-75.

Krauss M, Mueller N, Luke D. Interorganizational relationships within state tobacco control networks: A social network analysis. Prev Chronic Dis. 2004;1(4): 1-25.

Krieger N. Theories for social epidemiology in the 21st century: An ecosocial perspective. Int J Epidemiol. 2001;30(4): 668-677.

Kumaranayake L, Watts C. Resource allocation and priority setting of HIV/AIDS interventions: Addressing the generalized epidemic in Sub-Saharan Africa. J Int Dev. 2001;13(4): 451-466.

Labonte R, Schrecker T, Sanders D, Meeus W. Fatal Indifference: The G8, Africa and Global Health. International Development Research Centre. Ottawa. 2004.

Laterveer L, Niessne LW, Yazbeck AS. Pro-poor health policies in poverty reduction strategies. Health Policy Plann. 2003;18(2): 138-145.

Lloyd F Novick ; Gleen P Mays: Public Health Administration ; Principles for population based management" ; Jones and Bartlett Publishers;-2005

Locher AW, Didiion JA. Epidemic to endemic: The impact of HIV on health care policy and nursing practice. Policy, Politics & Nursing Practice. 2003;4(1): 62-70.

Mancini JA, Marek LI. Sustaining community-based programs for families: Conceptualization and measurement. Family Relations. 2004;53: 339-347.

Mathias RG. Death Sentence: Canada's Drug Laws. A public health framework for drug control in Canada. Monograph, Department of Health Care and Epidemiology, University of British Columbia. 2002.

Mayne J. Addressing attribution through contribution analysis: Using performance measures sensibly. Can J Program Eval. 2001;16(1): 1-24.

McCoy D, Sanders D, Baum F, Narayan T, Legge D. Pushing the international health research agenda towards equity and effectiveness. Lancet. 2004;364(9445): 1630-1631.

McDowell I, Spasoff R, Kristjansson B. Evaluation methods and practice: On the classification of population health measurements. Am J Public Health. 2004;94(3): 388-393.

McLaughlin, JA, Jordan, GB. Logic models: A tool for telling your program's performance story. Eval Program Plann. 1999;22(1): 65-72.

McLoughlin E, Fairweather. Influence of free trade on the politics of safety. Inj Prev. 2002; 8(1): 3-5.

Patrician Carroll; "Community Health Nursing: A Practical Guide"; Thomson Delonar learning; -2004

Philis E Schubert ; Janice E (EDT)" Community Health Nursing: Caring in action"; Thomson Delmor learning; -2003

Setting priorities in injury prevention: The application of an incidence based cost model. Inj Prev. 2002;8(1): 74-78.

Spasoff R A. (1999), Epidemiologic methods for Health Policy, Oxford University Press, new York, especially chapter 1 "Policy, Public

Policy and Health Policy", and chapter 7 "Policy Implementation" p. 169-173.

St Leger L. Health and nature - new challenges for health promotion. Health Promot Int. 2003;18(3): 173-175.

Stokols D. Translating social ecological theory into guidelines for community health promotion. Am J Health Promot. 1996;10(4): 282-298.

Stone D. Policy Paradox: The art of political decision-making. WW. Norton & Company. New York. 2002. p. 17-85.

Thompson D, Litthejohns LB, Smith N. Caught in the web: Piloting a methodology to assess community capacity in a rural heart health project. Can J Program Eval. 2000;15(2): 35-55.

Towner E, Dowswell T. Community-based childhood injury prevention interventions: what works? Health Promot Int. 2002;17(3): 273-284.

Vernon IS, Jumper-Thurman P. Prevention of HIV/AIDS in Native American Communities: Promising interventions. Public Health Rep. 2002;117(1): S96-S103.

Weed DL. Beyond black box epidemiology. Am J Public Health. 1998;88(1): 12-14.

Index

D

E

F